Behavioural Change

For Rani, Kali, Taran and Liam

Senior Commissioning Editor: Ninette Premdas
Project Development Manager: Katrina Mather
Project Manager: David Fleming
Design: Stewart Larking

Behavioural Change: An Evidence-based Handbook for Social and Public Health

Colette J. Browning

Associate Professor, School of Public Health, La Trobe University, Bundoora, Victoria, Australia

Shane A. Thomas

Professor, School of Public Health, La Trobe University, Bundoora, Victoria, Australia. Research Professor, Faculty of Health Sciences, University of Sydney, Lidcombe, NSW, Australia

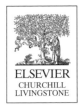

ELSEVIER
CHURCHILL
LIVINGSTONE

EDINBURGH LONDON NEW YORK OXFORD PHILADELPHIA ST LOUIS SYDNEY TORONTO 2005

CHURCHILL LIVINGSTONE
An imprint of Elsevier Limited

First published 2005

ISBN 0 443 07357 0

British Library Cataloguing in Publication Data
A catalogue record for this book is available from the British Library

Library of Congress Cataloging in Publication Data
A catalog record for this book is available from the Library of Congress

Notice
Medical knowledge is constantly changing. Standard safety precautions must be followed,
but as new research and clinical experience broaden our knowledge, changes in treatment
and drug therapy may become necessary or appropriate. Readers are advised to check the
most current product information provided by the manufacturer of each drug to be
administered to verify the recommended dose, the method and duration of
administration, and contraindications. It is the responsibility of the practitioner, relying on
experience and knowledge of the patient, to determine dosages and the best treatment for
each individual patient. Neither the Publisher nor the editors or contributors assume any
liability for any injury and/or damage to persons or property arising from this publication.

The Publisher

Working together to grow
libraries in developing countries

www.elsevier.com | www.bookaid.org | www.sabre.org

ELSEVIER   BOOK AID
            International   Sabre Foundation

ELSEVIER   your source for books,
            journals and multimedia
            in the health sciences
www.elsevierhealth.com

The
publisher's
policy is to use
paper manufactured
from sustainable forests

Printed in China

Contents

Contributors

Renee Bittoun
Director, Smokers Clinics
Central Sydney Area Health Service
Senior Research Fellow
Head, Smoking Cessation Unit
Woolcock Institute of Medical Research
Clinical Associate
Faculty of Medicine
University of Sydney, Australia.

Colette Browning
Associate Professor
School of Public Health
La Trobe University
Victoria, Australia.

Precilla Choi
Associate Professor
School of Human Movement, Recreation & Performance
Victoria University
Melbourne, Victoria
Australia

Helen Dixon
Centre for Behavioural Research in Cancer
Cancer Control Research Institute, Anti-Cancer Council of Victoria
Carlton, Victoria, Australia.

Connie Evashwick
Professor
Director and Endowed Chair
Center for Health Care Innovation
California Sate University Long Beach
Long Beach, California
USA.

Sally Fawkes
Research Fellow
School of Public Health
La Trobe University
Victoria
Australia.

Brian Fildes
Professor
Chair of Road Safety
Monash University Accident Research Centre
Monash University
Victoria
Australia.

Kenneth Mark Greenwood
Associate Professor
Acting Head of School
Director, Undergraduate Programs
School of Psychological Science
La Trobe University
Victoria
Australia.

Russell E. Glasgow
Senior Scientist, Clinical Research Unit,
Kaiser-Permanente Colorado
Denver, Colorado
USA.

Alun Jackson
School of Social Work
The University of Melbourne
Carlton
Victoria
Australia.

Vivian Lin
Professor
School of Public Health
La Trobe University
Victoria
Australia.

Helen Lindner
Senior Lecturer
School of Psychological Science
La Trobe University

Victoria
Australia.

Felicity Morris
School of Human Movement, Recreation & Performance
Victoria University
Melbourne
Victoria
Australia.

Marcia Ory
Professor, Social and Behavioral Health
Director, Active for Life National Program Office
School of Rural Public Health
The Texas A & M University System
College Station
Texas USA.

Professor Susan J Paxton
School of Psychological Science
La Trobe University
Bundoora
Victoria
Australia.

Marian Pitts
Professor
Director, Australian Research Centre in Sex Health & Society
La Trobe University
Melbourne
Australia.

Nicky Pronk
Research Fellow
Monash University Accident Research Centre
Monash University
Victoria
Australia.

Joseph Sharkey
Assistant Professor
School of Rural Public Health
The Texas A & M University System
College Station
Texas USA.

Professor Shane A. Thomas
Professor
School of Public Health

La Trobe University
Victoria
Australia.

Research Professor
Faculty of Health Science
University of Sydney
Lidcombe NSW
Australia.

John Toumbourou
Associate Professor
Centre for Adolescent Health,
University of Melbourne,
Parkville, Victoria
Australia.

Hal Swerissen
Associate Professor
Associate Dean, Regional Development
La Trobe University
Bendigo
Victoria
Australia.

Amanda Weeks
Monash Institute of Health Services Research
Faculty of Medicine, Nursing and Health Sciences
Monash University,
Clayton
Victoria
Australia.

Preface

It has been a privilege working with the authors on this book. We can genuinely say that the journey has been most pleasurable and we certainly know as a result of the journey a good deal more than when we started. We hope the reader also experiences this process of enlightenment as they progress through the text.

We wish to acknowledge the impetus for the production of the text through our interactions with John Prent. John is an official in the Department of Human Services in Victoria, Australia. On a number of occasions he related to us the difficulties confronting officials and service providers in selecting and designing appropriately evidence-based interventions from the research literature. His rigorous and systematic questioning was in no small part a key influence in our wish to bring about this text.

One of the major things we have learned from our review is that the issues confronting the translation of research evidence into viable and sustainable intervention programs is in itself a worthy area of research endeavour. We are particularly pleased with the efforts of our authors in addressing this issue and we are most grateful to Marcia Ory and her colleagues for providing an important contribution to this discussion in this book. We also consider that John Toumbourou's contribution in this volume linking theory, intervention design and practice is a model for all of us to aspire to.

The use of systematic reviews to inform research and practice is a major feature of the last decade's progress towards higher quality health and human services programs. However, we consider that we have shown that the technology and usefulness of systematic reviews such as those lodged in the Cochrane Library still have a way to go before they can be used 'off the shelf' by practitioners to design their programs. As we have noted in our concluding chapter, most systematic reviews do not include information such as unit cost that is basic to program design and funding decisions. We can and need to do better through the design and application of protocols that reflect the needs of program funders and practitioners as well as researchers.

On a sad note one of our authors, Precilla Choi, died before the publication of this book. We wish to warmly acknowledge her scholarship and pay tribute to her contributions to the field of women's health.

Colette Browning
Shane A. Thomas

Melbourne 2005

CHAPTER 1

Introduction

Colette Browning
Shane A. Thomas

CHAPTER CONTENTS

INTRODUCTION

Many public and social health programs have at their heart the goal of modifying people's behaviour. These programs may be targeted at the individual, group and population level. There is a huge research literature concerned with behaviour change across a large number of behavioural domains. The following question is of pivotal interest to people designing behaviour change programs:

What is the best way to achieve sustainable behaviour change for people with this issue? Our primary goal in this book is to attempt to answer this question across a broad range of behavioural domains by providing a wide-ranging review of the best evidence and practices available to achieve behaviour change. The specific behaviour change domains covered by this book include:

- Eating and nutrition.
- Sexual health and behaviour.
- Drugs and alcohol use.
- Physical activity and exercise.
- Smoking prevention and cessation.
- Depression.
- Insomnia.
- Problematic gambling.
- Crash and injury prevention.
- Management of chronic disease.

Each of these areas has a major impact upon our society and the public health and human services designed to address them. However, the book is not just a review of these areas. It includes chapters on models of behaviour change and establishing the effectiveness of health promotion programs, a chapter on enhancing the application and sustainability of health promotion programs and a chapter dealing with practical suggestions as to how to incorporate evidence into the design and delivery of health services.

Since the commencement of this project we were under no illusions as to the scope of the challenge we set ourselves and our co-authors in this task. Each of these areas in their own right, for example smoking, drugs and alcohol, has a very large research literature that includes contributions from many disciplines. The assembly and critique of these literatures and our attempts to integrate the findings from them has been truly a daunting task.

Yet this book is needed for several purposes. The first purpose is to respond to a growing demand in the health sciences and public health disciplines to provide evidence-based teaching and advice about how to promote behaviour change for individuals and populations. We and our colleagues are actively involved in research and teaching in behaviour change and while there are many excellent academic resources, because of the size and scope of the literature they are frequently focused on only one behaviour change domain and/or have a somewhat narrow disciplinary orientation. The second purpose is to respond to the growing demand for information about how to design high-quality behaviour change programs among the tens of thousands of program managers and workers who have the practical task of designing effective programs based upon an often incomplete and outdated knowledge of the current evidence base for this work. A major impetus for the development and production of this book was our participation in the facilitation of research development meetings with senior staff in an Australian state government agency involved in the funding of major health and human services programs. The managers posed the question 'So what do you know about behaviour change that we could use in the design of our programs? We urgently need this knowledge.' Their portfolios included the domains covered in this book.

FRAMEWORK FOR THE BOOK

Because of the wide variety in domains covered by this book and the varied disciplines of the authors conducting the reviews, it was important that some degree of communality in approach was employed in the reviews. Figure 1.1 shows the framework that was used by the authors in writing each of the specific behavioural domain chapters. For each of these chapters, a discussion of incidence and prevalence of each behaviour is presented followed by the evidence for the effectiveness of interventions reviewed in terms of the level of the intervention (community, group, individual) and in terms of its durability (immediate impact, 12-month and lifetime outcomes).

For each of the behavioural domains the following questions were addressed:

- What is the scope of the problem within the international communities?
- What approaches are typically used to prevent or treat it?
- What is the evidence as to the most effective approaches to prevention and treatment?

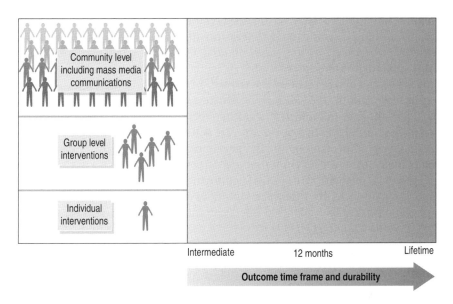

Fig. 1.1   Framework for levels of interventions and durability.

- What is the performance of these approaches in terms of prevention/diversion and full or partial recovery for the short and long term?

OVERVIEW OF CHAPTER CONTENTS

In Chapter 2, Browning and Thomas provide an overview of the models of behaviour change and health promotion underpinning the interventions reported in the subsequent chapters. This chapter draws together themes concerning health promotion and behaviour change for individuals and populations, and addresses the social and structural factors in behaviour change. In Chapter 3, Lin and Fawkes address the issue of the nature of evidence and effectiveness in health promotion using health promotion in developing countries to illustrate the problems of applying the principles of evidence-based medicine.

The following ten chapters focus on the specific behavioural domains: Eating and nutrition (Dixon and Paxton); Sexual health and behaviour (Pitts); Drugs and Alcohol use (Toumbourou); Physical activity and exercise (Morris and Choi); Smoking prevention and cessation (Bittoun and Browning); Depression (Lindner); Insomnia (Greenwood); Problematic gambling (Jackson); Crash and injury prevention (Fildes and Pronk) and self management of chronic disease (Weeks and Swerissen).

The chapter on eating and nutrition focuses on eating behaviours that have a negative impact on health: under-nutrition, over-nutrition leading to obesity and disordered eating patterns such as anorexia nervosa. Prevention interventions are examined according to the three types suggested by the WHO: universal, selective and targeted prevention. Dixon and Paxton examine the epidemiology of dietary behaviour and nutrition in developed and developing countries and the various dietary and body weight recommendations detailed by governments and the WHO. They present a multi-factorial model of the determinants of dietary behaviour including the roles of food policies and legislation, mass media, local community initiatives, family practices and individual factors. Various public health dietary behaviour interventions are reviewed including social marketing approaches and worksite, school-based and primary care settings. The chapter also includes a discussion of interventions for the prevention and treatment of obesity and public health interventions for disordered eating.

Interventions to improve sexual health and reduce high-risk sexual behaviours are examined by Pitts. She discusses the characteristics of successful sexually transmissible infection interventions. The role of the A (abstinence), B (Behaviour change), C (condom use), of prevention aimed at the individual is contrasted with the more recent C (condoms), N (needles) and N (negotiating) approach, particularly as applied to HIV prevention. Group intervention approaches including peer education are discussed using modification of sexual risk for HIV among men, interventions to reduce HIV and STI risks among young homeless people, occupational interventions, and cervical cancer prevention interventions as examples. The chapter also includes examples of interventions directed at the community level including mass media campaigns and multi-component interventions.

Toumbourou examines interventions to prevent harm related to alcohol and drug use by integrating developmental and motivational theories. The scope and major determinants of substance misuse are examined. He discusses the development of substance misuse in terms of four motivations (escaping developmental stress, self-managing body and spirit, conforming to norms and individuating identity) and their moderating influences. For each major motivation the types of individual, group and community interventions are evaluated.

In the chapter on physical activity, Morris and Choi address the issue of declining levels of physical activity despite most people understanding the importance of activity to health. They explore the factors associated with inactivity including sociodemographic, lifestyle and environmental factors and personal barriers. The types of interventions reviewed focus on active living or lifestyle programs that focus on individuals changing their daily routines rather than specific exercise prescriptions. Primary care-based interventions and community interventions are highlighted.

Bittoun and Browning examine smoking as an addictive behaviour and the effectiveness of the various approaches to smoking cessation. The mechanisms involved in nicotine addiction and withdrawal are discussed along with individual differences in withdrawal symptoms. Interventions including nicotine replacement and other pharmacological interventions, and group and community interventions among others are reviewed in terms of their efficacy.

The chapter on depression describes the symptoms of depression and the classification systems for the diagnosis of depression. Lindner discusses the causes and consequences of depression together with an examination of the epidemiology of the condition. The burden of co-morbidity of depression with physical illness as well as gender differences in the prevalence of depression are highlighted. Treatment modalities including pharmacological and psychological therapies and broad educational approaches are described and evaluated. The role and effectiveness of these approaches at the individual, small group and community levels are discussed.

Insomnia causes serious social and public health problems but has had little recognition as a public health issue. Greenwood discusses the current behavioural interventions for insomnia including sleep hygiene, stimulus control therapy, sleep restriction therapy, and cognitive therapy. While noting the extensive literature on the efficacy of current cognitive behaviour therapy approaches to insomnia for individuals and small groups, the chapter focuses on less common approaches such as self-help treatment, mass media approaches and community interventions which may be more effective in addressing the problem in larger numbers of individuals.

In the chapter on problematic gambling Jackson points out that there are knowledge gaps and contention in the underlying causes of the target behaviour. He further argues that because there are various types of problem gamblers and models to explain their behaviours, measures of behaviour change in the various intervention types vary. The chapter discusses issues related to the definition and measurement of problematic gambling and the related problem of estimating prevalence. The prevalence in various subpopulations, including adolescents, ethnic communities and women is highlighted. Problematic gambling intervention models are presented as well as a discussion of the methodological issues involved in determining problematic gambling intervention outcomes. Individual treatment approaches (the predominant intervention type in this area) including psychoanalytic formulations, self-help approaches, behavioural and cognitive therapies, controlled gambling, multi-modal therapies and pharmacological interventions are discussed in terms of their operation and effectiveness. A model of the influences on gambling behaviour and outcomes is presented as a way to target interventions.

Fildes and Pronk examine road crash and injury prevention. They point out that the improvement in road safety over the last 50 years has been primarily due to the adoption of an evidence-based approach. The chapter examines interventions in terms of three approaches: engineering, enforcement and education; and three levels of intervention: individual, group and community. Individual interventions discussed include motor vehicle sanctions and rehabilitation programs for recidivist offenders. Road safety educational programs targeted to specific groups including older people and company employees and broad community interventions such as speed enforcement and mass media campaigns are examined. The chapter also includes a discussion of changing philosophies in road safety approaches from the traditional transportation model where safety is '... a tradeable commodity against mobility' to models arising from Europe that place safety as a health issue and includes notions of sustainability. The merits and challenges associated with adopting these new approaches are discussed.

Weeks and Swerissen evaluate interventions focusing on self-management of chronic illnesses and participatory models of care. Characteristics of chronic illnesses are discussed as well as the experience and social, psychological and economic impacts of chronic illness. The concept of self-management is described and the underlying behaviour change models that have been used to inform self-management interventions are highlighted. The chapter includes an evaluation of the strategies and techniques used in the teaching of self-management skills, a comparison of professional and peer-led intervention programs and an analysis of the effectiveness of chronic illness self-management programs.

Following the chapters that focus on specific domains for intervention, Ory, Evashwick, Glasgow and Sharkey address the issue of translational public health program research that focuses on identifying strategies for application and sustainability of evidence-based programs in different settings and in diverse populations. In the concluding chapter, we summarize the evidence from the previous chapters and present an epistemological framework for evaluating behaviour change interventions.

The content framework proposed to the authors provided a useful structure within which to organize the work from the highly diverse domains and disciplines included within this book. However, as we note in our final chapter, despite the vast array of published evidence available, there remain many common gaps in the knowledge base across these domains and many deficiencies in our behaviour change achievements. Broadly, the sustainability of behaviour change interventions is not as well known as it should be. Most studies, perhaps reflecting the funding preferences of research funding bodies, have a short time-span. Yet we know from those relatively few studies with a longer-term orientation that the sustainability of many behaviour change programs is relatively short-lived.

We also note in our final chapter that the design and reporting of outcomes from many studies, including those with the so-called 'gold standard' of a randomized controled trial (RCT), are a major concern. We observe that most studies do not include information that is basic to the evaluation of the scientific integrity of the study let alone the possibility of actually incorporating the study's results into an actual program to deliver services. Our call is not a lame one of 'more research is needed'; rather it is a call for 'better research is needed' along with 'better reporting of the research'. It is not that collectively we have lacked the resources to make substantial inroads into addressing the behaviour change problems that are endemic to the human condition, but we certainly need to structure these efforts more systematically and less chaotically if we are to make the best difference possible. Those people with serious and avoidable health problems and those who pay for them demand our best efforts.

CHAPTER 2

Models of behaviour change and health promotion

Colette Browning
Shane A. Thomas

INTRODUCTION

The aim of this chapter is to describe the dominant models of behaviour change and health promotion that underpin many of the interventions presented in this book. Whole books have been devoted to an examination of the strengths and weaknesses of the various models of behaviour change and for a more detailed description the reader is referred to Conner & Norman,[1] DiClemente, Crosby & Kegler,[2] Glanz, Rimer & Lewis,[3] Norman, Abraham & Conner,[4] Prochaska & DiClemente[5] and Rollnick, Mason & Butler.[6] While behaviour change models focus on the individual determinants of health, and health risk and protective behaviours, health promotion models focus on the role of social, economic, cultural and environmental influences on health and illness. Again the reader is referred to the following authors for a detailed examination of health promotion approaches: Baum[7]; Egger, Spark & Lawson[8]; Green & Kreuter[9]; Kreuter, Lenzin, Kreuter & Green[10]and Nutbeam & Harris.[11]

The impetus for a broader approach to the determinants of health beyond the role of individual behaviours was the Ottawa Charter for Health Promotion[12] that built on the Word Health Organization's 'Health for All' and the recognition that in order to improve the health of populations inter-sectoral action was necessary. The Charter defined health promotion as '. . . the process of enabling people to increase control over, and to improve, their health' (p. 1). It recognizes that health promotion should be incorporated in all policy sectors, as health is a '. . . resource for everyday life' (p. 1). Five strategies were set out in the Charter including building healthy public policy, creating supportive social and natural environments, strengthening community action and participation, developing personal skills and reorienting health services to reflect the shift in burden of disease towards chronic conditions, the ageing of populations and cultural diversity. An approach that recognizes the influence of individual, social, economic and environmental factors in health and wellbeing acknowledges the multiple opportunities for intervention and the complexity in designing interventions that translate into a variety of settings and communities (see Chapter 14).

Before we examine models of health behaviour change it is useful to discuss in more detail the determinants of health and illness as these perspectives underpin intervention design in public and social health. It is now well-recognized that health and illness are influenced by multiple determinants. Engel[13] developed the biopsychosocial model of illness in response to the limitations of the biomedical model. The model posits that it is necessary to incorporate biological, psychological and social (small group) explanations of the causes and treatment of disease. This perspective assumes that these factors influence and are influenced by each other. For example, a supportive friendship network may influence stress reactions while risk behaviours such as problematic gambling may impact negatively on family relationships. Similarly physical symptoms such as pain may contribute to negative self-beliefs about one's ability to manage illness, while increasing control beliefs can impact on pain perceptions. Later commentators incorporated the influences of social and health systems and the physical environments in which we live.[7,14-17]

From this broad perspective health and illness are influenced by:

- Biomedical factors, such as genetics, physiology and physical symptoms.
- Risk and protective behaviours, for example, smoking, drug misuse, physical activity and good nutrition.
- Psychological factors such as cognitions (beliefs, self-efficacy), stress, personality and motivations.
- Social (small group) factors such as social support, social networks, family relationships.
- Social and health system factors such as health policy, culture, employment and socioeconomic status.
- Physical environments (ecology), for example, the built environment, climate, and water and soil quality.

These factors also influence each other. For example, barriers to engaging in a protective behaviour such as physical activity for an older person may be poor access to safe walking environments, lack of family support to engage in the activity and low confidence (self-efficacy) in performing the activity.

Historically the biopsychosocial perspective reflects the changing patterns of illness and cause of death over the latter part of the last century. Reduced neonatal deaths and deaths from infectious diseases and increased prevalence of chronic illness influenced by an interaction between physiological, psychological, behavioural and social factors pointed to the necessity to move beyond the reductionist explanation embedded in the biomedical model where causes of illnesses focus on cellular and organ functioning. Nearly 30 years ago the US Centers for Disease Control noted that the causes of disease were explained by unhealthy behaviours (50%), human biology (20%), the physical environment (20%) and inadequate health care (10%).

As indicated above the broader social, cultural and physical environments in which we live and work also impact on health and illness. The socioeconomic determinants of health have been well documented.[15,18] The social gradient of health describes the observation that people who live in impoverished social and economic environments as evidenced by low levels of education, unemployment and inadequate housing are more likely to have lower life expectancy and higher rates of disease than those higher in socioeconomic status.[15] This relationship has been explained in terms of psychological processes such as stress, control over one's work or social environment, social cohesion, and investment by governments in the health of populations at critical time points, for example during childhood (for a review, see Turrell[18] and Wilkinson & Marmot[19]). The role of the physical environment (clean air and water, adequate food, the safety and accessibility of pedestrian, private and public transport and neighbourhood safety) in health was highlighted in the Ottawa Charter. McMichael's[16] book on the ecology of population health asserts that ' ... the health of populations is primarily a product of ecological circumstance: a product of the interaction of human societies with the wider environment, its various ecosystems and other life-support process (pp. xiv–xv). He illustrates the influences of urbanization, pollution, demography and income distribution on the patterns of health and disease and concludes that managing these influences requires a systems approach and a commitment to sustainability by governments and individuals.

We now turn to models of individual behaviour change that underpin many of the interventions presented in the following chapters.

MODELS OF INDIVIDUAL BEHAVIOUR CHANGE

The main behaviour change models can be classified as social cognition models (for example the Health Belief Model and the Theory of Planned Behaviour) and stage models (for example the Stages of Change Model (or Transtheoretical Model) and the Precaution Adoption Process Model). Most models incorporate perceived behavioural control or self-efficacy concepts as a predictor of action. Social cognition models assume that the individual evaluates the benefits and costs of a health action. By determining the factors (for example, attitudes, norms, self-efficacy) that impact on this decision it is assumed that we can predict the likelihood that a person will act. Interventions using this approach aim to increase the likelihood of the action occurring and individuals are assumed to move along a continuum of behaviour change.[20] In contrast, stage theories assume that people can be classified according to a discrete stage and can move between stages to achieve the desired behaviour. The aim of interventions using a stage approach is to tailor the intervention to the specific stage of change.[5] In this section we will provide an overview of the models that have been tested most widely in the literature: the Health Belief Model, the Theory of Planned Behaviour, the Stages of Change Model and Self-Efficacy. These models are also discussed in some of the chapters that follow as they apply to specific behavioural or problem domains.

Health Belief Model

The Health Belief Model assumes that the perceived threat of a bad health outcome is a result of an individual's evaluation of the perceived seriousness of and susceptibility to that health problem.[21] If an individual judges that they may contract an illness or that illness has serious consequences then they are more likely to engage in health actions to avoid the illness. The perceived costs (barriers) and benefits associated with taking preventive actions, as well as health motivation, moderate the decision to take preventive action. Demographic and personal factors also influence perceived susceptibility, perceived severity, health motivation, perceived benefits and perceived barriers and cues to action such as doctor's advice or mass media health campaigns can influence preventive actions. The model provides a common sense way of understanding why people do or do not engage in healthy actions but ignores the influence of social factors and emotional responses on behaviour.

Table 2.1 shows the components of the Health Belief Model as applied to a man with high cholesterol and at risk for heart disease. His doctor (cue to action) has prescribed a cholesterol-lowering drug that he must take each day (action). His doctor has also provided him with a low cholesterol diet to follow (action). The man understands that having high cholesterol is not healthy and that changing his diet would reduce his risks for heart disease (perceived susceptibility) but he is not convinced that heart disease would be a problem for him. 'Doctors can always fix you' (perceived severity). He is confident that he can follow the drug regimen but is unsure about the new diet. The man lives alone and travels a lot for his job and tends to eat take-away foods, or if he cooks, his meal consists of meat and fried food. He does not believe he could follow the diet suggested by the doctor: 'I am not good cook' (perceived barrier). In this case, the doctor would need to help the man understand the effects of heart disease, that is, increase his knowledge about the severity of the condition and the value of prevention to his health and quality of life. Additional support and strategies would need to be provided to assist the man with shopping and cooking according to the new diet and selecting healthier alternatives if eating away from home.

The Theory of Reasoned Action/Planned Behaviour

Ajzen and Fishbein's model, the Theory of Reasoned Action, asserts that intentions precede actions.[22,23] Intentions are determined by two attitudes: the intrinsic value of the action and the social appropriateness of the action. A later development of the model, the Theory of Planned Behaviour, incorpo-

Table 2.1   Components of the Health Belief Model applied to a man with high cholesterol and at risk for heart disease

Individual influences on beliefs and motivation	Beliefs, motivation and cues to action	Action
Demographic variables Male aged 45 years who lives alone	*Perceived susceptibility* High cholesterol and understands that this is a risk factor for heart disease	Follow drug regimen Change diet
Personal characteristics Hardy personality	*Perceived severity* Knowledge of effects of heart disease is low Health motivation: Low motivation to change diet	
	Perceived benefits Lower cholesterol levels, weight loss and reduced risk of heart disease	
	Perceived barriers: Travels a lot for work and cooking skills poor	
	Cues to action Doctor's advice Father died of heart attack at 55 years of age	

rated perceived behavioural control (influenced by skills, information and barriers) as an added component.[24] Interventions based on this model attempt to change beliefs and increase perceived control. A recent systematic review of the application of the model in behaviour change interventions found that about two thirds of the interventions were effective in changing behaviour but concluded that the evidence for the usefulness of the model is limited.[25] Like the Health Belief Model, the Theory of Planned Behaviour has been criticized for not incorporating broader social and structural influences on behaviour and focusing on perceived rather than actual control.[1]

In the next example the Theory of Planned Behaviour is applied to a young man to promote safe sex. The young man holds a negative attitude towards condom use (attitude to target behaviour). The social norm within his peer group is that condom use is not relevant to them. They do not perceive that they are at risk for sexually transmissible diseases. However his mother is aware that he is sexually active and has provided condoms to him (subjective norms regarding target behaviour). He is unsure about how to discuss this issue with his partner and is not confident about how to use condoms (perceived control of target behaviour). His mother has asked him to talk about the issue with the school welfare officer. The welfare officer would need to challenge negative attitudes to condom use by presenting information to challenge them, and demonstrate that condom use will decrease his chances of developing STDs. She would also need to develop his skills in negotiation and communication with his partner and increase his confidence in being able to use condoms.

Self–efficacy

Self-efficacy beliefs are important components of behaviour change models and have been shown to predict behaviour change.[26] Self-efficacy is behaviour specific and describes the confidence one has in achieving a specific outcome. For example, high self-efficacy to start exercising is predictive of actually starting an exercise program.

Health behaviour change interventions that incorporate self-efficacy focus on convincing the person that they have the personal resources required to act in the required manner. Changing self-efficacy for a particular behaviour, however, needs to proceed in small steps. Lorig's[27] work on chronic illness self-management (see Chapter 13) uses behavioural contracting to help people set goals for behaviour change that are consistent with a high self-efficacy to achieve those goals. For example, if you want a person with arthritis to increase the use of relaxation to manage their pain you need to ask them what they are 100% confident of achieving in a given week (high self-efficacy). In the case of a person who has never practiced relaxation before, behavioural contracting could be used to successively approximate the target behaviour and improve self-efficacy. For example if the target behaviour is to engage in a half-hour of progressive relaxation each day, in the first week the target may be to engage in this activity for ten minutes, three times a week. This would be negotiated with the person in a way that ensured that for the target behaviour in that week, the person was 100% certain that he/she could achieve their goal. Initial targets need to be lowered until the person is 100% certain that they can achieve the target behaviour. In the second week, the person's self-efficacy should be improved based on successfully achieving their goals from the previous week. At this point the relaxation goal for the second week can be increased. This procedure is repeated over successive weeks and as success occurs, self-efficacy increases.

The Stages of Change Model

The transtheoretical model of behavioural change proposed by Prochaska & DiClemente has four central tenets.[5,28] First, people move through stages to achieve change. Second ten processes have been identified that help people to change and maintain their behaviour and processes need to be tailored to the stage of change.[5,29] Third, thoughts (decisional balance) need to be shifted so that the positive aspects of the target behaviour outweigh the negative aspects of the target behaviour. Self-efficacy is the fourth component of the model and incorporates confidence in maintaining the new behaviour and resisting the temptation to relapse.

The stages in this model include pre-contemplation (the person is not practising nor planning to practise the target health behaviour and decisional balance is negative), contemplation (the person is not practising but is considering the practice of the target health behaviour and decisional balance remains negative), preparation (the person is preparing actively to initiate the behaviour), action (the person adopts the target health behaviour and decisional balance is positive) and maintenance (the person maintains the target health behaviour for an extended period and decisional balance remains positive). Processes of change include consciousness-raising, dramatic relief, self re-evaluation, environmental re-evaluation (all used at the contemplation stage to move the person to the preparation stage) counter-conditioning, reinforcement management, self-liberation, social liberation, helping relationships and stimulus control (all used in the action phase to promote maintenance).[29] Identifying at what stage the person is at helps identify their motivational readiness to change and the intervention and processes of change can be tailored to suit the individual.[29]

Table 2.2 shows the components of the Stages of Change Model as applied to increasing physical activity. To apply this model one needs to be able to

Table 2.2   Components of the Stages of Change Model as applied to increasing physical activity

Stage of change	Processes of change
Pre-contemplation Not considering increasing physical activity levels	Elicit positive and negative aspects of target behaviour(s) and provide simple information (*consciousness-raising, dramatic relief*)
Contemplation Thinks about increasing physical activity levels	Motivate and elicit commitment Enhance self-efficacy Identify physical activity classes (*social liberation*)
Preparation Consults doctor and visits local gymnasium	Identify goals and plan start date and type of physical activity. Use social support (*helping relationships*) Use *stimulus control*
Action Joins local gym	Review goals and suggest coping strategies for fatigue, discomfort, lack of motivation etc. Praise high self-efficacy Use *reinforcement management, counter-conditioning and stimulus control*
Maintenance Has visited gym three times a week for 6 months	Review coping strategies and reassess goals and physical activity type

Adapted from Dunlap and Barry[31] and Jordan and Nigg.[32]

identify the stage of change through a short questionnaire and the processes that the person uses with respect to physical activity.[30] For example, does the person read articles to learn more about physical activity (*consciousness raising*)? Does the person believe that physical activity will make them healthier (*self re-evaluation*)? Including tailored processes of change that affect physical activity assists the person to move from the current stage of change to the next one.

The models discussed above have been used widely (and with varying success) across the various domains reviewed in the following chapters.

References

1. Connor M, Norman P, eds. Predicting behaviour: Research and practice with social cognition models. Philadelphia: Open University Press; 1995.
2. DiClemente RJ, Crosby RA, Kegler MC. Emerging theories in health promotion practice and research: Strategies for improving public health. San Francisco: Jossey-Bass; 2002.
3. Glanz K, Rimer BK, Lewis FM, eds. Health behaviour and health education: Theory, research and practice, 3rd edn. San Francisco: Jossey-Bass; 2002.
4. Norman P, Abraham C, Conner M, eds. Understanding and changing health behaviour: From health beliefs to self-regulation. London: Harwood Academic Publishers; 2000.
5. Prochaska JO, DiClemente CC. The transtheoretical approach: Crossing traditional boundaries of change. Homewood, IL: Dorsey Press; 1984.
6. Rollnick S, Mason P, Butler C. Health behaviour change: A guide for practitioners. Edinburgh: Churchill Livingstone; 2000.
7. Baum F. The new public health: An Australian perspective, 2nd edn. Melbourne: Oxford University Press; 2002.
8. Egger G, Spark R, Lawson J. Health promotion strategies and methods. Sydney: McGraw-Hill; 1990.
9. Green LW, Kreuter MW. Health promotion planning: An educational and ecological approach, 3rd edn. Mountain View, CA: Mayfield Publishing Company; 1999.
10. Kreuter MW, Lenzin NA, Kreuter MW, Green LW. Community health promotion ideas that work. Sudbury, MA: Josh & Bartlett; 2003.
11. Nutbeam D, Harris E. Theory in a nutshell: A practitioner's guide to commonly used theories and models in health promotion. Sydney: National Centre for Health Promotion; 1998.
12. WHO. Ottawa Charter for Health Promotion, 1986.
13. Engel G. The need for a new medical model: A challenge for biomedicine. Science 1977; 196:129–136.
14. Graham H, ed. Understanding health inequalities. Buckingham: Open University Press; 2000.
15. Marmot MG, Wilkinson RG. Social determinants of health. Oxford: Oxford University Press; 1999.
16. McMichael T. Human frontiers, environments and disease. Cambridge: Cambridge University Press; 2001.
17. WHO. Active ageing: A policy framework. Geneva: WHO; 2002.
18. Turrell G. Income inequality and health: In search of fundamental causes. In: Eckersley R, Dixon J, Douglas B, eds. The social origins of health and illness. Edinburgh: Cambridge University Press; 2001.

19. Wilkinson R, Marmot M. Social determinants of health: The solid facts, 2nd edn. Copenhagen: WHO; 2003.
20. Weinstein ND, Sandman PM. The Precaution Adoption Process Model and its application. In: DiClemente RJ, Crosby RA, Kegler MC, eds. Emerging theories in health promotion practice and research: Strategies for improving public health. San Francisco, CA: Jossey-Bass; 2002:16–39.
21. Rosenstock IM, Strecher VJ, Becker MH. Social learning theory and the health belief model. Health Education Quarterly 1988; 15:175–183.
22. Ajzen I, Fishbein M. Understanding attitudes and predicting social. Englewood Cliffs, NJ: Prentice-Hall; 1980.
23. Sheppard BH, Hartwick J, Warshaw PR. The theory of reasoned action: A meta-analysis of past research and recommendations for modifications and future research. Journal of Consumer Research 1988; 15:325–339.
24. Ajzen I. The theory of planned behaviour. Organizational Behaviour and Human Decision Processes 1991; 50:179–211.
25. Hardeman W, Johnston M, Johnston DW, Bonetti D, Wareham NJ, Kinmonth AL. Application of the theory of planned behaviour in behaviour change interventions: A systematic review. Psychology and Health 2002; 17(2):123–158.
26. Bandura A. Self-efficacy: Thought control of action. New York: Freeman; 1994.
27. Lorig K. Patient education: A practical approach, 3rd edn. Thousand Oaks, CA: Sage; 2000.
28. Prochaska JO, Velicer WF. The transtheoretical model of behaviour change. American Journal of Health Promotion 1997: 12:38–48.
29. Burkholder GJ, Nigg CC. Overview of the transtheoretical model. In: Burbank PM, Riebe D, eds. Promoting exercise and behaviour change in older adults. New York: Springer; 2002:85–146.
30. Nigg CR, Riebe D. The transtheoretical model: Research review of exercise behaviour and older adults. In: Burbank PM, Riebe D, eds. Promoting exercise and behaviour change in older adults. New York: Springer; 2002.
31. Dunlap J, Barry H. Overcoming exercise barriers in older adults. http://www.physsportsmed.com/issues/1999/1010-15-99/dunlap.htm; 1999.
32. Jordan PJ, Nigg CR. Applying the transtheoretical model: Tailoring interventions to stages of change. In: Burbank PM, Riebe D, eds. Promoting exercise and behaviour change in older adults. New York: Springer; 2000:181–207.

CHAPTER **3**

Achieving effectiveness in health promotion programs: Evidence, infrastructure and action

Vivian Lin
Sally Fawkes

INTRODUCTION

Interest in health promotion effectiveness stems from a concern to find and use the best approaches to improving health and decreasing health differentials between and within population groups. High quality and systematic approaches to undertaking, documenting and evaluating health promotion programs have the potential to enhance opportunities to share experiences, to scale up successes, and to improve the evidence base for health promotion. However, as a relatively new area of public health practice, there is still debate about how best to undertake evaluation that is appropriate to the different forms of practice, although significant work is underway to change this situation.[1]

It is perhaps not surprising that an evidence base of effective health promotion interventions has been slow to develop. Contemporary health promotion represents a complex process, 'the purpose of which is to strengthen the skills and capabilities of individuals to take action, and the capacity of groups or communities to act collectively to exert control over the determinants of health.'[2] Health promotion programs target determinants of health over which individuals might have some control (health behaviours, use of health services) and those outside the control of individuals (macro-level factors such as social, economic, physical and environmental conditions, and the provision of health services). To bring about changes in this web of health determinants requires a highly developed set of techniques for interventions and evaluation.

Basic forms of health education, involving face-to-face educational approaches engaging individuals and groups, have an important place in health promotion, but they have been augmented by sophisticated social marketing strategies that exploit the mass media and mobile communications technologies to convey health messages to the public. Complementing health education are complex interventions that change social, economic and physical environments so they support norms and practices conducive to good health. These include legislation and regulation, and professional, organisational and community development. The challenge for evaluation is not only to produce evidence but also scale up effective interventions.

This chapter discusses the contrasting nature of evidence and effectiveness in medicine and in health promotion. A framework for achieving program effectiveness is then offered to show what is required for programs to be effective and where the evidence base fits. A review of effectiveness of health promotion in developing countries will illustrate health promotion in practice and the difficulties of ensuring effectiveness. The chapter concludes with a checklist for ensuring program effectiveness and suggestions for moving forward.

EVIDENCE OF EFFECTIVENESS

The nature of evidence

The term 'evidence' is used in various ways. While a dictionary might define it as a fact that leads to a conclusion, the term has come to be used in academic worlds, health-care settings and public policy to mean information which is derived from rigorous research.[3] The nature of that research remains a matter for debate.

Importance of evidence–based practice

There are a number of reasons why the notion of evidence-based practice is important[4]: it is crucial to know whether interventions are doing more good than harm; where resources become scarce, there is increasing competition between programs and services and demand for cost-effectiveness considerations in investments; the costs and benefits of different approaches should be considered so that the best option and use of funding is adopted; people who make the decisions about interventions, and those who are affected by the decision, should know the strengths, limitations, and gaps in the available evidence.

There has been a general commitment, domestically and internationally, to program evaluation since the 1960s, as pressure increased to demonstrate how funds were being used in health and social programs.[5] Concern for a more rational approach to the adoption of innovations in clinical medicine in the 1970s,[6] based on a commitment to cost-effectiveness in health services and programs, led to the concept of and practices supporting evidence-based medicine (EBM). Today, EBM is important from the perspective of both cost and quality.

Evidence of effectiveness in clinical medicine

EBM is defined as the 'conscientious, explicit and judicious use of current best evidence in making decisions about the care of individual patients'.[7] Reflecting Archie Cochrane's original vision, evidence for the use of specific clinical procedures and drug treatments is best generated by synthesising published, primary research based on particular research methods, with preference for randomized controlled trials (RCTs). Being able to attribute changes to a particular intervention is a key issue in producing evidence. The production of evidence of effectiveness is a five-step process that can feed into collections of systematic reviews:

1. Intervention.
2. Evaluation of intervention.
3. Published paper or report on intervention (primary research).
4. Systematic review of multiple papers or reports (secondary research).
5. Evidence of effectiveness of an intervention.

Systematic reviews of existing evidence are important tools for use by policy-makers, decision-makers and practitioners. They aim to give a thorough, unbiased search of the relevant literature, explicit criteria for assessing studies and structured presentation of the results. Their value lies in their attempt to avoid the bias that comes from single studies, while distilling the essential learnings for application in policy development, program planning and investment decisions.[8] Tools for developing, collecting and disseminating systematic reviews of public health and health promotion include the Cochrane Collaboration (www.cochrane.org), the Campbell Collaboration (www.campbell.gse.upenn.edu), The Guide to Community Services (www.cdc.gov) and the National Health Service Centre for Reviews and Dissemination (www.york.ac.uk/inst/crd/). Developing and applying these tools have illuminated theoretical and practical issues about evidence, centred around the hierarchy of evidence used to judge the strength of effectiveness and the types of outcomes to be assessed.

EBM strengthened progressively in the 1980s and 1990s and has led to the pursuit of information about effectiveness of all health interventions that allow judgements to be made about their potential adoption.

Levels of evidence

In EBM, randomized controlled trials (RCTs) are ranked as the highest quality, most robust method for attributing causes, as they control for bias in order to generalize. As shown in the designation by National Health and Medical Research Council (NHMRC) of levels of evidence in the area of clinical medicine,[9] a systematic review of all RCTs relevant to a research question (especially concerning drug treatments or clinical techniques) is therefore at the top of a hierarchy of study design and levels of evidence (see Table 3.1).

Problems and issues in applying standards of evidence for clinical medicine to health promotion

Applying the hierarchy of evidence for clinical medicine to health promotion is not straightforward, even though it is a tool for critical thinking and careful consideration of what may be good quality evidence. For a start, the goals and methods of health promotion differ from clinical medicine. For example, health promotion is not only about changing the behaviour of individuals but changing behaviour and environments of organizations, communities and societies. Furthermore, health promotion interventions might be simple (such as a health education program for individuals in a general practice setting) or complex (such as multi-strategy programs to bring about change in communities). Since Speller et al. argued that health promotion is 'at risk from the application of inappropriate methods of assessing evidence' and 'over-emphasis on outcomes of individual behaviour change and pressure on resources',[10] there is now wide agreement that new ways of assessing evidence of effectiveness of health promotion are required to fit the nature of health promotion.

Table 3.1   Levels of evidence[9]

Level of evidence (highest to lowest)	Type of research design
Level I	Evidence obtained from a systematic review of all relevant RCTs
Level II	Evidence obtained from at least one properly designed RCT
Level III–1	Evidence obtained from well-designed pseudo-RCTs (alternative allocation or some other method)
Level III–2	Evidence obtained from comparative studies (including systematic reviews of such studies) with concurrent controls and allocation not randomized, cohort studies, case–control studies, or interrupted time series with a control group
Level III–3	Evidence obtained from comparative studies with historical control, two or more single arm studies, or interrupted time series without a parallel control group
Level IV	Evidence obtained from case studies, either post-test or pre-test/post-test

EVIDENCE OF EFFECTIVENESS IN HEALTH PROMOTION

Innovations in three related areas are currently being developed and can improve the ways in which evidence of health promotion effectiveness is assessed:

- Research design and methods.
- Focus of program evaluation.
- Intervention outcomes.

Research design and methods

Systematic reviews need to include a broader range of studies and research methods. The concept of controlled trials in RCTs is neither practical nor appropriate for establishing evidence of effectiveness in multi-level, multi-strategy programs, such as healthy cities initiatives. Both ethical and practical constraints limit their value: 'To make sense of the controlled trial, two communities would need to be very near to identical. Even if such communities were found, it would not be possible to stop all initiatives in a community so that it remains as a control.'[11] What might be more important is to understand particular populations and to observe changes over time in communities. Combining qualitative and quantitative methods will produce a more complete representation of program implementation. Criteria for assessment of qualitative research are under development so that this form of research evidence can also be systematically reviewed.[8]

Focus of program evaluation

Effectiveness of health promotion programs is related to both program design and also the quality of program implementation. Evaluation of processes plays an instrumental role in revealing the circumstances and experiences of program implementation that affect whether a program will succeed in achieving its objectives. Evaluation produces knowledge and insights that help explain program successes and failures and are needed to replicate and disseminate programs.'[12] They are important for sharing lessons but less available (i.e. less likely to be funded or published), and therefore less able to be accounted for in assessments of evidence.

Intervention outcomes

A significant amount of work has been done internationally to identify appropriate outcomes for health promotion programs and on developing suitable evaluation methods and tools to measure effects of health promotion.[13] These efforts have been important for accumulating an evidence base for health promotion.

Health promotion outcomes should reflect the multi-method approach of health promotion. These methods include awareness-raising activities, provision of health information and advice, lobbying and advocacy, professional training and development and community development. Behaviour change might be one type of outcome, but not the only or indeed the most important one, and moreover, behaviour change might be contingent on other factors such as changes in social attitudes and practical opportunities to behave in certain ways.

Successful health promotion programs produce measurable changes to health status and quality of life months or even decades after interventions have occurred. Consequently, intermediate outcomes must be identified and measured. These will be observable changes that can be directly related to the health promotion intervention and which in turn lead to health status and social outcomes (when a program is implemented properly).

Nutbeam argues that the evaluation of health promotion interventions should consider three sets of outcomes.[14] His conceptual model, presented in Figure. 3.1 illustrates the links between health promotion actions, effects resulting from these actions (health promotion outcomes and intermediate health outcomes) and the longer-term changes in health and wellbeing. Ideally, programs tested for effectiveness will be able to deliver predictable changes at each

Health and social outcomes	Social outcomes measures include: quality of life, functional, independence, equity	Health outcomes measures include: reduced morbidity, disability, avoidable mortality	
Intermediate health outcomes (modifiable determinants of health)	Healthy lifestyles measures include: tobacco use, food choices, physical activity, alcohol and illicit drug use	Effective health services measures include: provision of preventive services, access to and appropriateness of health services	Healthy environments measures include: safe physical environment, supportive economic and social conditions, secure food supply, restricted access to tobacco and alcohol
Health promotion outcomes (intervention impact measures)	Health literacy measures include: health-related, knowledge, attitudes, motivation, behavioural intentions, personal skills, self-efficacy	Social action and influence measures include: community participation, community empowerment, social norms, public opinion	Healthy public policy and organizational practice measures include: policy statements, legislation, regulation, resource allocation, organizational practices
Health promotion actions	Education examples include: patient education, school education, broadcast media and print media communication	Social mobilization examples include: community development, group facilitation, targeted mass communication	Advocacy examples include: lobbying, political organization and activism, overcoming bureaucratic inertia

Fig. 3.1   Outcome model for health promotion.[14]

of these levels. The model has been discussed in international forums in relation to its usefulness in framing a national minimum data set for health promotion in developed and developing country contexts. To date, the model has been applied in a number of countries for this purpose, including UK, Iceland, Estonia, France and Canada, while the health promotion foundation in Switzerland uses the model to evaluate their organization and projects they fund.

In this model, the most immediate focus is on evaluation of health promotion actions. Their immediate outcomes include changes in three main domains[12]:

1. Health literacy (health-related knowledge, attitude, behavioural intentions, interpersonal skills).
2. Social mobilization (community participation, community empowerment, social norms and public opinion).
3. Healthy public policy and organizational practices (policy statements, legislation, regulation, resources allocation, organizational practices).

The achievement of intermediate health outcomes (related to determinants of health) comes sometime later and cover[12]:

- Healthy lifestyles (tobacco use, physical activity, food choices).
- Healthy environments (safe physical environment and supportive economic and social conditions).
- Effective health services (provision of preventive services, access to and appropriateness of health services).

These factors lead to changes in health and social outcomes (morbidity, mortality, disability, dysfunction) resulting quite some time after an intervention, so tracing these changes to the effect of the intervention can be very difficult. Many other factors not associated with the intervention might influence health outcomes yet be difficult to identify and monitor. Particularly with short-term funding, programs can be in jeopardy if the intermediate outcomes of health promotion initiatives are not identified and valued, and their predicted links to longer term health outcomes explained carefully. As an area of national and local investment, health promotion can also be at risk if meaningful proof of impact cannot be demonstrated in time frames relevant to those who can provide technical and political support.

Rychetnik and Frommer's schema for evaluating evidence on public health interventions[15] represents a step forward in thinking about how health promotion effectiveness could be assessed. It accounts for 'the complexity of public health practice and the diversity of evaluations that are conducted in public health settings.'[15] It does this by accounting for:

- Contextual factors that might have played a critical role in interventions.
- Issues about evaluation – whether the timing of the evaluation related to project development and implementation or if it was done separately.
- Who did the evaluation and why.
- Whether the design and conduct of the evaluation was suitable to produce credible evaluation results.

SYSTEM FOR ACHIEVING PROGRAM EFFECTIVENESS

More than evidence is needed for programs to work. Existing evidence about what works – how and in what contexts – provides the basis for effective programs. However, evidence alone does not lead to effectiveness. The many elements required for program implementation and to build the evidence base for health promotion are captured in the following framework for achieving program effectiveness (Table 3.2).

Weaknesses in any of these domains will reduce the ability of programs to achieve their objectives. On the other hand, strengthening each of these aspects in a planned and comprehensive way is necessary to maximize the impact of health promotion programs. While efficacy requires technical knowledge, leadership skills become important in planning and implementation. The elements of this model will be explored in more detail in the following sections. Specific comments will be made about achieving program effectiveness in developing countries.

Efficacy

Improving the evidence base will require efforts in three main areas: availability of evidence; assessment of evidence about appropriate program design; and forms of evidence. Efficacy is the first dimension of the effectiveness equation, and this is the conventional focus for consideration of evidence-based practice. Efficacy studies answer the question: *Do we know what works and how it works?* This is the traditional realm of 'evidence'.

While programs may have been shown to work in one context, evidence from intervention research is still needed that examines how to design and

Table 3.2   A framework for achieving health promotion program effectiveness

Effectiveness =	Efficacy +	Planning +	Implementation
	Theory ('evidence')	Policy, planning and financing framework	Appropriate targeting
			Sufficient coverage
		Organizational structures and resources	Skilled actions
			Community ownership
		Workforce and community capacity Monitoring and evaluation	

*Adapted from Lin V and Fawkes S. 'Effectiveness of health promotion in changing environment and lifestyles in developing countries of the Western Pacific Region : A review and a proposed framework: Technical paper prepared for WHO Workshop on Capacity Building for Health Promotion. Manila, Phillipines, 5-8 November 2002.

make the program work in other contexts and with different populations. Intervention research that demonstrates the outcomes and costs of a program under *ideal conditions* to assess efficacy is a necessary prerequisite for research that tests the ability of a program to modify determinants of health in *natural conditions in a variety of contexts*. However, the ethical standards of research might preclude particular types of interventional research and therefore the types of evidence available to review.

While there are case studies of practice in specific contexts,[16] there is a relatively poor evidence base for health promotion programs in developing countries and resource-poor communities and health systems. This is related to a range of inter-connected factors:

- Divergent theories inform health promotion, such as: sociology, anthropology, economics, psychology, and political science. This makes the design and application of traditional experimental methods of interventional research difficult.
- The resources and capacity for interventional studies are limited.
- Programs may not be implemented successfully.
- Even if programs are implemented successfully, there is a history of poor documentation of the process and results of programs and activities. As a result, their value and/or harm is not known.
- Funding of projects tends to be short-term, limiting the range of opportunities for evaluative research. Funding is frequently directed to services rather than research and evaluation.

There is systematic bias inherent in the bodies of health promotion evidence. Countries that are well represented in the literature have well-developed systems for evaluation, peer review and publishing; good research conditions[17]; specific linguistic capacities and Western cultural and philosophical traditions.[18] In order to publish studies, researchers depend on a favourable resource environment that facilitates research into specific study questions. They also need access to training to develop the skills necessary to conduct research. Furthermore, they depend on access to the peer review and publication processes to make their work available for scrutiny and debate. At any stage of the research process, from framing the study question to producing research findings, there may be obstacles in the way of producing insight into important public health questions.[19]

Resource and technical capacity is weak in many developing countries and resource-poor health systems for recording, gathering and analysing the information required for monitoring health indicators and evaluating health changes over time at district levels.[20] As a consequence, process and impact outcomes from programs are not available to inform policy and practice. Inadvertently, developed country and Westernized models of problem solving might be adopted. Furthermore, developed countries are not able to benefit from the experience in developing countries and resource-poor communities in implementing low-cost programs in community settings.

The types and forms of evidence available clearly raise issues about applicability of evidence. Communities differ in their socioeconomic make-up, cultural disposition, ethnic mix, community resources, and any number of other factors which shape health beliefs and behaviours. The current evidence base about efficacy may not address the variations across all communities. For this evidence base to be successfully applied requires an understanding about conditional effectiveness – that is, under what circumstances would the interventions remain efficacious.

Infrastructure

The failure of program implementation (depicted in Fig. 3.2) and the inability to scale up programs to increase their reach and impact, can often be traced to

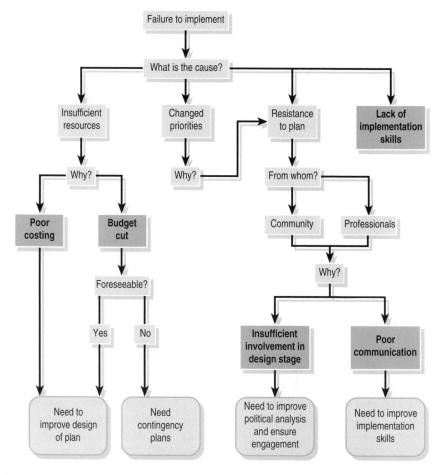

Fig. 3.2   Failure of implementation model. Adapted from Green A. An introduction to health planning in developing countries. Oxford: Oxford University Press; 1999.

symptoms of poor planning processes, weak infrastructure and inadequate capacity[21]:

- Responsibilities, strategies or plans are not clearly written or communicated or are difficult to understand.
- Lack of appropriate management controls and incentives.
- Lack of coordination.
- Lack of mechanisms for resolving difficulties in implementation.
- Resistance to implementation at the ground level, for example where the process has not been participatory[22] or where the values of the people responsible for implementation diverge.
- Workforce issues, such as lack of staff, inadequate training or skills, or staff changes.
- Lack of resources allocated to implementation.
- Emergence of new priorities.

Developing countries and resource-poor communities, in particular, face complex challenges in creating and sustaining national and local infrastructures and capacity for implementation in planned and comprehensive ways. Important underlying issues include:

- The robustness, priorities and 'planning horizon' of organizations that support health promotion.
- The ability of organizations to harness an adequate workforce and resources, and predict their availability.
- The variety and reliability of financing arrangements in place for health promotion and rules governing them.
- An emphasis on program delivery rather than monitoring and, especially, evaluation.

Four key aspects of infrastructure and capacity can be identified and used to assess health promotion program implementation capacity. These are:

1. Policy, planning and financing framework.
2. Organizational structures and resources, including commitment, competencies, structures for networks, communication, planning, decision-making.
3. Workforce and community capacity.
4. Monitoring and evaluation.

Policy planning and financing

An explicit and stable policy, planning and financing framework for health promotion is essential if programs are to be sustained adequately over time to produce results. Evidence about the efficacy of programs, and evaluations of their effectiveness play a critical role in securing policy support. Such data help to 'refocus policy and expenditure priorities on interventions that have been shown to work, rather than on programs that are well-established or well-marketed.'[23]

As with health promotion programs, there are social, cultural and historical as well as technical issues involved in the design of policy and financing frameworks. A framework with four inter-related dimensions for evidence-based purchasing of health promotion programs in New Zealand illustrates how these issues can be captured in four effectiveness criteria to frame policy[24]:

- Scientific dimension – rules of evidence. Provide scientific evidence of need and effectiveness.
- Organizational dimension – Governmental objectives, Treaty of Waitangi. Fit policy frameworks and be consistent with treaty-based obligations.
- Sociocultural dimension – equity. Be sensitive to social and cultural needs.
- Health promotion dimension – Ottawa Charter. Adopt recognized health promotion principles.

A framework such as this helps resources to be allocated and managed through the entire cycle of implementation and evaluation, even if process evaluation is producing ambiguous results or if there are emerging issues competing for attention and resources.

Organizational structures and resources

It has been argued that countries benefit from having dedicated 'driving forces' within and outside of government to promote health.[25] Three types of organizational structures[25] are commonly seen internationally in health promotion initiatives:

1. Government-led structures.
2. Independent structures.
3. Networks and professional associations.

Governments are uniquely placed to model and encourage quality, values and ethics in health promotion. Government-led structures have important forms of authority and opportunities for leadership that enable them to establish innovative structures *within* government and *between* government and external bodies to promote health.

Strong government backing of health promotion – led by Ministries of Health – is vital to the successful creation of partnerships across government sectors to form healthy public policy and between government and non-government or private sectors. Working across sectors is more feasible with formalized structures invested with decision-making capabilities, such as high-level committees. Appropriate sector representatives sit at the same table to drive research, analysis, action and evaluation relevant to health promotion.

Independent structures based on democratic processes are playing increasingly important roles in health promotion across the world. In some countries they offer new prospects to realize the health promotion principle of engaging people to increase control over the factors that affect their health. They provide shelter from short-term budget imperatives, enabling health promotion programs to continue through changes of government and policy. This group of organizations includes: independent, publicly funded health promotion institutions and non-government health promotion institutions.

Independent organizations are important because they provide knowledge, views, resources and networks that differ from government and other entities. They often operate on the principles of democracy, have close connections to communities, and might even be controlled by communities. They contribute a public voice on health matters in debates, agenda setting for policy and action. The potential of independent organizations to exercise influence is strengthened if they have capacity across the following areas[26]:

- Planning and consultation to enable a strategic approach to be developed.
- Credibility drawn from sources such as grass-roots connections, open and independent approaches, expertise, and a strong track record.
- Leadership.
- Networks and proactive building of relationships.
- Skills and resources for identifying, obtaining, analyzing and synthesizing relevant information.
- Internal and external communication processes, including using the media effectively.
- Ability to manage multiple roles and cope with multiple demands.
- Resources that do not limit influence and independence (human, financial and physical resources).
- Critical reflection skills to foster change in direction and strategy as necessary.

Networks and professional associations have similar types of organizational resources available to influence agenda-setting and drive action, such as: expertise in technical and political arenas; access to decision-making processes and leaders; flexibility in responding to issues and forming joint working relationships with government and other entities; and international relationships with peer organizations. Networks and associations of professionals operating at regional, national and international levels offer some capacity to advance action on health issues by engaging in debate, enquiry and advocacy.

While it is crucial to build new infrastructures that support effective health promotion, it has been argued that better and more imaginative use can be made of existing structures by 'identifying the potential of such structures and by adopting creative approaches that will bring other sectors into mutually beneficial partnerships.'[25] This strategy has particular relevance in resource-constrained conditions.

Workforce and community capacity

As well as organizational structures and resources, successful implementation of programs relies on a critical mass of skilled people to transfer program experiences and learnings to new issues and contexts. The health promotion skills of health workers and community members are complementary. Technical skills of a national health promotion workforce can be systematically developed through training and education and enriched by experience. Building the capacity of communities to play ongoing roles in health promotion[27] is equally important: 'developing skills and capacities in communities to affect the issues and decisions that affect their health is what health promotion is all about'.[28] Where workers develop skills more formally, communities learn 'on the job', through participating in decision-making and action.

A vital aspect of capacity is leadership; leaders in health promotion have to be identified and cultivated both from within the workforce and communities. Common to all leaders are appropriate values, ethics and practice skills. Among other important qualities, leaders need to be able to harness opportunities and negotiate the political milieu of health promotion, which in a number of countries may be uncertain.

All countries or jurisdictions and health systems should aim to develop a human resource strategy that articulates how the capacity of the workforce and communities can be developed for health promotion. For example, workforce capacity could be systematically enhanced in cost-effective ways through a combination of these approaches:

- Integrating health promotion in basic curricula for all health professionals.
- Providing on-site training and mentoring with more experienced and qualified personnel.
- Accessing training modules and programs from around the world via new technologies to raise the level of knowledge and skill.
- Contracting with training institutions to offer professional development programs, exchanges and mentoring.

Monitoring and evaluation

Monitoring occurs during program implementation. It uses the most relevant indicators and other milestones to provide feedback about the implementation process that can assist in making decisions that keep program implementation 'on track'. Alternatively, adjustments that are required to improve implementation or when repeating the program can be identified.

The types of information that are of interest arise at different stages of planning and implementing programs; from harnessing inputs, to conducting programs, to assessing changes in determinants of health, health status and quality of life. Systems – comprising structures, skills, technologies and other resources – need to be in place at program and organizational levels ('micro' level) and community and country levels ('macro' level) to gather the required information for planning and policy purposes.

The information model in Fig. 3.3 builds on Nutbeam's model of assessing health promotion outcomes and shows the types of information required to support health promotion programs. The model illustrates that implementation of programs relies on the provision of adequate resources, funding and information from the beginning of an initiative, including resources and information for evaluation (for example baseline data), through to longer-term evaluation of the outcomes of the intervention. While the model

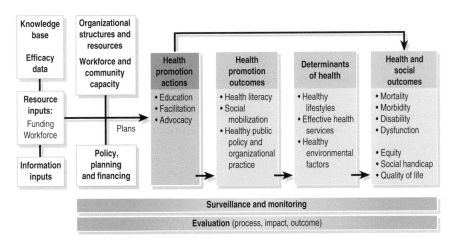

Fig. 3.3   Information model for monitoring and evaluating health promotion. Adapted from National Public Health Partnership. A Planning framework for public health practice. http://www.nphp.gov.au/ppi/planning/planfrwk/ accessed 8 July 2002 and Nutbeam.[14]

appears linear, in fact it has a dynamic quality that features the production and use of information at a number of points.

Monitoring systems should be based on minimum data sets in order to promote learnings about health promotion programs across countries and help make comparisons where appropriate. Associated with information about primary prevention, early detection, treatment and health promotion programs, a minimum data set can shed light on the impact of particular programs in reducing disease incidence. The approach can also drive capacity building to strengthen a country's ability to detect and analyse required information. Areas for national and local investment can be discovered by the gaps in data.

There are some prevailing problems in implementing minimum data sets across countries, given the variation among countries in the quality of data collected and the varying standards of health information available.[29] Health information may not be available due to inadequate skills, poor technical and technological support to develop and use local health information systems and lack of resources to gather and communicate data.

Problems in monitoring programs are often accompanied by problems evaluating programs. Many of the same types of resources are required for evaluation: technical knowledge about what data to collect, how and when; systems for collecting, analysing and communicating data; and resources that support both the workforce and evaluation processes. The evaluation of health promotion programs is frequently judged to be difficult, complex and often executed poorly.[30] Reasons for this include:

- The difficulty of attributing causality to a program, because of the length of time between an intervention and its effects[30] or 'interference' caused by other factors influencing outcomes.

- The likelihood that when implementing health promotion programs, general principles and strategies are applied rather than standardized procedures or protocols.[23]

Despite these difficulties, it is necessary to encourage a culture shift in developing countries and resource-poor health systems that brings evaluation into the range of normal practice, leads to appropriate resourcing over the required timeframe to reveal results, and is conducted to the best ability of the workforce using the available tools. In addition to resource commitment for evaluation, some of the key challenges for evaluation practice are:

- Using evidence more systematically in the planning of activities.
- Improving the definition and measurement of outcomes (categories such as changes to determinants of health, health outcomes, health promotion outcomes).
- Choosing an evaluation intensity that 'fits' with requirements and existing knowledge.
- Adopting evaluation designs that are appropriate for the intervention, making optimal use of quantitative and qualitative methods.

Action

Implementation is the third dimension of the effectiveness equation. Making detailed plans for disseminating efficacious programs is insufficient if implementation is not carried out well. Successful implementation builds on the evidence base and sound planning, and relies on:

- Targeting the program to the right population group/setting.
- Achieving adequate coverage by the program of sufficient numbers of the target population.
- Ensuring that those involved have the skills to implement the program in accordance with the design specification, or adjust the program design to local contexts.
- The program be actively supported and sustained by the community in which it is implemented.

Targeting a program

In planning a program, populations affected by a health issue are described and quantified. A distinction between a general population approach and targeting specific groups in higher risk categories is important. Targeting a general population might make good statistical sense in public health terms, as there is a measurable overall impact or lowering of risk across a given population. However, the aim might be to use the techniques of health promotion to make a difference to the health potential of *specific* groups, who might be at higher risk, such as socially disadvantaged groups.

An example can highlight this aspect of implementation. Developing a program to educate the whole population, via mass media channels, of the benefits of a low-fat diet to reduce heart disease risk is an appealing approach. Indeed, widespread uptake of the recommendations could lead to a measurable lowering of risk across the whole population. However, this result might be achieved by a significant reduction in risk in those communities who were least at risk.

An alternative or complementary approach is to target settings associated with the groups at higher risk in order to change the environmental conditions in which food choices are made and develop relevant personal skills. Useful settings would include schools, workplaces and marketplaces. Those communities who are affected by the issue of heart disease as well as stakeholders relevant to the issue can become active agents in changing products as well as the social, cultural and economic environments in which food choices are made.

Achieving sufficient coverage with the program

Attention also needs to be given to achieving adequate coverage of the program, that is, ensuring access by the target groups in sufficiently large numbers to achieve an impact. In statistical terms, a program that leads to small changes across a large population will have more effect than one that produces a large change in a small population. Effort needs to focus on scaling-up, or broadening the coverage of, health promotion programs so that more people can access the intervention. For example, this might involve the expansion of pilot settings projects (such as healthy schools) to engage the full network of settings in a country or region.

The reach of a program can be monitored during program implementation to provide information about the extent to which adequate population sizes or environments are being accessed by the program. This feedback can be used to refine strategies to increase coverage, and maximize the impact of the program on health.

Diffusing the program, to increase access, is a social and cultural process rather than a technical one. Organizations and communities might not automatically accept a program as beneficial for them.[31] Planning for successful program implementation involves analysis of a range of factors in advance of committing resources. The extent to which an innovation is adopted may be related to any or all of the following factors[32]:

- Values of organizations.
- Information available about innovations that would match perceived needs.
- Prevailing conditions.
- Timing.
- Perceived obligation to engage in change.
- Anticipated positive and negative consequences.

Implementation is a dynamic process, marked by ongoing negotiation between the parties, rather than being a rational, logical sequence. Rigorous analysis of program diffusion factors will assist in preventing implementation failure.

Employing skilled actions

A program can only achieve intended outcomes if it is implemented by health workers, communities and partner organizations in ways that are consistent with the evidence about what makes a program work. Variations in implementation can arise when personnel are not adequately trained and experienced in a specific program. This can lead to the failure of programs to bring about the changes expected and to achieve their objectives. Successful program implementation involves a range of skills and the insights gained through experience, so that actions can be carried out according to program specifications and adapted to changing conditions. The workforce engaged to manage the process of implementation requires not only skills but also access to appropriate resources (such as audiovisual equipment and communications technology) so that their skills can be used effectively.

Activities that support effective action include:

- Intervention protocols that specify how to implement the program.
- Models of optimal organizational structure that support programs.
- Development of evaluation criteria from the outset.
- Monitoring program adoption through process evaluation techniques.

Creating community partnerships

Research has demonstrated that 'the stronger the representation of the community and the greater the community involvement in the practical activities of health promotion, the greater the impact and the more sustainable the gains'.[33] Engagement of communities features in all WHO regional guidelines for healthy settings and in policies and guidelines for promoting health.[34] On its own, support for programs conducted by government or other agencies does not constitute community ownership; programs must also be cultivated, adapted and their effect sustained by the community. The development of community ownership starts early in the process of program planning, at the point of assessing and identifying needs. This early engagement sets the scene for community participation in agenda setting, policy-making, implementation and monitoring, and evaluation.

Developing countries have considerable experience (though largely undocumented) in generating community ownership of health promotion programs, and expertise to share.[18] Communities are more likely to become and remain engaged when a range of conditions are met:

1. Hardship arising from strained economic conditions does not prevent participation.[18]
2. Issues are relevant to them. When needs assessment and data gathering processes involve a community, the information base for program development is more likely to be owned by the community. Issues will be identified that are relevant and a high priority for communities. This process establishes a sound basis for longer-term working relationships between

community members and health services or other health promoting organizations.

3. Suitable and durable types of processes, structures and organizations are set up that make participation possible and rewarding. These include committees, cooperatives, coordinating councils, volunteer networks, forums, peer programs and civic activities. Local level projects such as healthy settings projects provide access by community members to structures that value their contribution and welcome involvement.

4. Participation can produce community leaders who carry the values and interests of the wider community. The main reward for leaders will be 'getting the job done', but incentives and rewards from valued social institutions and groups can help them develop further skills, roles and influence.

The main benefit of creating community ownership is that programs are better resourced to achieve their objectives. The process of creating ownership contributes to building the skills, resources, problem-solving capacity and experience of communities. This expanded social capital results from community members interacting with groups and social institutions during the processes of program development and implementation. It is a vital community asset that can be drawn on in addressing other issues and 'multiply health gains'.[35] Social capital has also been associated with good governance, economic prosperity, a range of health measures including infant mortality and some health conditions, for example deaths from stroke, accidents and suicides.[18]

Enhancing implementation capacity can occur in a range of mutually supportive ways – as a result of the conduct of specific programs; building on the experience of specific programs; and more systematically through investments in basic types of capacity – structures, skills, and resources. The absence of these is likely to lead to partial or complete failure of programs to achieve the necessary coverage to make an impact and to be implemented according to the program design. The prospect of scaling up even successful programs is weak without the necessary structures, skills and resources to do so.

EFFECTIVENESS OF HEALTH PROMOTION IN CHANGING ENVIRONMENT AND LIFESTYLES IN DEVELOPING COUNTRIES

A review of recent health promotion efforts in the developing countries of the Western Pacific Region illustrate some of the challenges in achieving health promotion effectiveness, including the accumulation of the evidence base. Countries in the Region have undertaken projects addressing a diverse range of health-related issues over many years, with the support of WHO and international aid agencies including AusAID,[36] World Bank,[37] Asian Development Bank[22] and non-government organizations such as Red Cross.[38] More recently, the settings approach to health promotion has been adopted as a popular and useful way to bring about changes in communities that support health.

In Vietnam, the concept of 'safe communities' has been successfully applied and achieved with 'remarkable results': injury prevention/safe community implementation is considered the 'duty' of the whole community, local authorities and citizen committees, and is incorporated into local plans. To establish efficacy, however, the program needs to establish more pilot models in other localities and expanded to a national scale.[39] The Healthy Lifestyle Campaign in Malaysia has given many health issues (cancer, nutrition, safety, child health, hygiene, HIV/AIDS, heart health) high national visibility by the campaign since 1991. Evaluation of the project[40] has recommended a shift from this short-term health promotion campaign to a long-term strategic health promotion program and evaluation approach.

In general, formal evaluations of issues-based and settings-based projects to assess their effectiveness are limited. A 1999 review of the settings approach in the Western Pacific Region[41] identified the need for:

- Strong institutions with a clear policy mandate around health.
- Skill development of the workforce to implement healthy settings.
- More data from process, impact and outcome evaluations that demonstrates what works (or doesn't work), how and why.
- Enhanced evaluation and documentation about local settings projects and mechanisms for their effective diffusion.
- Mobilizing and coordinating resources.

A 2002 review of reports from the WHO country missions reveals both strengths and weaknesses across healthy settings projects. Among its achievements, the settings approach has:

- Generated public and institutional visibility and political support for action on health.
- Inspired shared visions as a basis for collective action. For example, the Healthy Islands vision emphasises the experience of children, the centrality of ecological balance and the role of oceans in wellbeing.
- Added value to or reformed existing local infrastructures and mechanisms for health planning and action. For example, many healthy cities projects have facilitated broader participation at the local level multi-sectoral coordinating structures that bring together key players to mobilize commitment, resources, networks and integrated, multi-level actions to address multiple risks to health and improve conditions for health.
- Developed general and specific skills of workers at all levels so that they can implement the approach in their setting. For example, schools in many countries have trained teachers, parents groups and community organizations connected to schools in the principles and practice of health-promoting schools.
- Created alliances and partnerships between stakeholders, including community members, in an effort to secure broader commitment, ensure representation of key interests and expand the range of influence settings have in achieving change.
- Fostered sustainability, with communities remaining involved and continuing to participate in and resource action.

Reviews and a small number of independent research projects have been undertaken in relation to a range of settings: cities, islands, schools and workplaces. They provide further descriptive data about the implementation status of settings projects in the Region and are discussed in the following section.

The Healthy Cities approach has matured from the original concepts described in the mid-1980s[42] and is arguably one of the most significant settings for health promotion interventions. Achievements in implementing the concept have been accomplished at national and local levels[43,44] in Cambodia, China, Fiji, Laos, Malaysia, Mongolia, Papua New Guinea, Philippines and Vietnam. Countries' capacity to plan and implement healthy cities projects have strengthened in various ways[45] by putting into place national coordination structures and national guidelines that provide technical support to cities. Multi-sectoral structures at national and local levels have been established, project coordinators have been appointed, some resources have been mobilized and many activities in physical, social and economic spheres have been undertaken. Countries have developed mechanisms for advocacy, communication and networking as part of national networks.

Despite these achievements, some key areas need strengthening for the concept to lead to measurable changes in environments and lifestyles. At the national level in countries, weaknesses and gaps have been identified in: policy, leadership, organizational structures, guidelines, resources, personnel and support for information dissemination through networking. There are weaknesses in the processes that link top–down and bottom–up activities to build the legitimacy, infrastructure and sustainability for healthy cities. At the local level, policy and investments are needed to boost action in a number of areas. These are[1]:

- Leadership, as well as good planning processes, to secure resources.
- Engagement of stakeholders in planning, implementation and evaluation of healthy cities projects to mobilize commitment, improve priority setting and encourage cross-sectoral action.
- Ways to enrich community involvement through local settings require particular attention.[2]
- Training and raising awareness of many different stakeholders (government and non-government organizations, profit and not-for-profit organizations, and the community) through workshops, seminars, study visits and other dissemination mechanisms.[3]
- Development of resource capacity to support specific local initiatives.[4]
- Strengthening documentation and reporting of project implementation.

The Healthy *Islands* concept was spawned from Healthy Cities. Understanding of its implementation has been developing since the Yanuca Island Declaration of Health in the Pacific in the 21st century was proclaimed in 1995, through Ministerial meetings,[46] the Regional action plan and release of implementation guidelines. Accomplishments in Fiji, Papua New Guinea and Samoa have included establishing infrastructure (cross-sector committees, budgets, project management teams), training, and production of guidelines. The WHO Healthy Islands database will help to facilitate research, evaluation and information sharing, and contribute to strengthening the basis for assessing effectiveness.[47]

Health Promoting *Schools* are cost-effective sites for interventions that aim to improve the health of children and adolescents, and influence the health of teachers. Achievements by schools in the Region are developing consistency with research findings that good quality health promoting school programs[48]:

- Strengthen the curricula around health.
- Enhance schools' geographical, psychosocial, physical and organizational environments.
- Lead to improved water and sanitation facilities in the community.
- Facilitate links between schools and medical, dental and counselling services for preventive initiatives such as health checks and crisis support.
- Nurture partnerships between the school, parents, health sector and local community agencies.
- Implement school policies in key areas to maximize the health of students.

Healthy *Workplaces* reinforce occupational health and safety standards, but move beyond this to change physical, organizational and community environments so that they protect and promote the safety, health and wellbeing of workers. The model has been applied or adapted in China, Fiji, Malaysia, Mongolia, Papua New Guinea, Republic of Korea, Vietnam and some other sites.[49–51] Initiatives have been created in the following areas[52]: workplace policies for health and safety; organizational environment (how work is designed and organized); physical environment, for example water and sanitation facilities; lifestyles and personal health skills; health services; and wider social environment. Assessments of activities suggest that the healthy workplace approach is useful in reducing: the incidence of work-related injuries; diseases and related health-care costs; risk behaviours (such as cigarette smoking); and levels of sick leave.[50] Successful initiatives have been characterized by: participation by all staff in all phases; project management based on the problem-solving cycle of needs analysis, setting priorities, planning, implementation, continuous monitoring and evaluation; integration of programs into the normal life of organizations; and comprehensiveness of approaches to include individual-directed and environment-directed measures.

For all settings, there is a significant need for an evidence base for the healthy settings approach to be built from high quality monitoring and evaluation.

Effectiveness of health promotion in developing countries

This brief review of health promotion program implementation in developing countries in the Western Pacific Region points to a range of cross-cutting conclusions.

In general, high-quality published evaluations of health promotion programs are rare in the Region. While findings about short-term achievements can be located, access to comprehensive evaluation data through all stages of a program is limited. Consequently, an adequate evidence base is yet to be developed to aid the expansion of specific programs across a variety of social, cultural and economic contexts.

Available information from existing evaluation activities suggests that a number of programs that focus on settings, issues and capacity building merit continued support, but the technical quality of monitoring and evaluation activities needs strengthening. Provision of technical know-how by the WHO and partner organizations is increasing the number and frequency of completed program evaluations in the Region, which should help to shed light on the effectiveness of the full range of health promotion programs in the Region.

Some of the key areas for action emerging from the review include the following:

- A more systematic use of existing evidence (including literature and local knowledge) is required in planning and implementation.
- More documentation is needed in all programs (i.e. monitoring and evaluation products) to foster an evidence base of what does and does not work in specific contexts.
- Isolated pilot projects in particular contexts and with specific populations are most useful when they are comprehensively evaluated in terms of their effectiveness. Scaling up of projects on a national basis should be staged to build on the experiences and outcomes of pilot projects.
- More active dissemination/transfer of successful programs within a country and across communities is necessary to achieve impact.
- There need to be two tiers of policy, infrastructure and inter-sectoral engagement for settings projects to be sustainable and have momentum: national and local.
- Programs need to be linked to broader systems (especially education and health) as well as community-based organizations to be able to draw in necessary expertise and resources and link programs to other initiatives.
- Training programs in technical areas and leadership skills would help to boost the use of existing resources and structures for health promotion.

CONCLUSION

Notable achievements have been made by many health promotion programs around the world since the 1990s. There has also been considerable activity in a number of countries to strengthen national and local structures, capacity and partnerships for health promotion. However, the effectiveness of health promotion programs in bringing about desirable changes in environment and lifestyles is largely unknown. Initiatives to support improved effectiveness deserve to be given priority, particularly given the rapidity of demographic, epidemiological, social, and economic transitions occurring across the Region.

Table 3.3   A checklist for ensuring health promotion effectiveness

Framework element	Checklist
Efficacy	Literature search and systematic review conducted
	Program evaluations reviewed
Infrastructure	Policy authority in place
	Funding secure and adequate
	Organizational commitments assured
	Workforce skills developed and adequate
	Key stakeholders engaged
	Information system in place for monitoring and evaluation
Action	Target groups specified, quantified, and reachable
	Population coverage specified and achievable
	Community commitment gained
	Implementation protocol in place
	Feedback reporting mechanisms in place

An achievable first step towards improving effectiveness is to ensure that the planning process of all programs secures the requirements for successful implementation and evaluation. A checklist is proposed that distils the key requirements for ensuring program effectiveness (see Table 3.3).

From ensuring that *individual programs* apply existing evidence and are evaluated, other advances need to occur so that results of program evaluations can be disseminated and aggregated to contribute to the body of health promotion evidence. Reforms of supporting information systems (local and national) are needed to produce model projects, case studies, systematic reviews of effectiveness in priority areas, and regional guidelines. These rely on good quality monitoring and evaluation of *all programs*.

Existing structures, organizations, workers, resources and activities provide a good basis for the further development of systems to enhance program implementation and health promotion effectiveness. Active links with centres of excellence for health promotion evaluation will be important sources of know-how and legitimacy for countries and health systems to move forward. Engagement of new partners in strategic aspects of program development and implementation, such as leadership training, would strengthen the overall capacity to build evidence about effectiveness and to ensure effective outcomes.

References

1. International Union of Health Promotion and Education. The evidence of health promotion effectiveness. Shaping public health in the new Europe. 2nd edn. Brussels: European Commission; 2000.
2. International Union of Health Promotion and Education. The evidence of health promotion effectiveness. Shaping public health in the new Europe, 2nd edn. Brussels: European Commission; 2000.

3. Lin V, Gibson B. Evidence-based health policy: Problems and possibilities. Melbourne: Oxford University Press; 2003.

4. Frommer M, Rychetnik L. A schema for evaluating evidence on public health interventions. Melbourne: National Public Health Partnership; 2002.

5. Thorogood M, Coombes Y. Evaluating health promotion. Practice and methods. New York: Oxford University Press; 2000.

6. Sackett DL, Richardson WS, Rosenberg W, Haynes RB. Evidence-based medicine. New York: Churchill Livingstone; 1997.

7. Sackett D, Rosenberg W, Gray JM, Haynes R, Richardson W. Evidence based medicine: what it is and what it isn't. British Medical Journal 1996; 312:71–72.

8. Jackson S, Edwards R, Kahan B, Goodstadt M. An assessment of the methods and concepts used to synthesise the evidence of effectiveness in health promotion: a review of 17 initiatives. Canadian Consortium for Health Promotion Research; 28 September 2001.

9. National Health and Medical Research Council. A guide to the development, implementation and evaluation of clinical practice guidelines. Canberra: Commonwealth of Australia; 1999.

10. Speller V, Learmonth A, Harrison D. The search for evidence of effective health promotion. British Medical Journal 1997; 615(7104):361–363.

11. WHO Regional Office for the Western Pacific. Regional guidelines for developing a healthy cities project. Manila; March 2000.

12. Nutbeam D. Health promotion effectiveness – the questions to be answered. In: International Union of Health Promotion and Education. The evidence of health promotion effectiveness. shaping public health in a new Europe. Part 1: Evidence book, 2nd edn. Brussels: European Commission; 2000.

13. Rootman I, Goodstadt M, Hyndman B, McQueen DV, Potvin L, Springett J, et al. Evaluation in health promotion. Principles and perspectives, 1st edn. Copenhagen: World Health Organization; 2001.

14. Nutbeam D. Health outcomes and health promotion – defining success in health promotion. Health Promotion Journal of Australia 1996; 6(2):58–60.

15. Rychetnik L, Frommer M. A schema for evaluating evidence on public health interventions. Version 4. Sydney: University of Sydney; April 2002.

16. Hughes J, McCauley AP. Improving the fit: adolescents' needs and future programs for sexual and reproductive health in developing countries. Adolescent Reproductive Behaviour in the Developing World 1998; 29(2):233–246.

17. Editorial. Enabling research in developing countries. Lancet 2000;356(9235):1043.

18. Gillies P. Effectiveness of alliances and partnerships for health promotion. Health Promotion International 1998; 13(2):99–120.

19. Kavanagh A, Daly J, Jolley D. Research methods, evidence and public health. Australian and New Zealand Journal of Public Health 2002; 26(4):337–342.

20. Chung SA, Shapiro CM. Editorial. Journal of Psychosomatic Research 1999; 46:1–2.

21. Bryson J. Strategic planning for public and nonprofit organisations. San Francisco: Jossey-Bass; 1995.

22. Asian Development Bank. Fighting poverty in Asia and the Pacific. World Wide Web: http://www.adb.org accessed 5 October 2002.

23. Legge D. The evaluation of health development: the next methodological frontier? Australian and New Zealand Journal of Public Health 1999; 23(2):117–118.

24. Rada J, Ratima M, Howden-Chapman P. Evidence-based purchasing of health promotion: methodology for reviewing evidence. Health Promotion International 1999; 14(2):177–187.

25. Moodie R, Pisani E, Castellarnau MD. Infrastructures to promote health: the art of the possible. Technical paper prepared for the 5th Global Conference on Health Promotion, Mexico City, Mexico, June 2000.

26. Nathan S, Rotem A, Ritchie J. Closing the gap: Building the capacity of non-government organisations as advocates for health equity. Health Promotion International 2002; 17(1):69–78.

27. Yajima S, Takano T, Nakamura K, Watanabe M. Effectiveness of a community leaders' programme to promote healthy lifestyles in Tokyo, Japan. Health Promotion International 2001; 16(3):235–243.

28. Hawe P. Capacity building: for what? NSW Public Health Bulletin 2000 March:22–23.

29. WHO Regional Office for the Western Pacific. Cancer database for the Western Pacific Region. Essential features and data analysis. Manila: WHO Regional Office for the Western Pacific; 1999.

30. Nutbeam D. Evaluating health promotion – progress, problems and solutions. Health Promotion International 1998; 13(1):27–44.

31. Denis J, Hebert Y, Langley A, Lozeau D, Trottier L. Explaining diffusion patterns for health care innovations. Health Care Management Review 2002;27(3):60–73.

32. Davis H. Management of innovation and change in mental health services. Hospital and community psychiatry 1978; 29: 649–658.

33. Gillies P. WHO Working Paper. The effectiveness of alliances and partnerships for health promotion. In: Fourth International Conference on Health Promotion; Geneva: WHO; 1997.

34. NSW Health Department, Aboriginal Health and Medical Research Council of New South Wales. New South Wales Aboriginal Health Promotion Program: Directions Paper. Sydney: NSW Health Department; 2001.

35. Hawe P, Noort M, King L, Jordens C. Multiplying health gains: the critical role of capacity building in health promotion. Health Policy 1997; 39:29–42.

36. AusAID. Key aid sectors. Health.World Wide Web: http://www.ausaid.gov.au/keyaid/health.cfm accessed 1 October 2002.

37. World Bank Asia and the Pacific. http://www.ifc.org/98ar/asia.pdf accessed 1 October 2002.

38. Red Cross, http://www.redcross.org.av. Accessed 1 December 2002.

39. Chuan LH, Svanstrom L, Ekman R, Lieu DH, Cu NO, Dahlgren G, et al. Development of a national injury prevention/ safe community program in Vietnam. Health Promotion International 2001; 16(1):47–54.

40. Heckert DK. Evaluation of healthy lifestyles and health promotion programmes. Mission report, Malaysia, 23 June–6 July 1999.

41. Lin V. Health protection and health promotion: harmonising our responses to the challenges of the 21st century. Manilla: WHO; 25 November 1999.

42. Tsouros A. The WHO Healthy Cities Project: a project becomes a movement. Copenhagen, Denmark: WHO; 1990.

43. WHO Regional Office for Western Pacific. Workshop on healthy cities: evaluation and future directions. Johor Bahru, Indonesia: WHO; 18–20 October 2001.

44. WHO Regional Office for Western Pacific. Regional Guidelines for Developing a Healthy Cities Project. Manila, Philippines: WHO; March 2000.

45. WHO Regional Office for Western Pacific. Workshop on Healthy Cities: evaluation and future directions. Johor Bahru; 18–20 October 2001.

46. WHO Regional Office for Western Pacific. The vision of healthy islands for the 21st Century. Regional implementation guidelines. Manila, Philippines: WHO; 2002.

47. Galea G. Mission report. Review of progress in a series of projects and plans of action related to HPR and NCD in the WR/South Pacific jurisdiction. Healthy settings. Manila: WHO; 2001.

48. Nutbeam D, St Leger L. Effective health promotion in schools. In: International Union of Health Promotion and Education. The evidence of health promotion effectiveness. Shaping public health in the new Europe, 2nd edn. Brussels: European Commission; 2000.

49. WHO Regional Office for the Western Pacific. The work of WHO in the Western Pacific Region. Report to the Regional Director. Manila, Philippines: WHO; 2001.

50. Chu C, Breucker G, Harris N, Stitzel A, Gan X, Gu X, et al. Health-promoting workplaces; international settings development. Health Promotion International 2000;15(2):155–167.

51. O'Byrne D, Yu S-H. WHO travel report summary. Visit to Beijing, Henan and Shanghai (People's Republic of China). Geneva: WHO; 7 July 1998.

52. WHO Regional Office for the Western Pacific. Regional Guidelines for the Development of Healthy Workplaces. Manila; 1999.

CHAPTER **4**

Eating and nutrition

Helen Dixon
Susan Paxton

INTRODUCTION

Eating behaviours that have a negative impact on health broadly take three forms in the Western world: (1) eating an inadequate selection of food to ensure optimum levels of nutrients; (2) consuming an excess of energy for the body's needs contributing to problems associated with obesity; and (3) disordered eating patterns, such as the use of extreme weight loss strategies and binge eating, associated with psychological problems. While it does occur, under-nutrition is not a major public health issue in most of the Western world. This chapter will consider first the nature of the health problems posed by these risk behaviours. It will then review the major findings and issues identified with population-based, public health prevention interventions in these areas. The World Health Organization[1] distinction between three different types of prevention intervention, universal, selective and targeted prevention, will be adopted. Universal prevention interventions aim to change the behaviour of the population at large and may include strategies such as legislation. Selective prevention aims to prevent the development of risk behaviours and symptoms in non-symptomatic individuals believed to be at risk. Targeted prevention aims to prevent the further development of early symptoms of the problem.

PUBLIC HEALTH NUTRITION

Epidemiology of diet–related diseases

Healthy dietary behaviour is important to achieving good nutrition and health throughout life. Poor nutrition impacts on children and infant's normal development and potential, it causes ill health in adults and contributes to the development of a range of chronic, life-threatening diseases.[2] Ischaemic heart disease, stroke, colorectal cancer and diabetes mellitus rank among the top ten leading causes of death in developed regions of the world and nationally within Australia. Poor dietary practices such as low consumption of vegetables and fruit and excessive intake of saturated fat are important risk factors for these major non-communicable chronic diseases.[3,4] Overweight and obesity, which are partly symptomatic of dietary factors, are also common underlying risk factors for major chronic diseases.[5]

Dietary factors and obesity also bear associations with a range of other health problems. For example, obesity is a risk factor for osteoarthritis, work disability, sleep apnoea and for other cancers such as cancer of the endometrium, kidney, breast (postmenopausal) and oesophagus.[4-7] In addition to health problems associated with excessive fat intake and low fruit and vegetable intake, other dietary factors are associated with disease risk. For example, calcium deficiency is a risk factor for osteoporosis.[8] Excess salt consumption is associated with increased risk of ischaemic heart disease and stroke.[9]

While the major diet-related illnesses affecting populations in developed countries tend to relate to nutritional excesses, in developing countries and among certain population subgroups in developed countries, nutritional deficiencies pose significant public health problems. For example, in Bangladesh and India, iron deficiency, vitamin A deficiency and iodine deficiency remain significant public health challenges.[10,11] In Australia, Aboriginal and Torres Strait Islander Australians are at greater risk of poor health due to inadequate nutrition compared to other segments of the population.[2] Food security refers to the capacity to access food of sufficient quality and quantity to enable unrestricted growth and development of all individuals at all times. Low incomes and environmental and social factors are thought to underpin issues of food insecurity experienced by many indigenous Australians.

Public health recommendations

The burden of chronic diseases is rapidly increasing in the developed and developing regions of the world.[4] Cardiovascular health, cancer control, and diabetes mellitus have been agreed on as National Health Priority Areas for

Australia.[12] While other lifestyle factors such as smoking contribute significantly to risk of non-communicable chronic diseases, dietary factors also play an important role. There tends to be convergence on the public health recommendations that can be made on the basis of epidemiological evidence. Encouraging healthy body weight, increased consumption of fruits and vegetables, and increased physical activity should help in prevention and treatment of diabetes, prevention of heart disease, and prevention of some cancers.

Various public health recommendations and strategies have been disseminated or implemented in an attempt to address the underlying causes of the preventable burden of diet-related disease and early death (e.g. see Ref. 4). The Dietary Guidelines for Australians specify dietary recommendations for adults,[3] children and adolescents.[13] There is broad agreement in international and national dietary guidelines, which emphasize the need to reduce dietary intake of fat (especially saturated fat), salt and refined sugars, and increase intake of wholegrain cereals, fruit and vegetables.

On average, Australians do not consume enough vegetables and fruit for optimal health.[2,14] National Nutrition Survey (1995) data indicated about half the adult population met the National Health and Medical Research Council's recommended '2 serves of fruit per day' and less than one-fifth of adults met the '5 or more serves of vegetables per day' recommendation.[15]

A common recommendation for adults has been that total fat should comprise about 30% of total energy intake, with a maximum of 10% of total energy intake coming from saturated fat.[3] National Nutrition Survey (1995) data indicated that adults' mean total fat intake and saturated fat intake slightly exceeded these recommendations.[15] Among adults, mean intake of total fats declined significantly between 1983 and 1995.[17] For children, total fat intake did not change significantly between 1985 and 1995.[17] During this period children's intake of fats added to prepared foods (e.g. butter) appeared to decline; however this was balanced out by an increased intake of fat from other sources such as cereal-based food and confectionery and 'health' bars.[17]

A common method of classifying body weight is based on the Body Mass Index or 'BMI', which is calculated as weight in kilograms divided by height in meters squared. According to World Health Organization[1] definitions:

- People with a BMI under 18.5 kg/m^2 are classified as underweight.
- People with a BMI of 18.5 to 24.9 kg/m^2 are classified as healthy weight.
- People with a BMI of 25.0 to 29.9 kg/m^2 are classified as overweight.
- People with a BMI of 30.0 kg/m^2 or higher are classified as obese.

The above definitions of overweight and obesity have been used in children. However, some researchers have developed more detailed assessments for children of different age levels (e.g. see Ref. 18).

Obesity is prevalent among adults and children in both developing and developed countries.[1] The fundamental causes of the obesity epidemic are sedentary lifestyles and high-fat, energy-dense diets. Being physically active and eating according to one's energy needs are both important to achieving healthy body weight.[313] The AusDiab survey found that the prevalence of overweight and obesity was almost 60% among Australian adults aged 25 and over.[20] Survey data for NSW and Victoria indicate that in 1997, over 20% of children were overweight or obese.[21] At the other end of the scale is the problem of underweight. People who are underweight are more prone to nutritional deficiencies.[15] The highest proportions of Australian adults who are underweight are aged 19–24 years, with more females than males underweight in each age group.[15]

Determinants of dietary behaviour

In reviewing methods of promoting changes in dietary behaviour, it is useful to consider factors that influence people's dietary behaviour. Figure 4.1 provides a conceptual model of social, economic and individual determinants of dietary behaviour. Dietary behaviour may be influenced by social and structural variables that influence people's capacity to access fresh, affordable and nutritious food. Environments, policies, social norms, and resources all exert influence. For instance, in some remote areas of Australia, high costs for refrigeration and food transport mean that fresh produce is more costly to consumers in these areas than in some other places in Australia where fresh produce is relatively cheap and accessible.[2] Food fortification (e.g. adding iodine to salt) is an important example of how changes at the food manufacturing level may facilitate people's capacity to access certain essential nutrients. Social and structural variables may also influence people's access to information about food and nutrition. For instance, concerns have been raised about the high prevalence of television junk food advertising to which children in Australia are exposed.[22] Exposure to food advertisements has been found to influence young children's food preferences.[23] If healthy diet messages do not receive similar television coverage in children's viewing times, this may mean that children receive more prompts to eat unhealthy foods than healthy foods via this medium.[108]

At the micro-level, individual factors such as knowledge, attitudes, skills, and age may all affect people's dietary behaviour. Models of individual health behaviour such as the Health Belief Model,[24] the Theory of Planned Behaviour,[25] and the Transtheoretical Model[26] may be used to inform health promotion and research aimed at identifying, assessing or modifying individual determinants of dietary behaviour. As a health-related behaviour, dietary behaviour is interesting, in that it is a biologically essential behaviour. Everyone needs to eat! The challenge for health educators is to encourage appropriate levels of consumption of nutritious foods. Typically this involves encouraging people to modify existing behaviour, such as eat less fat or eat more vegetables. Dietary behaviour, contrasts with health-risk behaviours such as smoking, where there is no safe level of tobacco consumption and the goal of health promoters is to discourage the behaviour of smoking altogether.

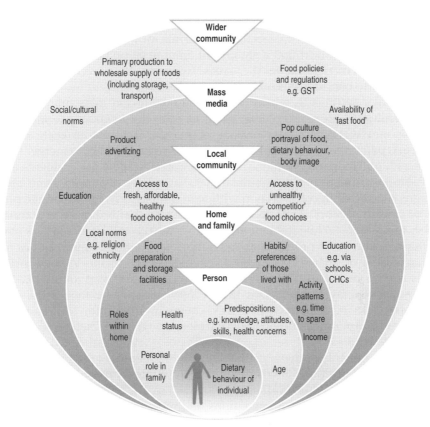

Fig. 4.1   Conceptual model of the determinants of individual dietary behaviour.

Public health nutrition interventions

Given the breadth of impact of dietary factors on health status, public health interventions promoting a balanced diet and healthy body weight are likely to afford multiple health benefits on the community.

Green and Kreuter[27] define health promotion as 'The combination of education and environmental supports for actions and conditions of living conducive to health'. The various factors influencing dietary behaviour draw attention to possible avenues for interventions to promote healthy eating. Efforts can be made to promote changes at different levels of influence (e.g. at the societal level, the organizational level, the community level, the family level or the individual level) that support healthy dietary behaviour among consumers. Education alone may be insufficient to bring about dietary change unless it is accompanied by appropriate policy and environmental changes.[28,29]

This section reviews public health nutrition interventions that have attempted to promote more healthy dietary practices among consumers, with a focus on interventions attempting to address dietary factors related to cardiovascular disease, cancer and type II diabetes prevention. These interventions have typically been aimed at promoting reduced consumption of fats, increased consumption of vegetables and fruits, or promoting healthy body weight. It is recognized that a significant amount of public health nutrition work has been carried out in other areas. However, it is beyond the scope of this chapter to consider this material here.

The major settings in which public health nutrition interventions have been conducted are mass media, point of sale, the food service industry, schools and worksites. Interventions employing new media such as the Internet, palm pilots and mobile phones are also beginning to emerge. Public health nutrition interventions have been carried out by governments and by non-government health organizations. There have also been some campaigns conducted in collaboration with food industry groups seeking to promote consumption of foods consistent with those that health organizations wish to promote. While the motives of the industry and health sectors may differ (i.e. pursuit of profit versus pursuit of health gain), opportunities for collaboration on shared objectives do exist. For example, in Victoria in the early 1990s, the '2 fruit and 5 veg every day' campaign was jointly funded and supported by public sector health agencies and the food industry.[30] Recently, Coles supermarkets' '7-a-day' campaign promoting fruit and vegetable consumption has been run in partnership with the Dieticians Association of Australia.[18]

The determinants of dietary behaviour highlighted in Fig. 4.1 draw attention to the various levels at which the impact of interventions may be monitored when conducting evaluation research. In the published evaluation literature on healthy diet interventions, the most frequently used outcome measures are of consumption of target foods or nutrients. Some interventions conducted in specific settings (e.g. schools, workplaces or primary care) have measured blood cholesterol or other markers of chronic disease risk. Interventions conducted in retail or food service settings have tended to use purchasing data on promoted food items as measures of impact. Measuring food consumption is challenging and researchers need to carefully select measures that are likely to be sufficiently sensitive to detect change, while being practically feasible and cost-effective to administer. Possible measures of impact are self-reported consumption (from direct surveys of consumers using food frequency questionnaires or other shorter questionnaires), use of biomarkers (e.g. blood cholesterol, carotin), physical measures (e.g. body mass index, waist measurement), or apparent consumption data (food disappearance or sales data from the food industry). It may also be relevant to assess cognitive and psychosocial correlates of dietary behaviour such as knowledge, attitudes and self-efficacy as intermediate markers of impact. For a review and analysis of evaluation measures used in nutrition education intervention research, see Reference 31.

When designing, implementing and evaluating dietary interventions, it is important to select appropriate intervention strategies that are likely to reach and facilitate change among the target audience and to use study designs and measurement instruments that have the capacity to detect impact should it occur. Several reviews have noted that many dietary intervention evaluations have been conducted with limitations to the study design or impact measures used, preventing firm conclusions being drawn from the results.[32-34] Ideally, evaluation methods should be designed alongside the development of the intervention. Publishing the results of well-designed evaluation studies in peer-reviewed journals enables other health researchers and practitioners to build on past experience in the field.

Literature reviews of good quality evaluation data from healthy diet interventions suggest that it is possible to achieve modest but significant improvements in outcome measures of impact. Long-term interventions in the general population have achieved reductions by 1 to 4% of energy intake from dietary fat; intensive interventions with highly motivated individuals have achieved reductions in fat intake and blood cholesterol of around 10%; interventions in supermarket and catering settings have shown increases between 1 and 4% in the market share of promoted items; passive manipulation of food menus has led to reductions in fat content of catered meals by 6 to 12 % of energy intake.[35] A number of interventions to promote fruit and vegetable consumption have achieved significant increases in consumption of these foods, with median differences between intervention and control groups indicating average increases in fruit and vegetable intake of 0.6 servings per day.[32] Given the generally small magnitude of change evident for those dietary interventions that have demonstrated impact, questions have been raised whether such efforts are justifiable or cost-effective. There is little published information concerning the cost-effectiveness of dietary interventions.[32] However, it has been argued that even small gains at the population level may amount to significant health gains.[36] For example, the Health Education Authority[35] argued that for every 1% reduction in blood cholesterol there should be a 2 to 3% lower risk of heart disease on a population basis.

Social marketing campaigns

Social marketing campaigns are a form of universal dietary intervention that has been conducted by both the food industry and the health sector. Social marketing campaigns are oriented towards consumers.[37] Research is conducted to identify target audiences' demographic, behavioural, psychological and media profile. Communications and strategies are tailored to reach consumers based on this research. Typically, products or messages are pre-tested with the target audience, and further research is conducted to evaluate the impact of the intervention once it is disseminated. Social marketing campaigns typically employ mass media promotions, which are reinforced by other community level interventions. In the diet area this has typically consisted of paid TV advertising, with some print or radio advertising, with other public relations events conducted to stimulate additional unpaid media coverage. Mass media promotions are then reinforced at the local level through promotions such as point of sale displays (often involving printed recipe leaflets or books) or sponsorship of sports or arts events.

A limitation of health industry campaigns is that they tend to have more modest budgets than industry-led campaigns. Consequently, the health sector has often run somewhat short media campaigns, with smaller budgets for creative advertising executions, and with less segmented target audiences than industry campaigns.[38] However, the strength of health sector involvement in campaigns is that they are generally well-regarded by the community as credible sources of health information and they are often able to make use of other communication channels less accessible to industry groups such as schools and community health centres. Collaboration between the health and industry sectors has given rise to the larger, more sustained social marketing campaigns run in this area.

A number of social marketing campaigns to promote awareness of dietary recommendations concerning fruit and vegetables and ultimately the increased consumption of these foods have been conducted nationally and internationally. The '5-a-day' program in the United States was a national, population-based nutrition initiative run in partnership between the US National Cancer Institute and the fruit and vegetable industry between 1989 and 1991.[39] Evaluation results indicate that the campaign raised public awareness that vegetables and fruit help reduce cancer risk, increased vegetable consumption and created an ongoing partnership between health and agribusiness.[40] In Australia, several state-wide social marketing campaigns aimed at promoting increased consumption of vegetables and fruit have been run. The 'fruit and veg with every meal' campaign ran in Western Australia from 1989 to 1993, and South Australia from 1990 to 1991. The '2 fruit and 5 veg every day' campaign ran in Western Australia from 1989 to 1993 and Victoria from 1992 to 1995. The 'Eat Well Tasmania' campaign ran in 1997. Where available, evaluation results indicate that these campaigns succeeded in promoting increased awareness of dietary recommendations for fruit and vegetables, with those campaigns that were sustained for a number of years (e.g. Victoria and Western Australia) detecting modest increases in reported vegetable and fruit consumption.[30,41,42] Those campaigns with larger media budgets that employed a comprehensive range of promotional strategies, and maintained a sustained presence over a number of years have yielded the strongest evidence of an impact on people's dietary behaviour. While available evidence suggests such interventions may impact on dietary behaviour, many evaluations of community-wide dietary interventions have only monitored dietary changes in a single community over time.[43] There is a need for randomized controlled trials to be conducted in this field to strengthen the evidence base.

Point of sale promotions

Point of sale promotions are able to reach diverse segments of society in large numbers, in a context where they make decisions about food purchases. They are commonly conducted in supermarkets or other food retail outlets. The most common forms of point of sale food promotions are recipe leaflets or poster displays alongside produce, product labelling, and in-store food demonstrations or tastings. These strategies have been employed in food industry and health industry point of sale promotions. Health industry promotions tend to focus on nutritional aspects of categories of foods, whereas food industry promotions tend to focus on promoting particular products.[38] Since the 1990s, health industry point of sale promotions have attempted to address behavioural as well as nutritional aspects of diet, through promoting the flavour, convenience or price of certain foods. These factors are important in influencing people's food choices.[44] Some point of sale promotions have been jointly funded by producer groups and health agencies (e.g. Coles '7-a-day' in Australia, '5-a-day' in the United States). The Heart Foundation's 'Pick the Tick' food approval program is a prominent example of promoting nutrition-related health information at the point of sale. Products with the tick have been independently tested and meet the Foundation's strict nutritional criteria for fat, salt, sugar and fibre content.[45] The aim of displaying the ticks on certain products is to enable consumers to quickly and easily make healthy food choices.

Point of sale promotions are often used as part of a broader promotion or campaign, and provide one avenue for reinforcing mass media messages at a local level. This means that when evaluating the impact of point of sale promotions, it can be challenging to isolate their effects from other influences. Most evaluations of point of sale interventions have used product awareness or sales data as measures of impact. Point of sale interventions appear to raise awareness, however there is a need for more research into the effects of such interventions on dietary behaviour.[43] Such interventions have also tended to be run for only a few months, with little long-term evaluation.

Supermarket interventions that promote the health benefits of particular brands (e.g. low sodium, cholesterol, calories or fat) at the place where the products are shelved or displayed have been found to increase sales of those products being promoted[46] – especially where shelf signs are supported by brochures and advertising.[35] Women with higher levels of education seem to be the most receptive to nutritional messages at point of sale.[38] Miller and Stafford[38] identified a number of factors that appear to contribute to the effectiveness of point of sale interventions: tailoring the message and type of promotion to the needs of target groups identified through research; using nutrition messages only when they are salient to the expressed needs of the target group (e.g. feeding children for young mothers); credible health agency endorsements; focus on taste, quality, value, convenience; seasonal promotion of fresh produce; meal solutions with recipes; interactive promotions. Certain aspects of the management of the promotion may contribute to effectiveness: regularly updating the promotion to sustain interest; achieving mutual agreement between store management and agency conducting promotion as to who is responsible for setting up, maintaining or implementing other aspects of the promotion; using professional merchandisers to set up and maintain displays.

Food service industry promotions

The food service industry includes restaurants, hotels and other settings where meals and snacks are served to consumers. The increasing trend among consumers towards takeaway food and dining out[3] means nutrition interventions conducted in food service settings are likely to be a promising means of reaching large numbers of people from diverse backgrounds in contexts where they select and consume food. Modifying the food service environment should help support and facilitate individual behaviour change and create social norms for more healthful eating practices. Nutrition interventions conducted in the food service industry have tended to focus on organizational or environmental strategies aimed at changing the nature of the food supplied (e.g. healthy catering policies for hotels), or on nutrition education and dissemination strategies aimed at influencing customer's knowledge, attitude and behaviour.[38] For example, labelling restaurant menus with nutrition information has been found to promote nutrition knowledge and selection of low fat or low cholesterol menu items among customers.[47] Passively manipulating the composition of food, instead of actively promoting healthier items has also been found to decrease the fat content of catered meals by 6 to 12% of energy intake.[35]

Miller & Stafford's[38] review of fruit and vegetable interventions conducted in the food service industry led them to conclude that the following elements contribute to effectiveness: basing programs on collaborative and behaviourally oriented models of change that consider organizational and environmental barriers to change; involving and developing a network of key stakeholders (e.g. working group to drive the intervention); involving food service staff in development and implementation of the intervention, and providing such staff with training and skills development; develop or modify policy that supports sale of target foods (e.g. cheaper pricing of healthier foods); modify menus, recipes and purchasing practices to support intervention goals; provide point of sale information that includes nutrient labelling and competitions/incentives (see also Ref. 46); negotiate feasibility of goals and changes sought; conduct intervention for a sustained period (12 months minimum); run food service intervention as a component of a broader multilevel campaign that includes mass media. The challenges in conducting food service interventions are that it can be difficult and time consuming to gain support for change (especially environmental/organizational change) from food service staff and management, developing appropriate training methods for staff may be difficult, and perceptions of the program as time consuming or costly may create resistance among management and staff.

School interventions

Schools are a popular setting for conducting selective health promotion interventions as they provide an avenue for reaching and impacting on the health behaviour of large numbers of children and teenagers with varied sociodemographic characteristics. Establishing healthful dietary practices early in life should be beneficial during childhood and later in life. School-based nutrition interventions have employed a range of strategies such as including nutrition education activities in the curriculum, introducing healthy canteen policies and working to involve the wider community, especially parents, in the interventions. The primary theoretical framework used has been social learning theory.[35] The majority of such interventions have been conducted in schools. However, some selective nutrition interventions targeted at teenagers have been conducted in other settings such as after-school programs, summer camps, community centres, libraries, and grocery stores.[48]

Some school-based nutrition interventions have demonstrated significant improvements in psychosocial correlates of healthy eating and increases in consumption of nutritious foods. Long-term, randomized, multi-contact interventions have achieved decreases in fat intake of between 2 to 3.5% of energy.[35] Reviews of school-based dietary interventions have tended to arrive at similar conclusions regarding features that appear to contribute to the efficacy of such interventions.[35,38,48–50]

The most effective interventions tended to rely on longer-term curriculum-based interventions, supported by teacher training, food service changes, health industry involvement, and parental or family involvement. A supportive school environment also appears to facilitate the impact of such interventions, whereas competing school priorities, and perceptions by teachers of the intervention as too demanding may act as barriers to implementation. Making food service changes at school canteens provides consistency between what is learned in class and the foods available to students at recess and lunchtime. Promising strategies include changes to menus or food pricing and training of food service staff. Reducing the price of low fat snacks at school cafeterias has been found to dramatically increase consumption of such foods.[44]

Children also appear to respond well to active participation in nutrition education activities such as cooking, supermarket tours, and taste testing. Involving parents and the wider community provides opportunities to reinforce school program messages outside of school. It is important that the strategies employed are developmentally appropriate to the children being targeted.[48] For example, family involvement appears to be particularly effective with younger children, and for older children, incorporating self-assessment and feedback into the program contributes to efficacy.[50] As with other public health interventions, using theory and research to inform the development of school-based nutrition interventions, providing adequate infrastructure and funding, conducting a sufficiently long and intense intervention, and evaluating the intervention's implementation and impact all appear to contribute to effectiveness. The Centers for Disease Control and Prevention[51] have published guidelines concerning strategies that are most likely to be effective in promoting healthy eating among school-age children.

Worksite interventions

Worksite interventions provide opportunity to access and impact on large numbers of people with diverse sociodemographic characteristics. As lower socioeconomic status tends to be associated with less healthful eating[52] worksites provide a promising channel for reaching blue-collar groups with selective nutrition interventions. Worksite nutrition interventions also provide opportunities to support individual dietary change by making changes in the environment, particularly food service changes in workplace canteens or cafeterias. Heimendinger et al.[53] proposed a model for worksite health promotion based on a review of worksite health promotion interventions on cancer prevention and theories of behaviour change applicable to such interventions. These authors argued strongly for the need to simultaneously address changes in individual behaviours and in the worksite environment.

Several reviews of worksite nutrition interventions have been conducted. Overall, evaluation evidence on worksite health promotion trials on diet and overweight indicates modest but positive effects on dietary behaviour.[43,54] Published studies indicate that such programs are feasible and that participants benefit in the short-term. However, limitations to many of the study designs (e.g. no control group, non-randomized designs, self-selection of high-risk or volunteer participants) limit the conclusiveness of evidence of impact.[55] Some published randomized controlled trials of worksite nutrition interventions have demonstrated significant improvements in psychosocial variables (e.g. dietary intake[56,57] and cardiovascular disease risk factors[58]).

The following factors appear to contribute to the effectiveness of worksite nutrition interventions: incorporating theoretical perspectives (e.g. community organization, socioecological model); being part of a comprehensive multilevel strategy campaign that includes mass media; training of worksite coordinators; targeting individual and environmental change to support and maintain change; food service changes (e.g. availability, access and competitive pricing of healthy food options, point of sale promotions); involving workers in development and implementation of the intervention; including family in the intervention strategy in order to carry the nutrition intervention beyond the worksite.[38,49] Reducing the price of low fat snacks at worksite food vending machines has been found to markedly increase consumption of such snacks.[44] Potential barriers to conducting worksite nutrition interventions include low recruitment rates for individually targeted strategies, low retention rates of workplaces and participants, and time and difficulty of involving management and workers in decisions about environmental initiatives.[38]

Primary care interventions

A number of selective and targeted nutrition interventions have been delivered in primary care settings either by nurses or general practitioners.[59,60] Providing educational materials with minimal contact has not been found to be very effective. However, more intensive, sustained and personalised interventions have demonstrated promising results, particularly those interventions targeted at people with increased risk (e.g. those with elevated cholesterol levels or who are already overweight). Such interventions appear to have had more success in reducing serum cholesterol levels than body mass index.[61] However, some randomized trials have achieved change on a range of outcome measures. For example, an intervention targeting overweight premenopausal women that included meal-replacements and general practitioner or dietician-led advice on lifestyle modification achieved significant reductions in percentage body fat, body mass index, waist circumference, insulin level and cholesterol levels.[62] An intervention involving nurse-administered health checks of urban adults in primary care resulted in significant reductions in self-reported saturated fat intake, blood pressure, cholesterol and body mass index, with benefits sustained over three years, especially for those who received annual health checks.[63] Targeting individuals at high risk may be advantageous because the intervention can be tailored to individuals, and subjects and health professionals may be motivated if a problem already exists. Studies conducted with populations at risk of (or diagnosed with) disease have observed greater changes in dietary fat and fruit and vegetable intake than studies conducted among the general population.[32] However, because those interventions targeting high-risk individuals have tended to be relatively intense, it is difficult to discern whether population or intervention characteristics are primarily responsible for the more marked outcomes achieved.

The benefits of conducting individually-oriented interventions need to be weighed up against the costs of screening and delivering them one-on-one compared to conducting universal interventions[36] for a discussion on the 'high-risk' versus population or universal approach to intervention). Interventions employing individual or group counselling to promote dietary change have demonstrated that it is possible to successfully change people's dietary behaviour, even by large amounts, 'We need to determine how best to leverage some of the successes of the individually randomized trials to community and public health settings'.[43]

Future directions

In reviewing public health nutrition interventions, a number of recurrent themes emerge. While much work has been conducted, there remains a need for well-designed evaluation studies to be conducted that include adequate sample size, control groups, documentation of intervention intensity and duration, use of appropriate measures of impact, and follow-up over time. To build the evidence base as to which dietary intervention strategies are the most effective, studies need to be sufficiently well-designed to detect change should it occur. There is also a lack of cost-effectiveness data available concerning dietary interventions.[32] Available research does highlight intervention characteristics that appear to contribute to efficacy. These include, using a theoretical basis to guide the intervention, targeting higher disease risk populations, using social support components in the interventions, using goal setting, small groups, participation in interactive activities with food, and the incorporation of family components.[32]

PREVENTION AND TREATMENT OF OBESITY: THE NEW PUBLIC HEALTH CHALLENGE

In 1997, a World Health Organization expert consultation on obesity declared that obesity should be regarded as today's principal neglected public health problem. They argued that it is essential that universal prevention interventions be developed to curb the obesity epidemic and the medical complications arising from it.[1] In Australia, the National Health and Medical Research Council[64] released a strategic plan for the prevention of overweight and obesity, which focuses chiefly on universal intervention strategies. It recommends a population-based approach involving efforts to change the macro-environment to enable people to make healthier food choices and undertake physical activity.

To date, more work has been done evaluating interventions targeted at those who are already overweight or obese than on universal interventions. Several reviews of targeted obesity interventions have been conducted. Among overweight and obese individuals, targeted interventions include dietary change, alterations in physical activity and behaviour modification.[1] A systematic review of randomized controlled trials[65] indicated that for obese children, family therapy and lifestyle modification appear to be effective in preventing and treating obesity. Among adults, the evidence is less clear, but indicates that behavioural therapy and multicomponent strategies may be useful. Non-behavioural methods of treating obesity, such as pharmacological intervention, may be successful initially, with subsequent regain of weight. For morbidly obese individuals surgery (e.g. gastric bypass) can be effective. Unfortunately, most overweight and obese people have difficulty maintaining weight loss in the long term.[66]

While it is generally agreed that prevention programs will stem the obesity epidemic more efficiently than weight-loss programs, to date relatively few prevention programs have been developed or implemented, there are limited high quality evaluation data available, and the success rates reported have been low.[5,67] Little rigorous evaluation of universal interventions has been carried out in larger populations.[68] Obesity prevention has been integrated into community-wide programs to prevent coronary heart disease, and while such interventions have been successful in reducing certain cardiovascular risk factors, they did not affect mean body mass index of the target populations. Some selective prevention directed at high-risk individuals (e.g. children with obese parents) has been conducted, with variable success.[68] Public health experts have argued that broad-based strategies with a strong emphasis on the environment are needed to control the obesity epidemic.[64] There is a need for further research and evaluation on well-designed interventions aimed at obesity prevention.

It is imperative that communications and other strategies used in any obesity prevention efforts avoid stigmatizing those who are already overweight and do not inadvertently perpetuate an unhealthily thin body ideal. Irving and Neumark-Sztainer[69] have recently proposed an integrated approach to the prevention of the spectrum of problems related to eating and weight (i.e. eating disorders, obesity, and unhealthy weight-loss practices) that includes personal, socioenvironmental and behavioural factors. They argue for primary prevention efforts to promote healthy attitudes and behaviours regarding food, physical activity, and body image and to reduce people's vulnerability to pressures (e.g. from peers, media, family) to engage in unhealthy behaviour.

PUBLIC HEALTH INTERVENTIONS FOR DISORDERED EATING

Epidemiology of disordered eating

The main eating disorders recognized include anorexia nervosa, bulimia nervosa and eating disorders not otherwise specified (EDNOS).[70] Anorexia nervosa is a self-starvation disorder that, while very serious, affects only a small proportion of the population in Western countries, approximately 0.3% of females and a smaller proportion of males.[70a] Bulimia nervosa is a disorder marked by regular binge eating of unusually large amounts of food in an uncontrolled manner, followed by compensatory behaviours such as fasting, excessive exercise and self-induced vomiting in healthy weight or overweight individuals. It is associated with poor body image, psychological distress, depression and low self-esteem.[71] This disorder has been estimated to affect 1.5–3% of adult females in Australia[72–74] and a smaller proportion of males. EDNOS is a diagnosis that captures a range of serious disorders of eating that do not fit these two diagnoses and have been estimated to affect over 3% of Western adults.[75] A further substantial proportion of the population use unhealthy weight loss behaviours and suffer from high levels of body dissatisfaction with resulting psychological distress and reductions in quality of life. These people are not usually given a diagnosis, and an accurate estimate is difficult to gauge. Taken together, eating disorders and related eating and body image problems are frequently occurring and associated with loss of both physical and mental health and high burden of disease.[76] Consequently, the importance of identifying effective public health interventions to counteract these problems is being increasingly recognized.[77]

Risk factors for disordered eating

The aim of prevention interventions for eating disorders is to modify causal risk factors for these problems and consequently reduce the likelihood of the disorders developing. There is strong evidence to indicate that the prevalence of eating disorders, especially of the bulimic type, occur more frequently in cultures in which there is a thin beauty ideal, and an abundant food supply as is the case in Western societies at the present time.[78] However, many women live in the presence of this social pressure but do not develop eating disorders. Thus, prior to a consideration of prevention interventions, an understanding of risk factors for eating disorders is required.

Proposed risk factors may be broadly categorized as cultural/social, psychological/behavioural or biological risk factors. Social environments that heighten risk include those that emphasize the importance of thinness, weight and shape, and may be family, peer, media, and some work and sporting environments.[78–81] Weight and shape teasing, a social pressure to be thin, is consistently observed to be a risk factor for disordered eating.[82,83] Psychological attributes that have been consistently observed to precede disordered eating in a potentially causal manner include body dissatisfaction,[82,84] internalization of the thin beauty ideal and a related strong belief in the importance of thinness[85,86] and perfectionist tendencies.[87,88] Other psychological attributes consistently associated with disordered eating, but not yet conclusively demonstrated to be causally related, include depression and low self-esteem[80] and high tendency to make body comparisons.[82,89–91] Self-reported dieting or use of extreme weight loss strategies are the major behavioural factors implicated in the development of disordered eating.[84,85] Biological risk factors may include a predisposition to a larger body size[80] and a genetic predisposition for eating disorders,[92] however, the mechanisms involved have yet to be clarified. Other variables have been proposed as risk factors, notably sexual abuse,[93,94] but have yet to be demonstrated to be consistent or specific risk factors for disordered eating.

While they differ in emphasis, most causal models of eating disorders are multivariate, and propose that a combination of the variables described above interact to contribute to the development or maintenance of eating disorders. The cognitive behavioural model of bulimia nervosa proposes that low self-esteem contributes to extreme concerns about weight and shape, and that these lead to dieting and to binge eating and finally to compensatory behaviours.[95] Stice[96] proposed one of the first multivariate models that delineated a role for sociocultural factors in addition to psychological factors. Later multivariate models of body dissatisfaction, dieting behaviour and disordered eating propose that a combination of depression, low self-esteem and a high value placed on thinness, contribute to greater body comparison leading to greater body dissatisfaction, dieting and finally disordered eating.[91,97] The notion of a causal pathway is important when considering prevention interventions, which are frequently implicitly or explicitly premised on the notion that intervening to change a risk factor upstream in the chain of causation will interrupt the causal chain to prevent disorder. For example, media literacy approaches are based on the notion that if a girl learns to question the authenticity of media presentations of women she will be less likely to feel the social pressure to conform to this ideal, will consequently not be so dissatisfied with her body, will not diet and will not develop disordered eating.

Prevention strategies and outcomes

In the eating disorder area, there have yet to be any universal prevention interventions or interventions that aim to make broad structural or legislative changes. However, selective prevention interventions in which adolescent girls have been involved, being a group generally at risk of disordered eating, have been conducted and evaluated. In addition, targeted prevention interventions for young women who already show early symptoms of poor body image and disordered eating have also been evaluated.[98]

Selective intervention programs have typically been designed for adolescent girls aged approximately 11–14 years, and conducted in school classroom settings[98] although one innovative program was conducted in a community girl-scout setting.[99] Most of the programs evaluated consist of 5–10 classroom sessions led by either an outside expert or usual class teacher. In these sessions activities and information are presented that aim to address the risk factors identified for disordered eating. These topics include: normal changes in body shape at puberty, cultural and subcultural pressures to be thin and unrealistic body shapes promoted in the media, media literacy in relation to manipulation of images in the media, suggestions for building positive body image, the importance of valuing non-appearance attributes, 'weightism', dangers of crash diets, healthy weight management and identifying non-hungry eating and the relationship between mood and eating.[98] While some are general programs,[100] others emphasize a particular risk factors such as the negative influence of the media[99] or low self-esteem.[101] While the important role of the family has been recognized, few programs have successfully engaged parents.[102] Rather than changing the risk environment in which most young women inhabit, most programs endeavour to impart coping strategies and information that will enable a young adolescent girl to manage the pressures to be thin and use extreme weight loss behaviours in a healthy way.

To date over 20 published controlled evaluations of selective intervention programs have included an assessment of an eating behaviour.[98,103] Immediately following the intervention, half report a positive effect of the intervention, though effect sizes are generally small. At a follow-up assessment this effect is frequently diminished.[98] These findings represent only a modest outcome for this style of prevention intervention and notably, there is no indication that interventions have reduced the incidence of actual eating disorder. Examination of the more successful programs suggests that those that are highly interactive are more likely to have a positive impact. It is likely that, at present, the counteracting social forces that encourage thinness and thereby support dangerous eating behaviours are too strong, pervasive and ongoing to be counteracted by relatively short-term prevention interventions. Interventions that change the attitudes of a whole subculture are likely to be more effective.[104] In addition, a better understanding of intervention messages that are credible and relevant to adolescent girls may add to the effectiveness of selective interventions.[105] Further, it is likely that ongoing intervention approaches that match developmental needs through childhood and adolescence will be required.[98]

Targeted programs that provide an intervention for young adult women in whom risk factors for eating disorder are already present, in particular poor body image, binge eating and use of extreme weight loss behaviours, appear potentially more successful in reducing risk factors.[98,103,106,107] Their greater impact may be due to young women with symptoms who volunteer to be involved being more motivated and cognitively able to make changes. The programs are also typically more intensive. Programs for young adults, however, are too late to prevent eating disorders that develop in adolescence.

While much has been learnt about issues in the prevention of disordered eating in the last decade, further creative ideas and research are required to establish effective prevention interventions. It is also vital to recognize that while the social pressures to conform to an unrealistic beauty ideal are so strong, prevention programs that address only the role of the individual are likely to be of only limited success.

CONCLUSIONS

Diet-related diseases have a detrimental health, economic and psychological impact on populations throughout the world. This chapter reviewed prevention interventions conducted in the fields of public health nutrition, obesity prevention and disordered eating. Various channels and strategies have been employed in interventions aimed at promoting healthy dietary behaviour or healthy body weight. Current thinking across domains indicates that prevention efforts need to address socioenvironmental as well as personal and behavioural factors if they are to succeed. Available research provides insight for public health practitioners as to the most promising approaches for preventing diet-related disease, and directs researchers to important topics that warrant future investigation.

References

1. World Health Organization. Obesity: Preventing and managing the global epidemic. Report of a WHO consultation. Technical Report Series No. 894 Geneva: World Health Organization; 3–5 June 2000.
2. Strategic Inter-Governmental Nutrition Alliance. Eat Well Australia: A strategic framework for public health nutrition. Canberra: National Public Health Partnership; 2001.
3. National Health and Medical Research Council. Dietary guidelines for Australian adults: A guide to healthy eating. Canberra: Commonwealth of Australia; 2003.
4. World Health Organization. Diet, nutrition and the prevention of chronic diseases: report of a joint World Health Organization/FAO expert consultation. In: World Health Organization Technical Report Series, No. 916. Geneva: Online [access August 2003]. Available from URL http://www.who.int/hpr/NPH/docs/who_fao_expert_report.pdf; 2003.

5. Visscher TL, Seidell JC. The public health impact of obesity. Annual Review of Public Health 2001; 22:355–375.

6. National Task Force on the Prevention and Treatment of Obesity. Overweight, obesity and health risk. Archives of Internal Medicine 2000; 160:898–904.

7. International Agency for Research on Cancer. Weight control and physical activity. Lyon: World Health Organization; 2002.

8. Heaney RP. Calcium, dairy products and osteoporosis. Journal of the American College of Nutrition 2000; 19(Suppl 2):83S–99S.

9. Law M. Salt, blood pressure and cardiovascular diseases. Journal of Cardiovascular Risk 2000; 7(1):5–8.

10. Ahluwalia N. Intervention strategies for improving iron status of young children and adolescents in India. Nutrition Review 2002; 60(5 Pt 2):S115–7.

11. Ahmed F. Vitamin A deficiency in Bangladesh: A review and recommendations for improvement. Public Health and Nutrition 1999; 2(1):1–14.

12. Australian Institute of Health and Welfare and Commonwealth Department of Health and Family Services. First report on National Health Priority Areas 1996. AIHW Cat. No. PHE 1. Canberra: Online [access 2003 December]. Available from URL http://www.aihw.gov.au/publications/health/frnhpa96/index.html; 1997.

13. National Health and Medical Research Council. Dietary guidelines for children and adolescents in Australia: A guide to healthy eating. Canberra: Commonwealth of Australia; 2003.

14. McLennan W, Podger A. National nutrition survey: Foods eaten Australia 1995 (Cat. No. 4802.0). Canberra: Australian Bureau of Statistics; 1999.

15. Marks G, Rutishauser H, Webb K, Picton P. Key food and nutrition data for Australia 1990–1999. Online [access 2003 June]. Available from URL http://www.sph.uq.edu.au/NUTRITION/monitoring/p5.htm; 2001.

16. National Health and Medical Research Council. Dietary guidelines for Australians. Canberra: Australian Government Publishing Service; 1991.

17. Cook T, Rutishauser I, Seelig M. Comparable data on food and nutrient intake and physical measurements from the 1983, 1985 and 1995 national nutrition surveys. Canberra: National Food and Nutrition Monitoring and Surveillance Project, Commonwealth Department of Health and Aged Care; 2001.

17a. World Health Organization. Obesity: Preventing and managing the global epidemic. Report of a WHO Consultation. Technical Report Series, No. 894. Geneva: World Health Organization; 2000.

18. Cole T, Bellizi M, Flegal K, Dietz W. Establishing a standard definition for child overweight and obesity worldwide: International survey. British Medical Journal 2000; 320:1240–1243.

19. World Health Organization. Obesity: Preventing and managing the global epidemic. In: World Health Organization Technical Report Series, No. 894. Geneva: Online [access December 2003]. Available from URL http://www.who.int/nut/documents/obesity_executive_summary.pdf; 1997.

20. Cameron A, Welborn T, Zimmet P, Dunstan D, Owen N, Salmon J, et al. Overweight and obesity in Australia: the 1999–2000 Australian Diabetes, Obesity and Lifestyle Study (AusDiab). Medical Journal of Australia 2003; 178(9):427–432.

21. Booth ML, Chey T, Wake M, Norton K, Hesketh K, Dollman J, et al. Change in the prevalence of overweight and obesity among young Australians. American Journal of Clinical Nutrition 2003; 77(1):29–36.

22. Hill J, Radimer K. A content analysis of food advertisements in television for Australian children. Australian Journal of Nutrition and Dietetics 1997; 54:174–180.

23. Borzekowski DL, Robinson TN. The 30-second effect: An experiment revealing the impact of television commercials on food preferences of preschoolers. Journal of the American Dietetic Association 2001; 101(1):42–46.

24. Rosenstock IM. Historical origins of the health belief model. Health Education Monographs 1974; 2:328–335.

25. Ajzen I. The theory of planned behavior. Organizational Behavior and Human Decision Processes 1991; 50:179–211.

26. Prochaska JO, DiClemente CC. Stages and processes of self-change: Toward an integrative model of change. Journal of Consulting and Clinical Psychology 1983; 51(3):390–395.

27. Green LW, Kreuter MW. Health promotion planning: An educational and ecological approach, 3rd edn. Mountain View, California: Mayfield; 1999.

28. Robertson A, Brunner E, Sheiham A. Food is a political issue. In: Marmot M, Wilkinson R. Eds. Social Determinants of Health. New York; Oxford: University Press; 1999.

29. Glanz K, Lankenau B, Foerster S, Temple S, Mullis R, Schmid T. Environmental and policy approaches to cardiovascular disease prevention through nutrition: Opportunities for state and local action. Health Education Quarterly 1995; 22(4): 512–527.

30. Dixon H, Borland R, Segan C, Stafford H, Sindall C. Public reaction to Victoria's '2 Fruit 'n' 5 Veg Every Day' campaign and reported consumption of fruit and vegetables. Preventive Medicine 1998; 27:572–582.

31. Contento IR, Randell JS, Basch CE. Review and analysis of evaluation measures used in nutrition education intervention research. Journal of Nutrition Education and Behavior 2002; 34(1):2–25.

32. Ammerman A, Lindquist C, Hersey J, Jackman AM, Gavin NI, Garces C, et al. Efficacy of interventions to modify dietary behavior related to cancer risk. In: Rockville, MD: Agency for Healthcare Research and Quality. Online [access 2003 September]. Available from URL http://www.ncbi.nlm.nih.gov/books/bv.fcgi?call=bv.View..ShowSection&rid=hstat1.chapter.35668; 2001.

33. Dixon HG, Janarthanan P, Kelly-Dalgety L. Compilation of unpublished Australian studies relevant to the acceptance of advice about food and nutrition. Melbourne: Centre for Behavioural Research in Cancer, Anti-Cancer Council of Victoria; 1999.

34. Estabrooks P, Dzewaltowski DA, Glasgow RE, Klesges LM. Reporting of validity from school health promotion studies published in 12 leading journals, 1996–2000. Journal of School Health 2003; 73(1):21–28.

35. Health Education Authority. Health promotion interventions to promote healthy eating in the general population – a review. Health Promotion Effectiveness Reviews: Summary Bulletin 6. London: Health Education Authority; 1997.

36. Rose G. Sick individuals and sick populations. International Journal of Epidemiology 1985; 14(1):32–38.

37. Maibach E, Holtgrave D. Advances in public health communication. Annual Review of Public Health 1995; 16:219–238.

38. Miller M, Stafford H. An intervention portfolio to promote fruit and vegetable consumption: Part 2 – review of interventions. Melbourne: National Public Health Partnership; 2000.

39. Heimendinger J, Van Duyn MA, Chapelsky D, Foerster S, Stables G. The national 5 a Day for Better Health Program: A large-scale nutrition intervention. Journal of Public Health Management Practice 1996; 2(2):27–35.

40. Foerster SB, Kizer KW, Disogra LK, Bal DG, Krieg BF, Bunch KL. California's '5 a day – for better health!' campaign: An innovative population-based effort to effect large-scale dietary change. American Journal of Preventive Medicine, 1995; 11:124–131.

41. Ejlak J, Seal J, van Velzen D. Eat Well Tasmania! End of year two survey 1997. Tasmania: Tasmanian Health Promotion Council, and Department of Community and Health Services; 1998.

42. Miller M, Pollard C, Paterson D. A public health nutrition campaign to promote fruit and vegetables in Australia. In: Worsely AW, ed. Proceedings of Food Choice Conference; 1996; University of Adelaide.

43. Bowen DJ, Beresford SA. Dietary interventions to prevent disease. Annual Review of Public Health 2002; 23:255–286.

44. French SA. Pricing effects on food choices. Journal of Nutrition. 2003; 133(3):841S–843S.

45. Heart Foundation: About us. Online [access 2003 December]. Available from URL http://www.heartfoundation.com.au/index.cfm?page=34; 2003.

46. Mayer JA, Dubbert PM, Elder JP. Promoting nutrition at the point of choice: a review. Health Education Quarterly 1989; 16(1):31–43.

47. Albright CL, Flora JA, Fortmann SP. Restaurant menu labeling: impact of nutrition information on entrée sales and patron attitudes. Health Education Quarterly 1990; 17(2):157–167.

48. Hoelscher DM, Evans A, Parcel GS, Kelder SH. Designing effective nutrition interventions for adolescents. Journal of the American Dietetic Association 2002; 102(3 Suppl):S52–63.

49. Glanz K. Behavioral research contributions and needs in cancer prevention and control: Dietary change. Preventive Medicine 1997; 26(5 Pt 2):S43–55.

50. Perez-Rodrigo C, Aranceta J. Nutrition education in schools: Experiences and challenges. European Journal of Clinical Nutrition 2003; 57(Suppl 1):S82–S85.

51. Centers for Disease Control and Prevention. Guidelines for school health programs to promote lifelong healthy eating. Journal of School Health 1997; 67(1):9–26.

52. Turrell G, Hewitt B, Patterson C, Oldenburg B. Measuring socio-economic position in dietary research: Is choice of socio-economic indicator important? Public Health Nutrition 2003; 6(2):191–200.

53. Heimendinger J, Thompson B, Ockene J, Sorensen G, Abrams D, Emmons K, et al. Reducing the risk of cancer through worksite intervention. Occupational Medicine 1990; 5(4):707–723.

54. Janer G, Sala M, Kogevinas M. Health promotion trials at worksites and risk factors for cancer. Scandinavian Journal of Work Environment and Health 2002; 28(3):141–157.

55. Glanz K, Sorensen G, Farmer A. The health impact of worksite nutrition and cholesterol intervention programs. American Journal of Health Promotion 1996; 10(6):453–470.

56. Abood DA, Black DR, Feral D. Nutrition education worksite intervention for university staff: application of health belief model. Journal of Nutrition Education and Behaviour 2003; 35(5):260–267.

57. Hebert JR, Harris DR, Sorensen G, Stoddard AM, Hunt MK, Morris DH. A work-site nutrition intervention: Its effects on the consumption of cancer-related nutrients. American Journal of Public Health 1993; 83(3):391–394.

58. Muto T, Yamauchi K. Evaluation of a multicomponent workplace health promotion program conducted in Japan for improving employees' cardiovascular disease risk factors. Preventive Medicine 2001; 33(6):571–577.

59. Woollard J, Burke V, Beilin LJ, Verheijden M, Bulsara MK. Effects of a general practice-based intervention on diet, body mass index and blood lipids in patients at cardiovascular risk. Journal of Cardiovascular Risk 2003; 10(1):31–40.

60. Neil HA, Roe L, Godlee RJ, Moore JW, Clark GM, Brown J, et al. Randomised trial of lipid lowering dietary advice in general practice: The effects on serum lipids, lipoproteins, and antioxidants. British Medical Journal 1995; 310(6979):569–573.

61. Thorell B, Svardsudd K. Intervention against ischaemic heart disease risk factors in primary health care in a semi-rural community. The population study '50-year-old people in Kungsor'. Scandinavian Journal of Primary Health Care 1994; 12(1):51–56.

62. Ashley JM, St Jeor ST, Schrage JP, Perumean-Chaney SE, Gilbertson MC, McCall NL, et al. Weight control in the physician's office. Archives of Internal Medicine 2001; 161(13):1599–1604.

63. Imperial Cancer Research Fund. Effectiveness of health checks conducted by nurses in primary care: Results of the OXCHECK study after one year. Imperial Cancer Research Fund OXCHECK Study Group. British Medical Journal 1995; 308(6924):308–312.

64. National Health and Medical Research Council. Acting on Australia's weight: a strategic plan for the prevention of overweight and obesity. Canberra: Australian Government Publishing Service; 1997.

65. Glenny AM, O'Meara S, Melville A, Sheldon TA, Wilson C. The treatment and prevention of obesity: a systematic review of the literature. International Journal of Obesity and Related Metabolic Disorders 1997; 21(9):715–737.

66. Sarwer DB, Wadden TA. The treatment of obesity: What's new, what's recommended. Journal of Women's Health and Gender-based Medicine 1999; 8(4):483–493.

67. Campbell K, Waters E, O'Meara S, Kelly S, Summerbell C. Interventions for preventing obesity in children. In: Cochrane Database of Systematic Reviews CD001871; 2002.

68. Muller MJ, Mast M, Asbeck I, Langnase K, Grund A. Prevention of obesity – is it possible? Obesity Review 2001; 2(1):15–28.

69. Irving LM, Neumark-Sztainer D. Integrating the prevention of eating disorders and obesity: feasible or futile? Preventive Medicine 2002; 34(3):299–309.

70. American Psychiatric Association. Diagnostic and statistical manual of mental disorders, 4th edn. Washington, DC: APA; 1994.

70a. Hoek HW, van Hoeken D. Review of the prevalence and incidence of eating disorders. International Journal of Eating Disorders 2003; 34(4):383–386.

71. Fairburn CG, Cooper Z, Cooper PJ. The clinical features and maintenance of BN. In: Brownell KD, Foreyt JP, eds. Handbook of eating disorders: Physiology, psychology and treatment of obesity, anorexia and bulimia. New York: Basic Books; 1986: 389–404.

72. Clayer JR, McFarlane A, Bookless C, Air T, Wright G, Czechowicz A. Prevalence of psychiatric disorders in rural South Australia. Medical Journal of Australia 1995; 163:124–129.

73. Hay PJ, Marley J, Lemar S. Covert eating disorders: The prevalence, characteristics and help-seeking of those with bulimic eating disorders in general practice. Primary Care Psychiatry 1998; 4:95–99.

74. Wade T, Heath AC, Abraham S, Treloar SA, Martin NG, Tiggemann M. Assessing the prevalence of eating disorders in an Australian twin population. Australian and New Zealand Journal of Psychiatry 1996; 30:845–851.

75. Hay PJ. The epidemiology of eating disorder behaviours: An Australian community-based survey. International Journal of Eating Disorders 1998; 23:317–382.

76. Mathers CD, Vos ET, Stevenson CE, Begg SJ. The Australian Burden of Disease Study: Measuring the loss of health from diseases, injuries and risk factors. Medical Journal of Australia 2000; 172:592–596.

77. Paxton SJ. Body image dissatisfaction, extreme weight loss behaviours: Suitable targets for public health concern? Health Promotion Journal of Australia 2000; 10:15–19.

78. Keel PK, Klump KL. Are eating disorders culture-bound syndromes? Implications for conceptualizing their etiology. Psychological Review 2003; 129:747–769.

79. Field A. Risk factors for eating disorders: An evaluation of the evidence. In: Thompson JK, ed. Handbook of eating disorders and obesity. New Jersey: John Wileysons; 2004:17–32.

80. Stice E. Risk and maintenance factors for eating pathology: A meta-analytic review. Psychological Bulletin 2002; 128:825–848.

81. Wertheim EH, Paxton SJ, Blaney S. Risk factors for the development of body image disturbances. In: Thompson JK, ed. Handbook of eating disorders and obesity. New Jersey: John Wiley&Sons; 2004:463–494.

82. Wertheim EH, Koerner J, Paxton SJ. Longitudinal predictors of restrictive eating and bulimic tendencies in three different age groups of adolescent girls. Journal of Youth and Adolescence 2001; 30:69–81.

83. van den Berg P, Wertheim EH, Thompson JK, Paxton SJ. Development of body image, eating disturbance and general psychological functioning in adolescent females: A replication using covariance structure modeling in an Australian sample. International Journal of Eating Disorders 2002; 32:46–51.

84. Stice E, Agras WS. Predicting onset and cessation of bulimic behaviors during adolescence: A longitudinal grouping analysis. Behavior Therapy 1998; 29:257–276.

85. Field AE, Camargo CA, Taylor CB, Berkey CS, Colditz GA. Relation of peer and media influences to the development of purging behaviors among preadolescent and adolescent girls. Archives of Pediatric Adolescent Medicine 1999; 153:1184–1189.

86. Fairburn CG, Stice E, Cooper Z, Doll HA, Norman PA, O'Connor ME. Understanding persistence of bulimia nervosa: A 5-year naturalistic study. Journal of Consulting and Clinical Psychology 2003; 71(1):103–109.

87. Vohs KD, Voelz ZR, Pettit JW, Bardone AM, Katz J, Abraham LY, et al. Perfectionism, body dissatisfaction, and self-esteem: An interactive model of bulimic symptom development. Journal of Social and Clinical Psychology 2001; 20:476–497.

88. Wade TD, Lowes J. Variables associated with disturbed eating habits and overvalued ideas about the personal implications of body shape and weight in a female adolescent population. International Journal of Eating Disorders 2002; 32:39–45.

89. Paxton SJ, Schutz HK, Wertheim EH, Muir SL. Friendship clique and peer influences on body image attitudes, dietary restraint, extreme weight loss behaviours and binge eating in adolescent girls. Journal of Abnormal Psychology 1999; 108:255–266.

90. Schutz HK, Paxton SJ, Wertheim EH. Investigation of body comparison among adolescent girls. Journal of Applied Social Psychology 2002; 32:1906–1937.

91. van den Berg P, Thompson JK, Obremski-Brandon K, Coovert M. The tripartite Influence Model of body image and eating disturbance: A covariance structure modeling investigation testing the mediational role of appearance comparison. Journal of Psychosomatic Research 2002; 53:1007–1020.

92. Bulik CM. Genetic and biological risk factors. In: Thompson JK, ed. Handbook of eating disorders and obesity. New Jersey: John Wiley; 2004:3–16.

93. Vogeltanz-Holm ND, Wonderlich SA, Lewis BA, Wilsnack SC, Harris TR, Wilsnasck RW, et al. Longitudinal predictors of binge eating, intense dieting, and weight concerns in a national sample of women. Behavior Therapy 2000; 31:221–235.

94. Wonderlich SA, Crosby RD, Mitchell JE, Thompson KM, Redlin J, Demuth G, et al. Eating disturbance and sexual trauma in childhood and adulthood. International Journal of Eating Disorders 2001; 30:401–412.

95. Fairburn CG. Eating disorders. In: Clark DM, Fairburn CG, eds. Science and practice of cognitive behaviour therapy. Oxford: Oxford University Press; 1997.

96. Stice E. Review of the evidence for a socio-cultural model of bulimia nervosa and an exploration of the mechanisms of action. Clinical Psychology Review 1994; 14:633–661.

97. Durkin SJ, Paxton SJ, Sorbello M. Mediational influence of internalisation and comparison tendency on the impact of media exposure on adolescent girls' body satisfaction. In: International Conference on Eating Disorders, New York; 2002.

98. Paxton SJ. Evidence-Based Health Promotion: Resources for Planning. No 6 Body Image. Research Overview. In: Department of Human Services, Victoria Online. Available from URL www.dhs.vic.gov.au/phd/ebhp/; 2002.

99. Neumark-Sztainer D, Sherwood NE, Coller T, Hannan PJ. Primary prevention of disorders eating among preadolescent girls: Feasibility and short-term effect of a community-based intervention. Journal of American Dietetic Association 2000; 100:1466–1473.

100. Steiner-Adair C, Sjostrom L, Franko DL, Pai S, Tucker R, Becker AE, et al. Primary prevention of risk factors for eating disorders in adolescent girls: Learning from practice. International Journal of Eating Disorders 2002; 32:401–411.

101. O'Dea J, Abraham S. Improving the body image, eating attitudes, and behaviors of young male and female adolescents: A new educational approach that focuses on self-esteem. International Journal of Eating Disorders 2000; 28:43–57.

102. McVey G, Davis R, Tweed S, Shaw BF. A program to promote positive body image with girls in grade 6 and their parents: A one-year follow-up evaluation. (Unpublished manuscript).

103. Stice E, Shaw H. Eating disorder prevention programs: A meta-analytic review. Psychological Bulletin 2004; 130:206–227.

104. Piran N. Prevention in a high risk environment: An intervention in a ballet school. In: Piran N, Levine MP, Steiner-Adair C, eds. Preventing eating disorders: A handbook of interventions and special challenges. NY: Brunner/Mazel; 1999:148–159.

105. Paxton SJ, Wertheim EH, Pilawski A, Durkin SJ, Holt T. Evaluations of dieting prevention messages by adolescent girls. Preventive Medicine 2002; 35:474–491.

106. Stice E, Mazotti L, Weibel D, Agras WS. Dissonance prevention program decreases thin-ideal internalization, body dissatisfaction, dieting, negative affect, and bulimic symptoms: A preliminary experiment. International Journal of Eating Disorders 2000; 27:206–217.

107. Zabinski MF, Pung MA, Wilfley DE, Eppstein D, Winzelberg AJ, Celio A, et al. Reducing risk factors for eating disorders: Targeting at-risk women with a computerized psycho-educational program. International Journal of Eating Disorders 2001; 29:401–408.

108. Coles Supermarkets. What is 7-a-day? Online (accessed 2004) Available from http://www.coles.com.av/7aday/what_is_content.asp/

CHAPTER **5**

Sexual health and behaviour change

Marian Pitts

INTRODUCTION

Sex has been studied in many different ways for a considerable time – sexual behaviours are but one aspect of sexuality. In this chapter I will examine the range of interventions associated with sexual behaviour. Many of these interventions have, as their goal, an improvement in sexual health, at the individual, community and societal level, and a reduction in 'high risk' sexual behaviours, of which, more later.

It might be useful to begin by a consideration of what constitutes good sexual health and even what constitutes 'sex'. The former has been defined and discussed in numerous meetings, often at the global level, hosted by the World Health Organization (WHO). The most recent WHO definition states:

'Sexual health is a state of physical, emotional, mental and social well-being related to sexuality; it is not merely the absence of disease, dysfunction or infirmity. Sexual health requires a positive and respectful approach to sexuality and sexual relationships, as well as the possibility of having pleasurable and safe sexual experiences, free of coercion, discrimination and violence. For sexual health to be attained and maintained, the sexual rights of all persons must be respected, protected and fulfilled'[1] (p. 1).

Thus sexual health is influenced by a complex web of factors ranging from sexual behaviour and attitudes and societal factors, to biological risk and genetic predisposition. It encompasses the problems of HIV and sexually transmissible infections (STIs), reproductive tract infections (RTIs), unintended pregnancy and abortion, infertility, cancer resulting from STIs, and sexual dysfunction. Sexual health can also be influenced by mental health, acute and chronic illnesses, and violence. Addressing sexual health at the individual, family, community or health system level requires integrated interventions by trained health providers and a functioning referral system. It also requires a legal, policy and regulatory environment where the sexual rights of all people are upheld, a situation that pertains in very few places in the world.

Addressing sexual health also requires an understanding and appreciation of sexuality, gender roles and power when both designing and providing services. Understanding sexuality and its impact on practices, partners, reproduction and pleasure presents a number of challenges as well as opportunities for improving sexual and reproductive health-care services and interventions. Validity of data collection, given researcher bias and difficulties in discussing such a private issue, also remains a problem in some settings that must be overcome if a greater understanding of sexuality as it is played out in various settings is to be achieved. Sexuality research must go beyond concerns related to behaviour, numbers of partners and practices, to the underlying social, cultural and economic factors that make individuals vulnerable to risks and affect the ways in which sex is sought, desired and/or refused by women, men and young people. Investigating sexuality in this way entails going beyond reproductive health by considering sexual health holistically and comprehensively. To do this requires adding to the knowledge base gained from the field of STI/HIV prevention and care, gender studies, and family planning, among others.

According to Mace, Bannerman & Burton[2] the concept of sexual health includes three basic elements:

1. A capacity to enjoy and control sexual and reproductive behaviour in accordance with a social and personal ethic.
2. Freedom from fear, shame, guilt, false beliefs, and other psychological factors inhibiting sexual response and impairing sexual relationship.
3. Freedom from organic disorders, diseases, and deficiencies that interfere with sexual and reproductive functions.

Thus the notion of sexual health implies a positive approach to human sexuality, and the purpose of sexual health care should be the enhancement of life and personal relationships and not merely counselling and care related to procreation or sexually transmitted diseases.

WHAT IS SEX?

The main issue of concern for planning and implementing interventions is to be clear about the range of behaviours encompassed by the term 'sex'. There has been a lack of standardization of terms in many areas of sex research. For example, in the tobacco field there are exact terms to define a smoker (for example, a daily smoker, aged 15 years and over), initially suggested by WHO and now used by many countries. This enables comparative analysis in a way that remains challenging for sex research. There are also significant issues concerning definitions.

Frequently 'sex' is linked solely with penetration, either vaginal or anal, but this narrow version of what constitutes a sexual act is not necessarily held by the general population, or by particular groups, such as 'young people'. The research evidence and anecdotal evidence concur that the definitions of sex are changing: studies in both the US and the UK[3,4] indicate that young people are more likely to view a wider range of behaviours as constituting 'having sex'.

Jeannin et al.[5] followed up a short telephone survey with interviews and confirmed that 12.5% of male respondents had included incidents of non-penetrative sex in their reports of sexual activity. Many would argue that these men were responding accurately and that it is concerning that 87.5% of male respondents did not include non-penetrative sex in their responses. It is also sometimes difficult to be explicit and specific in surveys to ensure that respondents and interviewers share an understanding of what is being asked about; this can be particularly problematic for research carried out with young people and in settings such as schools.

As indicated above, self-report is a major issue for sexuality research. Clearly there is much material related to sex that can only be obtained from the individuals concerned, and certainly cannot be observed first hand by the researcher. However, self-report carries with it inherent weaknesses such as social desirability bias. Smith et al.[6] reviewed the measurement of self-reported sexual activity (or lack of it) and identified cultural bias, poor recall and developmental issues as potentially problematic in establishing the accuracy of self-report.

Health outcome measures are potentially more promising. Those used frequently include birth rates and rates of STIs. However movement between centres or clinics, particularly for treatment of STIs mean that it is difficult to link such outcomes with specific programs or interventions, and there are naturally occurring fluctuations that make analysis and interpretation problematic.

THE EPIDEMIOLOGY OF SEX

There is no central depository for global sex data (in contrast to the World Health Organization's databank of health statistics). However, many countries do carry out surveillance that contributes to the epidemiology of sexual behaviours. If we consider HIV/AIDS: one of the most pressing and serious consequences of 'unsafe' sexual behaviour, the estimated number of people living with HIV in Australia is 20 580; 838 new diagnoses of HIV were made in 2003.[7] In the first quarter of 2004, there were 179 cases of chlamydial infection per 100 000 population, and 34 per 100 000 cases of gonorrheae. Certain STIs, most notably chlamydia, have increased rapidly in the last few years. This increase is likely to be the consequence both of increased infections and increased detection rates. It is clear from overseas data that routine and regular screening, for example for chlamydia, results in more infections detected and treated.

CHARACTERISTICS OF SUCCESSFUL STI INTERVENTIONS

McKay[8] carried out a review of a number of behaviourally effective interventions for HIV and STIs. He identifies some common characteristics of the more effective interventions. These include:

- **The incorporation of theoretical models of behaviour change.** This allows for a clearly defined set of intervention strategies to emerge and a better conceptualization of the targeted risk behaviours.
- **The incorporation of specific behavioural skills training.** It is very clear that providing factual information is a necessary, but certainly not sufficient, approach to achieving behavioural change.
- **Emphasis on facilitating consistent condom use.** Increased use of condoms and especially their use consistently has been shown to be the most effective target for prevention interventions.[9]
- **Helping to create a personal sexual health plan.** McKay identifies this element as particularly important for interventions aimed at sexual health clinic settings and at women at high risk for HIV/STIs.
- **Use of strategies that are community and culturally appropriate.** The common characteristics identified above need to be tailored and targeted to the specific needs of the group receiving the intervention. This will frequently require pre-intervention research to establish the existing social norms and behaviours for a particular group.
- **Involvement of peer educators and community opinion leaders.** Peer educators can be particularly effective for certain groups, for example for young people.

Interventions directed at the individual

Research into the prevention of HIV and other STIs has focused predominantly on the individual, in itself a conundrum given that sex usually involves more than a single person. In recent years, the ABC of prevention has come to dominate the area, particularly for those programs and interventions funded or supported from the United States. This catchy acronym stands for Abstinence, Behaviour change (or sometimes, Be faithful) and Condom use. The first and last of this triumvirate are fairly easily identified, (although see later discussion on the precise meanings of abstinence). The middle term has come to mean many different things in many different settings. In HIV prevention it tends to be equated with a reduction in the number of sexual partners – at its extreme it is known as 'zero grazing' in many parts of sub-Saharan Africa. It may also mean a change in particular sexual practices that can be riskier than others – unprotected anal intercourse, for example.

Abstinence

Abstinence is the most hotly debated topic in sex education at the moment. Abstinence can be defined in a number of ways; these include delaying first intercourse and maintaining abstinence at particular times. The focus is often on 'virginity', presumably meaning first vaginal intercourse, and this can lead us, and the young people exposed to these programs, to categorize other activities, e.g. oral sex as 'just experimenting' or 'not really having sex'.[10]

The US government has supported and funded abstinence education since 1996. Since the mid-1990s many schools in the US have adopted 'abstinence only' curricula in order to qualify for federal funding. These programs must teach that 'a mutually faithful monogamous relationship in the context of marriage is the expected standard of human sexual activity' and also to teach that sex 'outside' marriage can have 'harmful psychological and physical effects'. The evidence base for either of these value statements is as loose as for the WHO's definition of sexual health discussed earlier.

Defining and reporting abstinence can be particularly problematic. Stevens-Simon argues that reliance, inevitably, on self-report from young people, can mislead. For example, she re-examines Howard and McCabe's[11] report on a sexuality program for 'virginal teens and pre-teens'. This was a program introduced in Atlanta, Georgia to delay sexual involvement. The program's results included a reduction in the number of girls who became sexually active during the 8th and 9th grade. Howard and McCabe reported that the program reduced pregnancy rates by one third. However, they only included girls who reported themselves as sexually active in the denominator: 28 of 168 girls (16.6%) who took part in the program reported becoming sexually active during the time period, of these five (18%) became pregnant. In comparison, 19 of 70 girls (27%) who did not take the class became sexually active and three of these (16%) became pregnant. Howard and McCabe argue that if girls who were in the program had become sexually active at the same rate as those not in the program, then we would expect eight rather than five pregnancies in this group. Stevens-Simon argues for a different analysis – taking all the girls in the program as the denominator then five (3%) of the 168 program girls became pregnant compared with the (4%) of the 70 non-program girls. The intricacies of the analysis are some indication of the methodological and ideological issues associated with research in this area.

Most educators and programmers would agree that young people may not be cognitively or emotionally 'ready' for the challenges associated with sexual activity; we are rarely, however, specific, either about what the challenges are, or what the appropriate age for first sexual activity might be. What we know from our large-scale national cross-sectional studies such as The Australian Study of Health and Relationships (ASHR), is that age at first sex has been declining, for at least the last fifty years; and that for each generation many people feel that the age is too young.[12]

Periodic abstinence is fairly widely practised in certain areas of the world. Che et al.[13] estimate that in 2000 approximately 2.6% of all couples in the reproductive span were using periodic abstinence. The vast majority if these couples were living in less developed countries, and lifetime experience of periodic abstinence ranges from over 25% for women in Peru and Columbia to less than 5% in Egypt and Zimbabwe.

Be faithful or partner reduction

This component of the acronym is usually translated as monogamy, reductions in casual sex and multiple partners.[14] Sheldon also describes it as 'the neglected middle child of the ABC approach. Partner reduction has been identified as a key component in the success of Uganda and Thailand in reversing their rates of HIV'. In Uganda, the Global Programme on AIDS surveys found the proportion of men reporting one or more casual partners in the previous year dropped from 35% in 1989 to 15% in 1995; equivalent rates for women changed from 16% to 6%. Sheldon et al. also report that the proportion of men reporting three or more non-regular partners in the past twelve months fell from 15% to 3% during the same period. In both Thailand and Cambodia, the proportions of men reporting having paid for sex in the past year have shown equally large changes. Stoneburner and Low-Beer[15] compared evidence from Uganda with comparable data from Kenya, Zambia and Malawi. They conclude that: 'These findings suggest that reduction in sexual partners and abstinence among unmarried sexually inexperienced youth ... rather than condom use, are the relevant factors in reducing HIV infection' (p. 715).

Condom use

A major component in the prevention of HIV, condom use has increased dramatically in many countries in the last twenty years. In South Africa, free male condom distribution rose from 6 million in 1994 to 198 million in 1999.

ASHR data tell us that use of a condom at first sexual intercourse has risen from around 10% of those who report sexual debut in the 1950s to 79% of men and 76% of women who first had vaginal sex in the 2000s.[12] The proportion of people attending family planning clinics in the UK who chose condoms as their preferred method of contraception rose from 6% in 1975 to 36% in 1999–2000, according to a survey of National Health contraception services.

A review from the National Institute of Health in the United States demonstrated conclusively that condoms are effective against HIV when used consistently and properly.[16] The review estimates that the probability of HIV transmission per sex act can be reduced by as much as 95% by condoms and the annual incidence of HIV transmission between serodiscordant partners can be also be reduced by as much as 90–95%. However, condom use may be neither consistent nor reliable. Of any act, condom use requires the cooperation of two people, while its measurement has most frequently been by asking only one person. Condom use by an individual can vary both according to the other partner in the sex act, or by the circumstances of the sex act. For example, many studies have demonstrated that commercial sex workers, who use condoms consistently for their paying customers, are much less likely to use condoms in their 'private life'.[17] Similarly, research on gay men has indicated that condom use is high with partners met at sex on premises venues or saunas (45% protected anal sex), but less high if the sexual partner was met through friends (36%) and even less if the partner had been known for longer than twelve months (15%).[18]

ABC ... CNN?

In a recent twist to the ABC debate, there have been additional and alternative strategies suggested. The XV International AIDS Conference heard a debate entitled ABC versus CNN. Proponents of the latter approach say there is no better way to prevent HIV than by using condoms and giving clean syringes to intravenous drug users. Their philosophy is known as CNN, or Condoms, Needles and Negotiating Skills.

Robin et al.[19] reviewed sexual risk reduction programs that were conducted during the 1990s and had been evaluated. They focused on a number of outcome measures, most particularly condom use. They identified 24 articles meeting their inclusion criteria that identified 20 studies. These studies were conducted in a variety of settings. These included schools ($n = 9$), community-based venues ($n = 2$), clinics ($n = 2$) detention centres ($n = 2$). One took place in the participants' home and four had a combination of these sites. Sample sizes varied from under one hundred to more than 10 000 participants. Almost all studies used convenience sampling. Nine studies conducted only pre- and post-test measures; the longest post-test period was ten months. Nine studies carried out follow-up after twelve months. Most interventions were theory based, although many were based on a combination of social learning and social cognition theories. Of the twenty studies that were included, twelve reported positive effects, five had no effect and three had negative effects – these were also the shortest in duration. The majority of studies reporting positive effects targeted African-American young people.

INTERVENTIONS DIRECTED AT GROUPS

Peer education

Peer education has grown in popularity in recent decades. This has been especially the case among young people, where it is assumed that peers can be effective and persuasive communicators that have credibility and can use the right tone and language. Dunn, Ross et al.[20] cited by McKay point out the advantages of peer educators: 'Some adolescents may be more comfortable receiving sexuality-related information from peers than adults and peers may also have added credibility because of their perceived recent experience of the issues under discussion. An added advantage is that peer educators can increase their own knowledge and skills related to HIV/AIDS prevention in the process of training for and presenting such interventions.'[8] (p. 116).

A recent study by Caron et al.[21] evaluated the effectiveness of a Protection Express Program, based on the theory of Planned Behaviour and Interpersonal Behaviour.[22,23] Senior students at a Canadian high school were trained to deliver the program to junior secondary students. Respondents completed a questionnaire at baseline and nine months after receiving the program. Compared with controls, those who received the program showed clear attitude change with regard to postponing sexual experience and using condoms. However the groups did not differ with regard to condom use. Among the senior students who were peer educators, they were more likely to use condoms than their control, counter-parts. In this case it would appear that peer education was effective behaviourally for those involved in its delivery, rather than in those who received it, who demonstrated attitude changes, but few behavioural changes.

We will now examine interventions directed at particular target groups, of which the first concerns communities of gay men.

Modifying sexual risk for HIV among gay men

A Cochrane Review of interventions to modify sexual risk behaviours for preventing HIV among men who have sex with men (MSM) identified thirteen eligible studies.[24] Of these, seven were small group interventions, three were community level interventional and two were individual level interventions. In addition, one study reported on reduction in emotional distress after HIV testing and did not report behavioural outcomes. The interventions at the individual level were HIV prevention counselling,[25] or stress prevention training[26] and cognitive and behavioural self management training.[27]

At the level of small group interventions, there were relapse prevention workshops,[28] a four-session intervention led by trained counsellors[29] and small group lectures plus skills training.[30] The community level interventions included interventions in gay bars, including peer advocacy[31,32] and a peer-led program including outreach small groups and a publicity campaign.[33] In nearly all these interventions, the outcome measure was amount of unprotected anal sex occurring within a specified time period, usually six months.

Gay men adopted condom use during anal sex from very early on in the AIDS epidemic. This behaviour change has been identified as one of the most significant of any group, for any health behaviour. However, other strategies to increase the safety of sex have also been adopted by gay men. One such strategy is known as 'negotiated safety'.[34,35] The term 'negotiated safety' identifies an agreement between men to dispense with condoms in a committed HIV-negative relationship. Kippax identifies the safety aspects of this as follows:

- The sexual partners are in a regular relationship (difficult to define, as Kippax acknowledges).
- These sexual partners are antibody negative and aware of each other's status as negative – this necessitates adequate communication about HIV with one's partner.
- The sexual partners reach a clear and unambiguous agreement about the nature of their sexual practice within and outside their relationship. This negotiated agreement involves both agreement within the relationship and agreements beyond the relationship.

Kippax[35] describes the most common agreements as:

1. The men opt for no sex outside the relationship at all; that is they adopt mutual monogamy as a strategy.
2. The men opt for no anal intercourse outside the relationship and thus agree that any sex outside with casual partners is restricted to oral–genital sex, mutual masturbation or some other relatively safe sexual practice.
3. The men opt for anal intercourse outside the relationship, but agree that all such intercourse with casual partners is protected, that is that condoms are used 100% of the time (p. 96).

If these agreements are adhered to, then HIV transmission will not occur within the regular relationship.

There is still debate about the efficacy of negotiated safety strategies and their promotion. A campaign was run in New South Wales called 'Talk Test Test Trust ...Together'.[36] The campaign advised gay men to test, to be honest about the results, to test again in three months, then, if you are both still negative reach a clear mutual agreement ... etc. 'The Talk Test Test Trust ... Together' campaign was evaluated. Recall of the material was high; non-one understood the message to be – just give up condoms. Mackie[37] concluded: the campaign had 'added to gay men's understanding of how to negotiate unprotected sex within their relationships' (p. 36).

Three studies have measured compliance with the negotiated safety agreement.[38,39] Instances of non-compliance were recorded (around 10%). Elford et al.[40] in a study conducted in London, were concerned that men in regular relationships had taken on the first element, only to have unprotected anal intercourse (UAI) with regular partners; but had not necessarily understood the necessity of establishing HIV negative status first. Kippax[35] argues that: 'unprotected anal intercourse commonly occurs between men in regular relationships. The question that must be addressed is whether to lower the risk of such behaviour or attempt to change it. The evidence ... indicates that the former move may be the most appropriate and sensible one' (p. 96).

Interventions to reduce HIV and STI risks among young homeless people

Young people who are living away from the parental home are a varied group. Walters[41] suggests that the group includes:

> (a) runaways – those who have left home without a parent's or guardian's consent; (b) throwaways – those who are forced out of their homes; (c) system and foster care youth – those who leave problematic social service placements; (d) school dropouts – those who are exposed to and engage in risk behavior, but who may return to a residence to sleep; and (e) homeless youth – those whose families become homeless (pp. 188–189).

A study of homeless youth in New York City found that up to 26% were involved in 'survival sex'.[42] A comprehensive program targeting young homeless people in New York and focusing on HIV/STI prevention was carried out by Rotheram-Borus et al.[42] Young people at a residential shelter participated in an intensive HIV risk reduction program that targeted:

- Knowledge of HIV/AIDS through multimedia.
- Training related to emotional and behavioural strategies in HIV high-risk situations.
- The provision of health and welfare care.
- An individual counselling session addressing personal barriers to safer sex practices.

Self-report surveys were administered to the young people at the end of the intervention, and at three- and six-month follow-ups. Their responses were compared with young people at another, control, residential shelter. There was clear evidence of an increase in consistent condom use and a reduction in high-risk behaviours for the intervention group. There was also clear evidence of a dose-related effect – those young people, who had received the greater number of sessions had the greatest risk reductions. No changes were observed in levels of abstinence. This program has subsequently been developed as *StreetSmart*.

An occupational intervention

Jackson et al.[43] carried out a targeted intervention with long-distance truck drivers in Kenya. This occupational group is particularly at risk of STIs and HIV; the men have long days (and weeks) on the road away from home, they have disposable income, and truck stops are a magnet for many women selling sex. Jackson et al. set up an intervention comprising initial voluntary testing and counselling (VCT), STI treatment, group and individual counselling and condom distribution. They followed the truck drivers for 18 months. The outcomes were a significant reduction in extramarital sex and contact with sex workers, and a small reduction in incidence of STIs. However, there was no change in condom use. It was clear that the more travel a truck driver did, the more at risk he was. It was also the case that 25% of the original participants were lost to follow-up and that those with more travel were also more likely to be lost. There was no comparison or control group. Nonetheless, this integrated and targeted intervention is a good example of structural and behavioural interventions.

Interventions aimed at reducing the risk of cervical cancer

Shephard et al.[44] reviewed interventions for encouraging sexual lifestyle and behaviours intended to prevent cervical cancer. Cervical cancer is a common cancer, affecting women worldwide. Lifestyle behaviours that a woman engaged in relatively early on in her life are thought to play a significant part in the development of cervical cancer. In particular, we now know that the most significant risk factor for cervical cancer is HPV. The human papillomavirus, particularly the types most closely associated with cervical cancer (types 16 and 18) are transmitted sexually. The greater the number of sexual partners a woman has, the greater her risk of coming into contact with HPV. Many, if not most, men are asymptomatic with HPV. HPV is relatively common, and early onset of sexual activity is thought to increase the risk of HPV, since the cervix may be damaged at a time when it is still developing; similarly smoking may reduce immunity and the likelihood of clearing the virus. The combination of early onset of sexual activity and high rates of smoking are both associated with lower socioeconomic status, and we see that, in the UK, cervical cancer has a higher incidence among working class women.[45]

The review carried out by Shephard et al.[44] examined interventions to promote safer sexual behaviours, including condom use, reduction in the number of sexual partners and abstinence. All would be associated with a reduction in potential exposure to HPV and hence would constitute primary prevention of cervical cancer. Many of the reviews targeted at preventing HIV transmission would focus on very similar outcomes. However, many of these reviews either do not include women at all, or include only a relatively small number of women. In contrast, Shephard's review focused on interventions for sexually active and presexually active women between the ages of 13 and 64 years. Thirty studies met the rigorous inclusion criteria, of which 20 (66%) were excluded from data analysis for a number of reasons, including a lack of equivalence between intervention and comparison groups at baseline.

Of the ten remaining studies, all had a primary focus of improving sexual health, including HIV and other STIs. None explicitly had the aim to prevent cervical cancer. All studies included factual information (most often about HIV); many included the teaching of practical risk reduction skills that included correct condom use, and how to persuade a potential partner to use a condom. Role-plays, video presentations and other media were common features of the interventions.

The settings in which the interventions were delivered varied immensely; two featured prisons[46,47] four featured specialist health-care units such as STI clinics and one focused on a university college.[48] In all but this last study, the women were of low socioeconomic status. Eight of the studies were conducted in the United States, one was Canadian, and one was carried out in Bombay.

All ten studies reported favourable outcomes, most commonly, increased condom use during vaginal intercourse. Follow-up only averaged six months and so how long these effects might last is unclear. It is also of concern that condom use was the major targeted outcome since there remains some debate about the efficacy of condoms in reducing transmission of HPV – an issue that is 'hot' politically in the United States at the moment; see for example CDC recommendations for reducing risk of HPV infections that state: 'The available scientific evidence is not sufficient to recommend condoms as a primary prevention strategy for the prevention of genital HPV infection' (p. 4).

INTERVENTIONS DIRECTED AT THE COMMUNITY LEVEL

Behaviour Change Communication (BCC) has been developed as an interactive process with communities. The aim is to develop tailored messages using a variety of communication channels, promote and sustain individual, community and societal behaviour change with regard to HIV and maintain appropriate behaviours. Family Health International (FHI) promotes BCC and argues that when it is effective it can increase knowledge, stimulate community dialogue, promote attitude change, reduce stigma and discrimination, create a demand for information and services, and advocate and promote services for prevention care and support. BCC programs can also improve skills such as safe injecting, negotiating safer sex and developing confidence.

Mass media

Television is often portrayed as having potentially negative effects, particular on young people. Here we will review some attempts to use television constructively in sexual health education and in HIV prevention.

Young people in the United States between the ages of 14 and 18 are thought to watch an average of two and three quarter hours of television each day. It is estimated that the average primetime show contains six sex scenes per hour. In this context, the impact of a condom efficiency message televised in a program was assessed by Collins et al.[49]

An episode of the popular program *Friends* included a story of a condom failure. Rachel (she of the hair) experienced an unplanned pregnancy as a consequence of a single night of sex with her former boy friend, Ross. When told, he exclaims '*but we used a condom*'. The statement '*condoms are only 97% effective*' was included in the episode. This show was watched by an estimated 1.67 million 12–17 year olds in the United States. As part of a large-scale telephone survey, young people between the ages of 12 and 17 were asked if they regularly watched *Friends*. Those who did were then asked if they recalled the show when Rachel told Ross she was pregnant. Those who did were also asked about an unrelated event occurring in the same show. More than half of those who reported seeing the show interpreted the message as *'lots of times, condoms don't prevent pregnancy'*. In addition, those who were regular viewers were more likely to recall that Ross and Rachel had used a condom.

This is a good example of how mass media might ensure that health messages are conveyed to key audiences. However the authors of the paper also point out that the show aired opposite *Survivor* and many young people reported swapping back and forth between channels – mixed messages are a distinct risk!

Multi-component large-scale interventions

South Africa has become known for its population-based interventions to reduce HIV. Two of these, *loveLife* and *Soul City* are renowned for their innovative use of integrated programs of intervention. Both have well-documented websites. *Soul City* describes itself on its website (www.soulcity.org.za/02.01.asp) as: '... a dynamic and innovative multi-media health promotion and social change project'. Through drama and entertainment *Soul City* reaches more than 16 million South Africans. It has also been broadcast in many parts of Africa as well as Latin America, the Caribbean and South East Asia. *Soul City* examines many health and development issues, imparting information and impacting on social norms, attitudes and practice. Its impact is aimed at the level of the individual, the community and the sociopolitical environment.'

Every series since 1994 has included some content on HIV/AIDS. Each series comprises: a prime time television series, that consistently gains very high ratings, particularly in the under 25-year-old age group; a daily radio drama lasting 15 minutes; an advertising and publicity campaign; information booklets; an advocacy campaign; and an interactive website.

A second South Africa venture, developed in 2001 is *loveLife*. The *loveLife* program has three main components. These are:

- **Awareness and education:** *loveLife* uses a combination of television, radio, and outdoor media, such as billboards, taxis, and water towers, to encourage more responsible sexual behaviour. The media components are backed by printed educational materials and a national telephone help line. *loveLife* has developed a website (www.loveLife.org.za) as an interactive source for sexual health information.
- **Service development:** service provision for young people and separate from other public health services.
- **Outreach:** *loveLife* supplements existing successful sexual health education programs with the use of peer groups. They have established Y-Centres; these incorporate sexual health education, counselling, and care; partnership with a radio station; and a basketball court.

loveLife has been evaluated for brand-awareness and message-impact using a range of techniques. More than two-thirds of respondents could recognize the *loveLife* brand and, of those who recognized the brand, more than 80% described it as a program promoting sexual responsibility.

National campaigns

At the level of nations, two countries stand out as having been effective in reducing new HIV infections; these are Thailand and Uganda. Senegal is recognized as having successfully sustained a low rate of HIV, and the undoubted successes of Australia and New Zealand in limiting the spread of HIV should also be noted here. The shared characteristics of all these countries are high levels of commitment to behaviour change programs, most especially at the political level. In Thailand, the focus was primarily on increasing use of condoms among groups such as commercial sex workers and their clients, and army conscripts. Thailand's campaign to ensure 100% condom use in brothels was especially successful.[50] However, some of the structural issues that underpin the potential for an HIV epidemic remain unaddressed, for example the large number of women in the sex industry and the increasing incidence of HIV among injecting drug users in the region.

In the case of Uganda, the strong political leadership of President Musaveni ensured a multi-sectoral approach. Uganda's prevention programs focused primarily on young people and emphasized delayed first sex, reduction in multiple partners 'zero-grazing' and condom use. HIV prevalence among pregnant women in urban areas fell each year from its high point of 29.5% in 1992 to 11.25% in 2000.[51] The proportion of sexually active young people declined and the age of first sex increased by nearly two years.[52,53]

THE FUTURE OF SEX AND OF HIV

Piot and Bartos[51] sum up the challenges for future interventions to reduce the HIV pandemic:

> *For the foreseeable future, the solutions to AIDS will be developed in the complex territory formed at the intersection of politics, science and mass mobilization. The principal determinant of the future course of the HIV epidemic in Africa will remain African leadership, from village levels up (p. 212).*

This could easily be said of HIV elsewhere in the world and of STIs everywhere. The extent to which individual behaviour change is supported by structural factors and social contexts will determine success and good health for all.

More generally, sex is increasingly separated (divorced) from reproduction. New technologies will change our possibilities for reproduction, and for continued sex.

We will gather better and more comprehensive sources of data on sex and sexual health. It is not possible to plan interventions unless basic data are available, for example, there is no point planning sex education at the age of 15 if many young people are having sex at 13 years of age. Indeed, from our recent research we now know that 22% of young men and 13% of young women have had sex before the age of 16. Health facilities for AIDS, pregnancy, contraception and many other issues can also only be planned on the basis of epidemiological information.

Legislation will have to change in the areas of sex work and what kinds of sex are permissible. There are still, eight countries in the world with the death penalty for homosexuality: Afghanistan, Iran, Mauritania, Pakistan, Saudi Arabia, Sudan, United Arab Emirates, and Yemen. Numerous other countries, including parts of the United States, still have punitive sentences for engaging in 'homosexual behaviour'. There are still four countries with the death penalty for adultery: Iran, Pakistan, Saudi Arabia, and Yemen. Religions still have much to say about many aspects of sex, including masturbation, adultery, homosexuality, and birth control. There is little prospect of effective interventions to enhance sexual health in such contexts.

Interventions that acknowledge and celebrate the 'joy of sex' are likely to achieve more than those that seek to limit sexual behaviours and expression, not least because they will resonate with the pleasure and self-enrichment that many people associate with sex. In particular, we need to leave behind the moralism associated so consistently with sex; history tells us that, over centuries, attempts to limit sexual expression have regularly failed, and that poor sexual health is the inevitable consequence of the involvement of religious and other moral or civil authorities in the sexual lives of adults.

References

1. World Health Organization. Gender and reproductive rights, glossary, sexual health. Geneva: World Health Organization; 2002.
2. Mace DR, Bannerman RHO, Burton J. The teaching of human sexuality in schools for health professionals. Public Health Paper No. 57. Geneva: World Health Organization; 1974.
3. Sanders SA, Reinisch JM. Would you say you 'had sex' if...? Journal of the American Medical Association 1999; 281(3):275–277.
4. Pitts MK, Rahman Q. Which behaviors constitute 'having sex' among university students in the UK? Archives of Sexual Behavior 2001; 30(2):169–176.
5. Jeannin A, Konings E, Dubois-Arber F, Landert C, Van Melle G. Validity and reliability in reporting sexual partners and condom use in a Swiss population survey. European Journal of Epidemiology 1998; 14(2):139–146.
6. Smith TE, Steen JA, Spaulding-Givens J, Schwendinger A. Measurement in abstinence education: Critique and recommendations. Evaluation and the Health Professions 2003; 26(2):180–205.
7. National Centre in Clinical and Epidemiological Research. Annual surveillance report HIV/AIDS, hepatitis C and sexually transmissible infections in Australia. Sydney: University of New South Wales; 2003.
8. McKay A. Prevention of sexually transmitted infections in different populations: A review of behaviourally effective and cost effective interventions. Canadian Journal of Human Sexuality 2000; 9(2):95–120.
9. Maticka-Tyndale E. Reducing the incidence of sexually transmitted disease through behavioural and social change. Canadian Journal of Sexuality 1997; 6:89–104.

10. Whittaker DJ, Miller KS, Clark LF. Reconceptualising adolescent sexual behaviour: Beyond did they or didn't they. Family Planning Perspectives 2000; 32:111–117.

11. Howard M, McCabe JB. Helping teenagers postpone sexual involvement Family Planning Perspectives 1990; 22:21–26.

12. Rissel CE, Richters J, Grulich AE, de Visser RO, Smith A. First experiences of vaginal intercourse and oral sex among a representative sample of adults. Australian and New Zealand Journal of Public Health 2003; 27(20):131–138.

13. Che Y, Cleland JG, Mohamed MA. Periodic abstinence in developing countries: An assessment of failure rates and consequences. Contraception 2004; 69:15–21.

14. Shelton JD, Halperin DT, Nantulya V, Potts M, Gayle HD, King Holmes K. Partner reduction is crucial for balanced 'ABC' approach to HIV prevention. British Medical Journal 2004; 328:891–893.

15. Stoneburner RL, Low-Beer D. Population level HIV declines and behavioural risk avoidance in Uganda. Science 2004; 304:714–718.

16. National Institute of Health (NIH). Workshop summary: scientific evidence on condom effectiveness for sexually transmitted disease (STD) prevention. In: US Department of Health and Human Services Online [access 2004 July]. Available from URL www.niaid.nih.gov/dmid/stds/condomreport.pdf; 2000.

17. Ghys PD, Diallo MO, Ettiegne Traore V, Kale K, Tawil O, Carael M, et al. Increase in condom use and decline in HIV and sexually transmitted diseases among female sex workers in Abidjan, Côte d'Ivoire 1991–1998. AIDS 2002; 16:251–8.

18. Grierson J, Smith AMA, Wain D. Victorian Networks Study: Technical Report. Melbourne; 2003.

19. Robin L, Dittus P, Whitaker D, Crosby R, Ethier K, Mezoff J, et al. Behavioral interventions to reduce incidence of HIV, STD, and pregnancy among adolescents: A decade in review. Journal of Adolescent Health 2004; 34:3–26.

20. Dunn L, Ross B, Caines T, Howorth P. A school-based HIV/AIDS prevention education program: Outcomes of peer-led versus community health nurse-led interventions. Canadian Journal of Human Sexuality 1998; 7:339–345.

21. Caron F, Godin G, Otis J, Lambert LD. Evaluation of a theoretically based AIDS/STD peer education program on postponing sexual intercourse and on condom use among adolescents attending high school. Health Education Research: Theory and Practice 2004; 19(2):185–197.

22. Ajzen I. The Theory of Planned Behavior. Organizational Behavior and Human Decision Processes 1991; 50:179–211.

23. Triandis HC. Values, attitudes and interpersonal behavior. In: Page MM, ed. Nebraska Symposium on Motivation, Beliefs, Attitudes and Values. Nebraska: University of Nebraska; 1980:195–259.

24. Johnson WD, Hedges LV, Diaz RM. Interventions to modify sexual risk behaviours for preventing HIV infection in men who have sex with men. Chichester: John Wiley; 2004.

25. Rosser BRS. Evaluation of the efficacy of AIDS education interventions for homosexually active men. Health Education Research: Theory and Practice 1990; 5(3):299–308.

26. Perry S, Fishman B, Jacobsberg L, Young J, Frances A. Effectiveness of psychoeducational interventions in reducing emotional distress after human immunodeficiency virus antibody testing. Archives of General Psychiatry 1991; 48(2):143–147.

27. Kelly JA, St Lawrence JS, Hood HV, Brasfield TL. Behavioral intervention to reduce AIDS risk activities. Journal of Consultant Clinical Psychology 1989; 57(1):60–67.

28. Miller RL. Assisting gay men to maintain safer sex: An evaluation of an AIDS service organization's safer sex maintenance program. AIDS Education and Prevention 1995; 7 (Suppl):48–63.

29. Tudiver F, Myers T, Kurtz RG, et al. The talking sex project. Evaluation and the Health Professions 1992; 15(4):26–42.

30. Valdiserri RO, Lyter DW, Leviton LC, Callahan CM, Kingsley LA, Rinaldo CR. AIDS prevention in homosexual and bisexual men: results of a randomized trial evaluating two risk reduction interventions. AIDS 1989; 3(1):21–26.

31. Kelly JA, St. Lawrence JS, Diaz YE, et al. HIV risk behavior reduction following intervention with key opinion leaders of population: An experimental analysis. American Journal of Public Health 1991; 81:168–171.

32. Kelly JA, Murphy DA, Sikkema KJ, et al. Randomised, controlled, community-level HIV-prevention intervention for sexual-risk behaviour among homosexual men in US cities. Lancet 1997; 350:1500–1505.

33. Kegeles SM, Hays RB, Coates TJ. The Mpowerment project: A community-level HIV prevention intervention for young gay men. American Journal of Public Health 1996; 86:1129–1136.

34. Kippax S, Crawford J, Davis M, Rodden P, Dowsett G. Sustaining safe sex: A longitudinal study of a sample of homosexual men. AIDS 1993; 7:257–263.

35. Kippax S. A comment on negotiated safety. Venereology 1996; 2:96–97.

36. AIDS Council of New South Wales (ACON). Campaign overview of Talk, Test, Test, Trust ... Together. Sydney; 1998.

37. Mackie B. Report and process evaluation of the 'Talk, Test, Test, Trust ... Together'. Sydney: HIV/AIDS Education Campaign AIDS Council of New South Wales; 1996.

38. Kippax S, Noble J, Prestage G, Crawford J, Campbell D, Baxter D, et al. Sexual negotiations in the AIDS era: Negotiated safety revisited. AIDS 1997; 11:191–197.

39. Davidovich U, de Wit JBF, Stroebe W. Assessing sexual risk behaviour of young gay men in primary relationships: The incorporation of negotiated safety and negotiated safety compliance. AIDS 2000; 14(6):701–706.

40. Elford J, Bolding G, Maguire M, Sherr L. Sexual risk behaviour among gay men in a relationship. AIDS 1999; 3:1407–1411.

41. Walters AS. HIV prevention in street youth. Journal of Adolescent Health 1999; 25(3):187–198.

42. Rotheram-Borus MJ, Meyer-Bahlburg H, Rosario M, et al. Lifetime sexual behaviours among predominately minority male runaways and gay/bisexual adolescents in New York City. AIDS Education and Prevention Fall 1992; (Suppl):34–42.

43. Jackson DJ, Rakwar JP, Richardson BA, et al. Decreased incidence of sexually transmitted diseases among trucking company workers in Kenya: Results of a behavioural risk-reduction programme. AIDS 1997; 11(7):903–909.

44. Shephard J, Weston R, Peersman G, Napuli IZ. Interventions for encouraging sexual lifestyles and behaviours intended to prevent cervical cancer. Chichester: John Wiley; 2004.

45. Brown S, Vessey M, Harris R. Social class, sexual habits and cancer of the cervix. Community Medicine 1984; 6(4):281–286.

46. DiClemente RJ, Wingood GM. A randomized controlled trial of an HIV sexual risk-reduction intervention for young African-American women. Journal of the American Medical Association 1995; 274(16):1271–1276.

47. St Lawrence J, Eldridge GD, Shelby MC, Little CE, Brasfield TL, O'Bannon RE. HIV risk reduction for incarcerated women: A comparison of brief interventions based on

two theoretical models. Journal of Consulting and Clinical Psychology 1997; 65(3):504–509.

48. Ploem C, Byers ES. The effects of two AIDS risk-reduction interventions on heterosexual college women's AIDS-related knowledge, attitudes and condom use. Journal of Psychology and Human Sexuality 1997; 9(1):1–24.

49. Collins RL, Elliott MN, Berry SH, Kanouse DE, Hunter SB. Entertainment television as a health sex educator: The impact of condom-efficacy information in an episode of Friends. Pediatrics 2003; 112(5):1115–1121.

50. Rojanapithayakorn W, Hanenberg R. The 100% condom program in Thailand [editorial]. AIDS 1996; 10(1):1–7.

51. Piot P, Bartos M. The epidemiology of HIV and AIDS. In: Essex M, Mboup S, Kanki PJ, Marlink R, Tlou SD, eds. AIDS in Africa, 2nd edn. New York: Plenum Publishers; 2002.

52. Asiimwe-Okiror G, Opio AA, Musinguzi J, Madraa E, Tembo G, Carael M. Change in sexual behaviour and decline in HIV infection among young pregnant women in urban Uganda. Aids 1997; 11(14):1757–1763.

53. Mulder D, Nunn A, Kamali A, Kengeya-Kayondo J. HIV-1 seroprevalance in young adults in a rural Ugandan cohort. British Medical Journal 1995; 311:833–836.

CHAPTER 6

Alcohol and drug use: Theoretical integration of interventions to prevent harm

John W. Toumbourou

INTRODUCTION

The development of problems linked to alcohol and illegal drug use such as marijuana, heroin, cocaine, stimulants, analgesics, amphetamines and hallucinogens (substance use) has been extensively studied and efforts to reduce these problems have included a considerable investment in prevention, treatment and evaluation. Public health approaches have achieved notable successes such as reductions in alcohol-related road trauma.[1] Despite these efforts, substance use remains a major contributor to health and social problems. Illegal drug abuse expanded by 5.9% in the United States of America (USA) from 1992 to 1998, outstripping population and consumer price growth.[2] In 1998 the net costs to Australian society attributable to alcohol use was conservatively estimated at $A 7.6 billion while the use of illegal drugs were $A 6.1 billion.[3] In the same year net social costs attributable to alcohol use in the USA were estimated at US$ 184.6 billion[4] while the costs of illegal drug use were US$ 143.4 billion.[2]

A complex range of social, economic and individual determinants have been shown to motivate substance use behaviour.[5] To succeed, policies and programs need to mirror this complexity by coordinating responses across different service and policy domains to reduce the local determinants that give rise to these problems. To facilitate this complex coordination task simple theoretical frameworks must be distilled from the complex knowledge base.[6] The present chapter organizes alcohol and drug use interventions on the basis of their application to four major motivations for drug use: escaping distress, self-management and regulation, conforming to norms, and individuating identity. The range of intervention is considered including prevention activities aiming to reduce the antecedents motivating substance use, and treatment and harm-reduction interventions that aim to reduce escalation and maintenance of consequent problems.

A variety of behaviours has been identified in efforts to reduce substance use problems. Although the disorders of dependence and abuse are significant in clinical settings, there are considerable costs associated with substance use falling outside these diagnostic categories. Acute harms such as accidents and injuries can result through single episodes of alcohol intoxication while in the longer-term health can be compromised through regular consumption of excessive amounts of alcohol.[7,8] Alcohol-related harms are closely aligned with overall levels of community alcohol consumption.[9] Despite its overall negative impact, alcohol used in moderation can have health benefits in reducing cardiovascular disease in older populations and female strokes,[3] emphasizing the importance of setting specific behavioural targets in efforts to prevent harm.

First use of alcohol often occurs in childhood while use of illegal drugs arises largely in adolescence. In the Australian national school survey conducted in 1999 over three-quarters of students had used alcohol by age 12 and over 20% had drank in the past month. By age 17 over half (55%) were drinking on a weekly or more frequent basis[10] and a similar proportion (50%) had tried cannabis.[11]

Young adults experience high levels of acute harms associated with alcohol[12] and illegal drug use.[13] As early age use and regular adolescent use of alcohol,[14,15] cannabis,[16,17] and/or other illegal drugs[18,19] increases the likelihood of subsequent problems in adulthood, prevention efforts focus on preventing or delaying first use and reducing escalation to more frequent, higher quantity or polydrug use mixing different types of drugs.[20] Treatment programs typically focus on abstinence among dependent users or reductions in levels of use.

Longitudinal follow-up studies have established a considerable stability in patterns of substance use from adolescence into adulthood.[21] Figure 6.1 demonstrates the general stability of alcohol use in a sample of 3300 Australian youth followed from late high school into adulthood.[22] Youth drinking on at

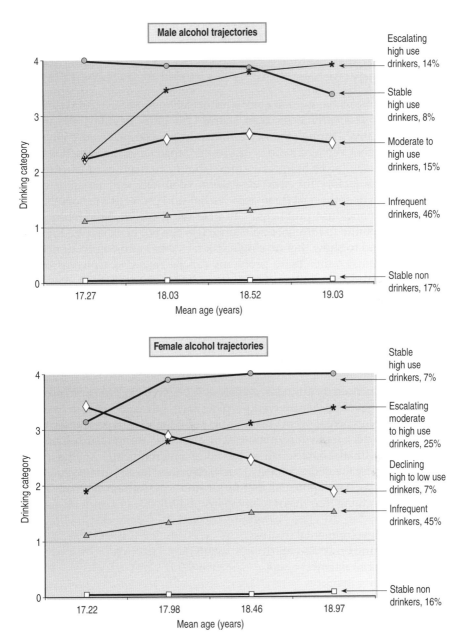

Fig. 6.1   Trajectories of alcohol use identified in Australian youth ($N = 3300$) followed from the last year of high school (wave 1) through to age 19 (wave 4). Drinking categories: 0 = Non-drinkers; 1 = Less than weekly drinkers; 2 = Low weekly drinking – within public health guidelines; 3 = Moderate weekly drinking (hazardous), 4 = High weekly drinking (harmful).[22] Reproduced with permission from Drug and Alcohol Review. http://www.tandf.co.uk/journals.

least a weekly basis in high school were more likely to subsequently escalate to drinking alcohol in amounts that risk harm.

EPIDEMIOLOGY

Per capita alcohol consumption among adults fell in most developed nations in the late 1980s and early 1990s then levelled off until the late 1990s when it increased slightly.[5] Through the 1990s youth alcohol use increased both in Australia and in other Western nations including Canada and the United States.[10]

Borrowing similar techniques to those that have been used to study risk and protective factors for heart disease, epidemiological researchers have been studying over the past three decades risk and protective factors that lead to youth substance use problems.[23] To date the theoretical model by which risk factors operate to influence substance use has not been clarified. Empirical studies tend to show that no single risk factor lies at the heart of developmental problems; rather these problems can be regarded to have complex causes or multi-determination. The more risk factors that persist over longer periods of time the greater the subsequent developmental impact.[24,25]

THE DEVELOPMENT OF SUBSTANCE MISUSE

To successfully guide interventions theoretical frameworks need to link practice with aetiological and intervention process research. Substance use is motivated behaviour influenced by attitudes, choices and preferences. The expressed motivations that treatment clients give to explain their substance use can be related to earlier developmental events that in turn point the way to prevention efforts. The extent to which motivation manifests in substance use and harm is modified by both individual characteristics, the local environmental setting (micro-processes) and by the wider context of social structural factors (macro-processes). In what follows developmental risk factor and intervention research is integrated by examining four major motivations underlying substance misuse:

- Escaping developmental distress.
- Self-managing body and spirit.
- Conforming to norms.
- Individuating identity.

Substance use motivated by developmental distress

The most severe and harmful substance use problems are associated with childhood backgrounds characterized by developmental problems that undermine healthy development and operate from prior to birth and through childhood. Early developmental risk factors appear to translate to social marginalization and emotional distress through social exclusion processes operating in families, schools and communities. The evidence linking early risk factors and substance misuse is summarized below.

In the New Zealand Christchurch cohort the small minority of youth (2.7%) experiencing the most severe behaviour problems had early childhood backgrounds characterized by in-utero insult (maternal smoking and drinking), birth complications, problems in infant care (low breast feeding, low infant care, poor parenting), and social instability through childhood (family breakdown and parental changes). The family backgrounds of these children were characterized by high levels of social disadvantage (teenage parents, low education, low income, sole parents) and social disconnection (low rates of church attendance, parent mobility).[26]

High rates of substance use problems among parents and other family members predict developmental problems and inter-generation substance misuse.[27–29]

Academic failure and truancy beginning in primary school and high rates of child behaviour problems can be linked to earlier developmental problems and are strongly predictive of subsequent substance misuse.[30]

Children with a higher cumulative number of early developmental risk factors have a greater likelihood of both substance misuse and also other problems including crime, health and mental health problems.[5,23]

Moderating factors

Widening economic divisions and family breakdown have left behind a large number of children living near or below the poverty line. The link between home ownership and wealth has created an increasing trend for poverty to be geographically segregated and this has exacerbated community and school risk factors for many children from vulnerable families.[31] This is unfortunate as healthy family, school, and peer social environments have the capacity to reduce the adverse developmental consequences of early temperament[32] and behaviour problems.[33]

Substance use motivated by efforts to self-manage body and spirit

Substance use is often an intentional activity that has functional motives relevant to feeling good, enhancing the body, or achieving spiritual connection. The discovery of new drugs has been linked to progress in the medical and pharmacological sciences that have as their aim the reduction of physical disease. Evidence for functional motivations for substance use include the following:

- Favourable attributions and expectations for the effects of substance use predicts intentions to use drugs and this in turn predicts substance use initiation.[34,35]
- High rates of adult substance use for functional purposes, e.g. coffee, painkillers, antibiotics, is associated with high rates of youth involvement in these activities. Youth who use coffee and pain killers tend to have high use of other substances such as tobacco, alcohol and illegal drugs.[36]

- In communities that overuse drugs for a functional purpose, self-efficacy for drug-free management of arousal, pain and health may be reduced. Low self-efficacy[37] and poor control of emotions[32] predicts substance misuse.
- Substances are explicitly used for instrumental purposes according to surveys of many groups. For example alcohol use is typically described as a method of lubricating social engagement. Young girls' dieting behaviour has been linked to tobacco and other substance use.[38] Use of steroids has been linked to efforts to enhance body shape and weight.[39] On the horizon are new drugs aimed at increasing intelligence.
- Substance use problems are unevenly distributed across occupational groups.[40] In some prominent cases substance misuse can be related to the functional role of drugs within the particular occupation. Prominent examples include stimulant abuse among transport workers and students, steroid and performance drug use among athletes, and excessive alcohol use in the alcohol industry.

Moderating processes

There is a genetic link modifying the impact of drugs on specific individuals and for some people the situational factors influencing the steps from initiation, through escalation to dependence are different. Severe drug problems may have a stronger genetic basis.[41] Society and culture influence attributions regarding the effects of drugs and the value placed on the effect of drugs. In many traditional cultures value has been placed on the use of drugs to transcend the material world. Within lower socioeconomic status groups a low sense of control over life has been associated with a greater emphasis on short-term pleasures.[42]

Substance use motivated by efforts to conform to social norms

Conformity is a general motivation behind the majority of alcohol and drug use. Conforming to social norms includes a variety of more specific motivations including the desire to achieve social inclusion, to achieve normal adulthood acceptance within a valued social group and obedience to the law. Factors indicating the operation of these influences include the following:

- Favourable attitudes to substance use are related to social bonding with others engaged in substance use.[43] Young people are more likely to initiate substance use where they perceive few risks through use and endorse prior intentions to use.[35]
- Rates of adolescent substance use are strongly linked to wider community norms[23] and parents' drug use.[32]
- Social norms are powerfully conveyed by laws and their enforcement. Laws and associated penalties relating to drug use are thought to influence individual attitudes and beliefs by expressing social disapproval of drug use.[5]

- Adolescent alcohol initiation is reduced where parents communicate clear rules against alcohol use.[44]
- The age at which it is legally permitted to purchase and use alcohol influences youth involvement in alcohol use.[45]

Moderating processes

Drug use motivated by conformity to norms is mediated by situational influences that determine the balance of social approval for a particular act of drug use. Easy availability and access to drugs, the balance of rewards associated with drug use, and the possibility of experiencing penalties influence substance use behaviour.[23] Although macro-forces such as the legal and illegal trade in drugs and changing cultural influences exert a pervasive influence on individual behaviour, their operation is often overlooked due to the difficulties in measuring individual-level variation.[46]

Substance use motivated by efforts to individuate identity

Industrial and technological sophistication has translated to social changes including a longer period young people spend in education postponing the responsibilities of work, marriage and children. Within the social form of individualism there is an increasing developmental requirement for youth to define a distinctive individual and peer identity and this appears to be motivating important aspects of youth involvement in illegal drug use. Although efforts to individuate may be a major motivation driving new patterns of drug use, its influence has been largely ignored in research and policy. The operation of globalization means that similar influences are also impacting young people internationally. The following community and individual indicators evidence the influence of the individuation motive:

- Families characterized by a balance of high demands for prosocial compliance together with good communication and nurture increase child competence and reduce involvement in substance use.[47]
- Youth with a weak identity status have higher rates of substance misuse.[48]
- Higher affiliation to peers rather than parents predicts norm violating substance use.[49] Initiation of substance use is reduced where adolescent–parent relationships are harmonious.[44,50]
- Youth who have high levels on measures of rebelliousness and unconventionality are more likely to engage in norm violating substance use.[23]
- The risk of initiating or escalating substance use shows a linear increase for siblings later in the birth order compared to those earlier in the birth order.[32]
- Liberalization of female gender roles has been associated with an increase in substance use and harm.[51]
- The rise to prominence of different and new patterns of drug use and new drug epidemics are often led by youth who express criticism of society and

wish to differentiate themselves and their generation.[35] New patterns of substance use are emerging in developing nations led by affluent middle-class youth breaking with tradition and influenced by Western values.[52]

Moderating influences

A young person may initially experiment with different lifestyles in an effort to individuate. By placing themselves within particular situational influences (e.g. gang involvement)[53] behavioural sequences can then unfold that move behaviour well beyond normative constraints. The influence of the individuating motive appears to be heavily influenced by policies and practices in families, schools, and the wider society. Individuating may be a higher motive on Maslow's need hierarchy emerging more strongly in the secure living conditions of modern societies.

In the next sections of the chapter the evidence base for the interventions that address these motivational pathways are reviewed (see Table 6.1 for a summary).

REDUCING DRUG USE MOTIVATED BY DEVELOPMENTAL DISTRESS

A growing range of interventions aim to reduce early age risk factors that undermine healthy development and to reduce the translation of developmental problems into social marginalization and substance misuse. Interventions tend to be targeted to individuals and communities that have high levels of developmental risk factors. To succeed interventions need to work long-term and to be well-integrated across different domains of socialization. In what follows intervention findings have been organized to differentiate individual, group and community interventions.

Individual interventions

Early years prevention

Early years prevention efforts aim to increase support to vulnerable families to prevent pre-birth exposure to maternal substance use and nutritional deficits and ensure infant needs are met for safety, stimulation, love and care. An important strategy developed by Olds and colleagues involved regular home visiting by a nurse from late pregnancy until the child's second birthday. A small experimental trial followed-up vulnerable families and found this strategy reduced rates of smoking and alcohol use for the mothers during pregnancy, leading to reductions in cigarette and alcohol-related cognitive impairment in the children as preschoolers. Follow-up of the children to age 15 revealed reductions in their early initiation of smoking and alcohol use.[54] Savings and returns to government have been estimated at around $5 for every $1 spent on the program over the first 15 years of the child's life. There is evidence that this strategy may not demonstrate benefits where it is applied more universally to include low-risk mothers.[31] The Perry Preschool

Table 6.1 Interventions addressing four motivational pathways to substance use, organized by level of intervention

Intervention target	Intervention level		
	Individual	Group	Community
Reducing developmental distress	Early years prevention** Preventative case management** Emotional competence training†	Behavioural parent education** Improving school environments** Informational and affective drug education*	Risk focused community prevention* Harm reduction strategies** Health promotion† Workplace testing* Restrictions on advertising†
Encouraging healthy self-management	Motivational interviewing* Pharmacotherapies*** Genetic counselling†		
Addressing normative conformity motives	Social competence counselling* Normative feedback***	Social influence drug education** Twelve-Step groups***	Controlling alcohol supply* Minimum age restrictions** Increasing the price of alcohol* Social marketing* Community mobilization** Police diversion†
Encouraging healthy individuation	Mentorship	Parent education** Family therapy** Peer intervention† Therapeutic community***	

Intervention evidence is summarized using the following legend adapted from Toumbourou et al.[126]:

†Innovation funding and formative evaluation will be required to settle an intervention model.

*An intervention model is emerging, process evaluation is warranted to achieve a safe and effective intervention process.

*An intervention manual has been documented and there is some evidence for early impact efficacy.

**Evidence for outcome efficacy (evidence from experimental and well-controlled small trials).

***Evidence for outcome effectiveness (efficacy can be maintained in real-world service delivery contexts).

program has encouraged intensive early preschool experiences combined with home visits for high-risk families.[55] A small experimental trial followed up children to age 27 and found development advantages that translate to a $6 saving for every $1 invested in the program.[31]

Preventative case management

Elevated early developmental risk factors increase the likelihood of crime. Given developmental deficits can result in complex and multi-faceted problems and treatment approaches have focused on coordinating a range of evidence-based interventions. The Multisystemic Treatment Program targeted court referred serious juvenile offenders. Treatment objectives were set in consultation with the offender and their family. Clinicians trained in evidence-based therapies were rewarded for attaining agreed outcomes relevant to family relationships, individual competencies, peer relationships, work, education, health and mental health. The program was effective in engaging families with complex problems and small well-controlled evaluations show reductions in crime and delinquency maintained after one to two years.[56] The net economic benefit is around $5 for each $1 invested.[57] A similar strategy for students evidencing poor school performance and substance misuse involved school counsellor assistance to achieve behaviour and academic improvement goals. An experimental trial revealed lower substance use after two years.[58]

Group interventions

Behavioural parent education

Interventions based on cognitive social learning and behavioural theories are now widely used in parent education programs aiming to prevent or reduce childhood problem behaviours. Such problems are an important manifestation of early developmental distress. These programs have been shown in small experimental trials to provide moderate improvements in parenting competencies and reductions in child behaviour problems.[59–61] There is only limited evidence of longer-term improvements.[62] Small improvements in child outcomes have been observed in short-term evaluations where intensive programs have been delivered to parents with drug problems.[63,64]

Improving school environments

Efforts to enhance teacher–student relationships and reduce negative school peer interactions appear to be important in reducing the translation of early developmental risk into social marginalization. The US Fast Track Program has included intensive individual and group components to enhance competencies in the early school years for children with a high number of developmental risk factors. A large experimental trial found moderate improvements in children's educational and social progress in Grade 3.[65] The Linking the

Interests of Families and Teachers Program supplemented classroom social competence training and parent components with playground behaviour monitoring to reinforce social skills. Students received individual rewards for positive social behaviours but an additional group reward was withheld if negative behaviours were not reduced. An experimental trial revealed reductions in school-ground aggressive behaviour, with effects particularly pronounced for the children who were most aggressive at baseline. Grade 5 students showed lower rates of delinquent peer involvement, lower arrests and less initiation of alcohol and marijuana use after three years. Large developmental benefits were also evident for younger cohorts.[33]

The Seattle Social Development Project (SSDP) combined teacher training in effective classroom management and instruction with student social competence and parent education components. An experimental trial revealed early increases in school retention and bonding, with effects also evident for low-achieving students. Long-term follow-up into early adulthood revealed moderate reductions in school failure, substance abuse and delinquency.[66] The program appears to offer differential improvements for the most vulnerable students from low SES backgrounds.[67]

Community interventions

Risk-focused community prevention

Communities That Care is a structured training and consulting program that has been widely implemented in the US to support community prevention planning. The program assists the formation of local community coalitions and facilitates these coalitions to develop and implement prevention strategies. Strategies are carefully tailored to address risk and protective factors implicated in the development of youth substance misuse and related problems. A youth survey is an important tool used to assess and monitor locally elevated risk factors and depressed protective factors. Evidence suggests the program elements can be implemented, and community trials have been proposed to evaluate the program.[68,69]

Harm reduction strategies

Accepting there are individuals strongly motivated to seek intoxication and release through substance use has led to pragmatic community strategies to reduce associated harms. There is evidence that thiamine supplementation of beer or to a less extent of bread can reduce the incidence of Korsakoff's syndrome among chronic alcohol users.[70] Vehicle and roadside engineering can reduce trauma in vehicle crashes. Changing ambulance operating codes can reduce mortality and morbidity in cases of drug overdose. Increasing access to needles and syringes has been important in reducing the spread of HIV among needle-users.[5] Safe injecting rooms and the clinical prescription of heroin have been used to reduce social alienation and harm associated with injecting drug use.[71] Provision of drug treatment services at a community level appears to reduce overall incidents of crime and violence.[72]

INTERVENTIONS ENCOURAGING HEALTHY MANAGEMENT OF BODY AND SPIRIT

There have been two main themes in efforts to address 'functional' motivations for substance misuse. On one hand a large investment is in place to create and market new drugs to help those who are experiencing problems with existing drugs. Prominent examples include a rising use of pharmacotherapies such as naltrexone to treat alcohol problems and methadone to treat heroin use. On the other hand are less developed efforts to encourage health and wellbeing through drug-free methods.

Individual interventions

Emotional competence training

Counselling approaches that aim to teach relaxation and anger management are relatively common. Although there are theoretical reasons to believe these programs may provide alternative means of achieving benefits sought through substance use, there has been little research.[73]

Motivational interviewing

Motivational interviewing is a counselling approach that guides the client to consider both benefits and problems arising from substance use. Alternative methods of achieving benefits and the importance of overcoming problems are examined in an effort to motivate action to reduce substance use. There is some evidence that this approach can increase the likelihood of treatment entry, but is probably insufficient on its own to encourage longer term benefits.[74]

Pharmacotherapies (e.g. methadone, nicotine replacement)

Systematic reviews of experimental trials suggest that disulfiram is not consistently effective as a treatment for alcohol dependence while acamprosate and naltrexone may offer some benefits.[75] Experimental trials support the use of methadone maintenance as an effective opioid substitution therapy and there are promising indications for the efficacy of buprenorphine and LAAM levomethadyl acetate. There are currently few pharmacotherapies treating drug abuse disorders other than opiate dependence.[76]

Genetic counselling

The emerging field of genetic counselling attempts to disseminate information on individual variation in genetic vulnerability to substance use impacts.

In time it is possible this field may be able to assist vulnerable individuals to avoid initiating particular forms of drug use. Proposals for wide-scale population screening face ethical and practical objections, but as knowledge in this area advances voluntary health screening or court mandated screening of targeted groups such as offenders may be feasible.

Group prevention

Informational and affective school drug education

Affective drug education programs include stress management components to increase self-efficacy for addressing difficult situations. There has been insufficient research to establish the extent to which such elements can improve drug education outcomes. Information programs target knowledge and beliefs about the social and personal consequences of using substances. This type of curriculum has been among the earliest school drug education programs and is almost universally included with other components. Reviews typically find that information is insufficient on its own to prevent substance use initiation.[77] More recent variants have incorporated harm-reduction information and evidence from an Australian experimental trial shows reductions in alcohol use and misuse after one year.[78]

Community prevention

Health promotion

Modern health promotion uses a range of policy and program strategies to improve population health. Many reports addressing national health priorities such as cancer, cardiovascular disease, mental health, and injury prevention explicitly target the reduction of tobacco use and excessive alcohol consumption.[79–81] In some cases health promotion programs have targeted more general health and wellbeing goals including social attitudes, and relationships.[82] Although there is growing recognition that antibiotics and analgesics are over-prescribed, strategies to reduce over-reliance on drugs to solve health and adjustment problems have not been a serious component in health promotion programs. Although there are theoretical reasons that health promotion emphasizing self-efficacy for health and wellness might reduce substance misuse, there is no evidence as yet to support this view.

Workplace drug testing

Requirements in many industries can lead to functional pressures to use drugs. Performance enhancing drug use by athletes and amphetamine use among transport drivers are examples. A variety of methods have been used to reduce drug use in the workplace.[40] Evidence is lacking to enable firm conclusions to be reached regarding the prevention benefits or health and safety advantages of workplace drug testing.[83] Programs to encourage alternative methods of achieving the functional benefits sought through substance use have been trialed in settings such as the transport industry, but there has been little controlled evaluation.

Restrictions on advertising

In many countries advertisers successfully link their products to the perception of positive benefits including popularity, status, and success.[52] Many countries have introduced legislation to ban or restrict the advertising of tobacco and alcohol products. Such restrictions probably make an important contribution to reducing substance use, although their aggregate influence has made evaluation difficult.[46]

INTERVENTIONS TO REDUCE SUBSTANCE MISUSE MOTIVATED BY NORMATIVE CONFORMITY

A variety of interventions has been developed to manage the influence of conformity motives on drug-related harm. A major challenge is to change the perceived prevalence and social rewards of substance use behaviours.

Individual interventions

Social competence counselling

Social competence programs aim to increase awareness and avoidance of social situations where pressure to use drugs may emerge. Resistance training aims to teach specific social competencies to enable youth to resist peer influenced drug use. When competently delivered these programs can result in small and short-term reductions in youth initiation of legal and illegal drug use.[77]

Normative feedback

Normative feedback programs aim to correct inflated estimates of levels of involvement in substance misuse. Brief counselling interventions have been designed to provide behavioural assessment of substance use, comparison against age norms and health guidelines and, where indicated, information on behaviour change strategies. Systematic review of well-controlled evaluations suggest that these interventions make a small but significant contribution in encouraging moderate alcohol consumption within primary health care settings.[5] Small samples of university students selected for heavy drinking patterns were randomly assigned to a similar intervention strategy. Follow-up after four years revealed small effects toward significantly better outcomes for the intervention group (33% drinking problems) compared to those allocated to the no-intervention control condition (45% problems).[84] A similar strategy involving tailored feedback on alcohol use in early high school has shown some short-term prevention benefits.[85]

Group interventions

Social influence school drug education

A number of school drug education programs have included social influence curriculum components aimed at developing general and peer resistance social competencies.[77] Reviews suggest these programs can reduce drug use initiation over one year, but there is little evidence for sustained effects over longer periods.[86,87] Some studies have found advantages for peer-delivered curriculum,[88] but such findings have not been consistent.[89] There is some evidence to suggest that behaviour changes have been associated with perceived improvements in social skills.[90] A competitive trial found that students randomly assigned to a drug education program challenging normative beliefs on substance use demonstrated significantly decreased alcohol use after one year.[91] Evidence from other evaluations also associates successful behavioural change with reductions in perceptions of the extent of peer and adult drug use.[92]

Twelve-Step groups

The use of group processes to encourage recovery from substance abuse and dependence is classically demonstrated within the 12-Step recovery movement originated by Alcoholics Anonymous (AA). The therapeutic elements within AA make important use of group, normative processes. A high standard of evidence supports the longer-term therapeutic effectiveness of AA as treatment for dependent alcohol users.[93] An Australian study evaluated treatment in Narcotics Anonymous groups finding that newly exposed members made important gains both in reducing substance use and in enhancing social support. Factors predicting better outcomes after one year included maintaining meeting attendance on at least a weekly basis and engaging in step-work and service roles.[94]

Community prevention

Legislation controlling alcohol manufacture and/or distribution

Government legislation and policies play an important role in codifying the consensus around social norms. In general citizens attempt to obey the law. Laws tend to be more effective where they are strongly enforced and likely to lead to punishment. International experience with government efforts to prohibit alcohol use suggests some success in reducing population-level consumption. The USA experience with prohibition resulted in net reductions in community alcohol use and associated harm. However, unintended consequences included the rise in the illegal alcohol economy. Scandinavian countries have a long history of government controlled alcohol monopolies and there is some evidence that these have been successful in reducing population levels of consumption and harm. Although laws and their enforcement may have important impacts there are ethical and pragmatic factors limiting the potential for controlled experimentation. High standard evaluation of these programs has tended to rely on time-series and descriptive research.[5]

There is little evidence with which to evaluate the success of legislative and law enforcement efforts aimed at illegal drug use and harms. Review of different international models for legislating the use of cannabis suggests little association with rates of cannabis use.[95] A recent analysis of Australian efforts concluded that supply reduction programs had been effective in reducing heroin availability and this was in turn associated with greater use of treatment services and lower mortality.[96]

Increasing the legal age for purchasing and consuming alcohol

US trend data associates older minimum ages for alcohol purchase and use with reductions in alcohol use and harms.[23,45,97] A large multi-site randomized trial of the enforcement of minimum drinking age laws in the US demonstrated a significant reduction in youth access to alcohol.[98]

Increasing the price of alcohol

Decreases in the price of alcohol appear to be associated with general increases in consumption while increases in price tend to lead to reductions in consumption, and harms.[99] This evidence has led to efforts to use the price of alcohol to control consumption. In Australia's Northern Territory the imposition of an alcohol levy to fund a range of prevention and treatment programs was associated with a 22% drop in per capita alcohol use and harms over four years.[100]

Social marketing

The mass media can be used to widely disseminate information about alcohol and other drugs and in some cases can influence attitudes and perceived norms.[101] The role these programs can play in preventing substance use initiation is unclear, although there is some evidence to suggest they may encourage less harmful substance use behaviours. A successful effort to use popular television episodes to introduce the concept of a 'designated driver' as a new social norm was reported in the USA. At the end of the program national polling revealed 64% of adults reported assigning a designated driver for events involving alcoholic consumption.[102]

Community mobilization

Community mobilization encompasses a broad range of practice aimed at reducing local social environmental influences that contribute to harmful substance use. Typically, activities aim to involve local people in the coordination and implementation of a range of complimentary prevention strategies to encourage local norms unfavourable to substance misuse. Programs strategies combining school and parent components with community mobilization to reduce the availability of alcohol and drugs have shown some small reductions over three years in tobacco and marijuana initiation,[103] escalation to regular marijuana use[104] and alcohol initiation while also reducing estimates of peer drug use.[105]

A community mobilization program run in California and South Carolina in the USA aimed to reduce harms associated with drinking.[106] Local organizations assisted with the coordinated implementation of the program that included training in responsible drink service, efforts to reduce drink driving, underage drinking and the access of minors to alcohol. A well-controlled evaluation associated the program with an increase in media coverage of alcohol-related trauma, a reduction in the sale of alcohol to underage decoys, a reduction in alcohol-related violence and a 10% reduction in alcohol-related vehicle accidents over five years. Economic evaluation suggested that just under $3 in health and social costs were saved through every $1 invested in the program.[107]

INTERVENTIONS ENCOURAGING HEALTHY INDIVIDUATION

Interventions to encourage healthy individuation involve social development experiences that identify and value individual strengths and encourage the contribution of these strengths in positive social activities.

Individual interventions

Mentorship

Mentoring programs typically involve non-professional volunteers spending time with individual youth in a supportive, non-judgemental manner while acting as role models. An evaluation of the Big Brothers/Big Sisters program found significantly less early age drug use among youth exposed to this mentorship program compared to youth that were randomly assigned to a waiting-list control group. Exposure to mentoring also demonstrated improvements in academic performance and family attachments.[108]

Group interventions

Parent education

The Social Development Model[43] organized knowledge of predictors of substance use and delinquency by modelling these behaviours as a competitive struggle for identity allegiance between antisocial and prosocial influences. Enhancing the attachment of young people to positive social influences such as families was conceptualized as important in reducing peer influenced drug use. A five-session, professionally led, parent-education program emerging from this model aimed to enhance positive parent–child interactions and effective family management. Relative to controls young people whose families were randomly assigned to the intervention showed increased family bonding and reduced alcohol use two years after the intervention.[109]

An Australian parent education program used adult learning principles to improve parents' skills for relating to adolescents. Parents and early high school students completed surveys in 14 schools targeted for intervention, with procedures matched in 14 control schools. Although only a minority of parents were recruited into the parent education groups, post-intervention findings demonstrated that benefits extended more broadly across families in the intervention schools. At the 12-week follow-up parents and adolescents reported a reduction in family conflict. Adolescents reported increased maternal care, less delinquency, and less substance use and the odds of transition to alcohol use were halved. Evaluation suggested that the substance use of respondents was influenced by their best friend's substance use. Improvements in troubled family relationships appeared to impact on a wide group of families linked through peer-friendship networks.[50]

Another Australian study investigated the intervention opportunity that can arise when parents initially recognise adolescent substance abuse. Parents in these situations often experience considerable distress, which can undermine effective responding. An eight-week, professionally led, group intervention encouraged healthy individuation.[110] High rates of depression among participating parents at pre-test (87% high symptoms) were observed to drop substantially over the course of the intervention (down to 24% after eight weeks). A small evaluation incorporating a wait-list control group revealed differential improvements for those exposed to the intervention in mental health, emotional independence, parental satisfaction and assertive parenting behaviours after 16-weeks.[111] The impact of these changes on youth substance abuse is not yet known.

Family therapy

The Iowa Strengthening Family Program[112] was targeted to all families within late primary school. Group interventions encouraged harmonious family relationships by developing communication skills and family management strategies for adolescents and parents in separated groups with reinforcement in combined sessions. An experimental trial suggested initially the program was about as successful as parent's education alone in discouraging alcohol use.[112] However, four-year follow-up data has suggested that benefits extend to reductions in youth hostile and aggressive behaviour.[113]

Perry and colleagues[114] evaluated the impact of the 'Slick Tracy Home Team' program, a set of activity books completed as homework tasks requiring parental assistance over the course of four consecutive weeks in Grade 6 (about age 11). The authors noted that the strategy of 'seeding' their program into school homework was successful in obtaining high rates of parental participation from a range of cultural backgrounds. At the end of Grade 6, families exposed to the intervention demonstrated increased communication regarding alcohol use, and children demonstrated lower initiation of smoking and regular alcohol use.

The 'Addicts and Families Project' was historically important in its use of a well-controlled evaluation to demonstrate the effectiveness of family therapy as a treatment for youth substance abuse.[115] The study demonstrated that, after six months, supplementing methadone treatment with family therapy reduced drug use in around two-thirds of cases. The adolescent's requirement for healthy individuation from the family of origin was an important theoretical construct guiding this intervention.

More recent programs have developed brief family therapy approaches.[116] The Functional Family Therapy approach has evidence as a strategy for reducing re-offending among voluntary and court-mandated adolescent offenders and has also been demonstrated to prevent offending among the younger siblings of targeted offenders.[117,118] Economic evaluation[57] estimated the net economic benefit at around $4 for each $1 invested. Process evaluation[119] has suggested a critical program component may involve reducing family out-group tendencies by reframing problem attribution away from individual blame (e.g. bad son) to focus on the concept of a mismatch in adolescent and parent needs.

Peer intervention

When properly coordinated, peer involvement may enhance the effectiveness of drug prevention programs.[120] However, evidence suggests that aggregating youth with antisocial behaviour[121] or selectively targeting programs in high-risk settings[122] can lead to increases in peer motivated substance use. Further research is required to establish the conditions under which peer interventions can contribute to reductions in substance misuse.

Therapeutic community

Therapeutic communities were first established in New York to address the heroin epidemic faced by that city in the early 1970s. Borrowing principles from the AA movement, critical treatment components involve the use of group principles to encourage a change in identity away from that of a drug user toward identifications such as 'peer-counsellor' or 'ex-addict'. Communities are typically organized according to peers who are at a similar 'level' in their recovery process. Better outcomes following treatment are predicted both by longer time in treatment and also by higher peer-status attainment.[123] A range of factors including the level of drug-free social support following treatment improve outcomes after three years.[123]

Community prevention

Police diversion

As police symbolize social authority, the way in which police respond to early adolescent behaviour can play an important role in identity development. Efforts within policing to divert youth offenders away from the legal system toward health and social services have included police–youth involvement programs[124] and the use of police in counselling and referral roles.[125] To date there has been little outcome evaluation examining these strategies.

SUMMARY, CONCLUSIONS AND FUTURE DIRECTIONS

In this chapter developmental and motivational theories have been integrated to organise knowledge of the predictors and effective interventions influencing substance use. Early developmental failure is associated with social and emotional distress later in life and this in turn has been linked to very extreme patterns of substance misuse. Prevention efforts aiming to improve conditions for healthy child development and to reduce the marginalization of disadvantaged children and youth have evidence to support their application in long-term efforts to address substance misuse. A major developmental challenge beginning in childhood is to teach appropriate strategies that can be used to effectively manage pain, arousal and physical health. In many families children are trained to manage these problems exclusively through the use of drugs such as painkillers and coffee. These early experiences can be linked to an increase in drug use to achieve functional ends such as enhancements to mood, body shape and physical performance. The rising dominance of pharmacological solutions to drug problems, the overuse of antibiotics and many aspects of substance misuse relate to functional motives. Enhancing competencies for drug-free management of body, mind and spirit may be a neglected strategy for addressing functional motives for substance misuse. Research is warranted to better understand the contribution functional expectations for substance use make in shaping the core beliefs that underlie individual attitudes and social norms.

From late childhood the social requirement to conform to existing family and community norms represents a major underlying motive explaining the considerable inter-generation stability in substance use. Reducing children's exposure to normative social pressures to use drugs, the enforcement of minimum drinking age laws and controls on the supply of alcohol and other drugs have each been shown to reduce substance use and related harms. Beginning in adolescence pressure to individuate and align with youth culture becomes an important motivation explaining inter-generation discontinuity in patterns of substance use. A growing range of interventions address social identification pathways to encourage healthy youth development.

Harmful substance use is not confined to disadvantaged communities.[18] Better assessment of the developmental pathways influencing motivations for substance misuse within specific communities can improve the local relevance, integration and coordination of prevention and treatment efforts.[6] Pathways to developmental distress may be more common in disadvantaged communities, while more affluent communities may require greater investment to encourage healthy individuation. Wider-scale national and state investment will be required to change current normative conventions that encourage substance misuse and to promote alternative means of achieving the functional benefits sought through substance use. Future research efforts should examine the synergistic benefits that may be achievable through the integrated delivery of intervention strategies to address the motivational profile of substance misuse within specific communities.

References

1. Moon L, Meyer P, Grau J. Australia's young people: Their health and wellbeing. Cat No. PHE 19. Canberra: Australian Institute of Health and Welfare; 1999.
2. Office of National Drug Control Policy. The economic costs of drug abuse in the United States, 1992–1998. Washington, DC: Executive Office of the President. Publication No. NCJ-190636, 2003:1–92.
3. Collins DJ, Lapsley HM. Counting the costs - Estimates of the social costs of drug abuse in Australia; National Drug Strategy Monograph series No. 49. Canberra: Commonwealth of Australia. 2002; 1998–9.
4. Harwood H. Updating estimates of the economic costs of alcohol abuse in the United States, update methods, and data. Bethesda, MD: National Institute on Alcohol Abuse and Alcoholism, National Institute of Health, Department of Health and Human Services; 2000.
5. Loxley W, Toumbourou J, Stockwell T, Haines B, Scott K, Godfrey C, et al. The Prevention of Substance Use, Risk and Harm in Australia: A review of the evidence. National Drug Research Institute and the Centre for Adolescent Health; Report prepared for the Commonwealth..
6. Arthur MW, Blitz C. Bridging the gap between science and practice in drug abuse prevention through needs assessment and strategic community planning. Journal of Community Psychology 2000; 28(3):241–255.
7. World Health Organization. International Guide for monitoring alcohol consumption and harm. Geneva, Switzerland: Substance Abuse Department, World Health Organization; 2000.
8. National Health and Medical Research Council. Australian alcohol guidelines: Health risks and benefits. Canberra: National Health and Medical Research Council; 2001.
9. Catalano P, Chikritzhs T, Stockwell T, Webb M, Rohlin CJ, Dietze P. Trends in per capita alcohol consumption in Australia, 1990/91 to 1998/99. Curtin University, Perth: National Drug Research Institute. National Alcohol Indicators Project Bulletin 2001; 4:1–4.
10. White V. Australian secondary students' use of alcohol in 1999. Canberra: Commonwealth Department of Health and Aged Care. National Drug Strategy Monograph 2001; 45:1–45.
11. White V. Australian secondary students' use of over-the-counter and illicit substances in 1999. Canberra: Commonwealth Department of Health and Aged Care. National Drug Strategy Monograph 2001; 46:1–61.
12. Heale P, Stockwell T, Dietze P, Chikritzhs T, Catalano P. Patterns of alcohol consumption in Australia, 2001. Perth: National Drug Research Institute and Turning Point Alcohol and Drug Centre. National Alcohol Indicators Bulletin 2001; 3.
13. Degenhardt L, Hall W, Lynskey M. The relationship between cannabis use, depression and anxiety among Australian adults: Findings from the National Survey of Mental Health and Well-Being. Social Psychiatry and Psychiatric Epidemiology 2001; 36(5):219–227.

14. Fergusson DM, Horwood LJ, Lynskey MT. The prevalence and risk factors associated with abusive or hazardous alcohol consumption in 16-year-olds. Addiction 1995; 90:935–946.
15. Guo J, Hawkins JD, Hill KG, Abbott RD. Childhood and adolescent predictors of alcohol abuse and dependence in young adulthood. Journal of Studies on Alcohol 2001; 62(6):754–762.
16. Coffey C, Lynskey M, Wolfe R, Patton G. Initiation and progression of cannabis use in a population-based Australian adolescent longitudinal study. Addiction 2000; 95(11):1679–1690.
17. Fergusson DM, Lynskey MT, Horwood LJ. The short-term consequences of early onset cannabis use. Journal of Abnormal Child Psychology 1996; 24(4):499–512.
18. Brook JS, Whiteman M, Finch SJ, Cohen P. Young adult drug use and delinquency: Childhood antecedents and adolescent mediators. Journal of the American Academy of Child and Adolescent Psychiatry 1996; 35(12):1584–1592.
19. Guy SM, Smith GM, Bentler PM. Adolescent socialization and use of licit and illicit substances: Impact on adult health. Psychology and Health 1993; 8:463–487.
20. Toumbourou JW. Preventing harmful drug use. West Melbourne: Australian Drug Foundation. Drug Info Clearinghouse 2003; 1:1–8.
21. Bachman JG, O'Malley PM, Johnston LD. Drug use among young adults: The impacts of role status and social environment. Journal of Personality and Social Psychology 1984; 47(3):629–645.
22. Toumbourou JW, Williams IR, Snow PC, White VM. Adolescent alcohol-use trajectories in the transition from high school. Drug and Alcohol Review 2003; 22(2):111–116.
23. Hawkins JD, Catalano RF, Miller JY. Risk and protective factors for alcohol and other drug problems in adolescence and early adulthood: Implications for substance abuse prevention. Psychological Bulletin 1992; 112(1):64–105.
24. Bry BH, McKeon P, Pandina RJ. Extent of drug use as a function of number of risk factors. Journal of Abnormal Psychology 2003; 91(4):273–279.
25. Newcomb MD, Felix-Ortiz M. Multiple protective and risk factors for drug use and abuse: Cross-sectional and prospective findings. Journal of Personality and Social Psychology 1992; 63(2):280–296.
26. Fergusson DM, Horwood LJ, Lynskey M. The childhoods of multiple problem adolescents: A 15-year longitudinal study. Journal of Child Psychology and Psychiatry 1994; 35(6):1123–1140.
27. Aronson M, Kyllerman M, Sabel KG, Sandin B, Olegard R. Children of alcoholic mothers: Developmental, perceptual, and behavioral characteristics as compared to matched controls. Acta Paediatrica Scandinavica 1985; 74(1):27–35.
28. Hans SL. Maternal opioid use and child development. In: Zagon IS, Slotkin TA, eds. Maternal substance abuse and the developing nervous system. California: Academic Press; 1992:177–214.
29. Singer L, Farkas K, Kliegman R. Childhood medical and behavioral consequences of maternal cocaine use. Journal of Pediatric Psychology 1992; 17(4):389–406.
30. Fergusson DM, Lynskey MT, Horwood LJ. Factors associated with continuity and changes in disruptive behaviour patterns between childhood and adolescence. Journal of Abnormal Child Psychology 1996; 24(5):533–553.
31. Mitchell P, Spooner C, Copeland J, Vimpani G, Toumbourou JW, Howard J et al. A literature review of the role of families in the development, identification, prevention and treatment of illicit drug problems. Melbourne: Commonwealth of Australia; 2001.

32. Williams B, Sanson A, Toumbourou JW, Smart D. Patterns and predictors of teenagers' use of licit and illicit substances in the Australian Temperament Project cohort. Melbourne: University of Melbourne; 2000.

33. Eddy JM, Reid JB, Fetrow RA. An elementary school-based prevention program targeting modifiable antecedents of youth delinquency and violence: Linking the interests of families and teachers (LIFT). Journal of Emotional and Behavioral Disorders 2000; 8(3):165–176.

34. Ajzen I, Fishbein M. Understanding attitudes and predicting social behavior. New Jersey: Prentice-Hall; 1980.

35. Petraitis J, Flay BR, Miller TQ, Torpy EJ, Greiner B. Illicit substance use among adolescents: A matrix of prospective predictors. Substance Use and Misuse 1998; 33(13):2561–2604.

36. Patton GC, Hibbert M, Rosier MJ, Carlin JB, Caust J, Bowes G. Patterns of common drug use in teenagers. Australian Journal of Public Health 1995; 19(4):393–399.

37. Newcomb MD, Huba GJ, Bentler PM. Life events and substance use among adolescents: Mediating effects of perceived loss of control and meaninglessness in life. Journal of Personality and Social Psychology 1986; 51:564–577.

38. French SA, Story M, Downes B, Resnick MD, Blum RW. Frequent dieting among adolescents psychosocial and health behavior correlates. American Journal of Public Health 1995; 35(5):695–701.

39. Irving LM, Wall M, Neumark-Sztainer D, Story M. Steroid use among adolescents findings from Project EAT. Journal of Adolescent Health 2002; 30(4):243–252.

40. Bush DM, Autry JH. Substance abuse in the workplace: Epidemiology, effects, and industry response. Occupational Medicine 2002; 17(1):13–25.

41. Glantz MD, Leshner AL. Drug abuse and developmental psychopathology. Developmental Psychology 2000; 12:795–814.

42. Farrington DP. Developmental criminology and risk-focussed prevention. In: Maguire R, Morgan R, Reiner R, eds. The Oxford handbook of criminology. Oxford: Clarendon Press; 2002.

43. Catalano RF, Hawkins JD. The Social Development Model: A theory of antisocial behavior. In: Hawkins JD, ed. Delinquency and crime: current theories. New York: Cambridge; 1996:149–197.

44. Kosterman R, Hawkins JD, Guo J, Catalano RF, Abbott RD. The dynamics of alcohol and marijuana initiation: Patterns and predictors of first use in adolescence. American Journal of Public Health 2000; 90(3):360–366.

45. Whitehead PC, Wechsler H. Implications for future research and public policy. Minimum-drinking-age laws: An evaluation. Washington DC: Lexington Books, Health and Company; 1980:177–184.

46. Chapman S. Unravelling gossamer with boxing gloves: Problems in explaining the decline in smoking. British Medical Journal 1993; 307:429–432.

47. Baumrind D. The influence of parenting style on adolescent competence and substance use. Journal of Early Adolescence 1991; 11(1):56–95.

48. Bishop DI, Macy-Lewis JA, Schnekloth CA, Puswella S, Struessel GL. Ego identity status and reported alcohol consumption a study of first-year college students. Journal of Adolescence 1997; 20(2):209–218.

49. Jessor R, Jessor SL. Theory testing in longitudinal research on marihuana use. In: Kandel DB, ed. Longitudinal research on drug use. Washington: Hemisphere Publishing Corporation; 1978:41–71.

50. Toumbourou JW, Gregg ME. Impact of an empowerment-based parent education program on the reduction of youth suicide risk factors. Journal of Adolescent Health 2002; 31(3):279–287.

51. Holdcroft LC, Iacono WG. Cohort effects on gender differences in alcohol dependence. Addiction 2002; 97:1025–1036.
52. Jernigan DH. Global status report: Alcohol and young people. Geneva: World Health Organization; 2001:1–57.
53. Battin SR, Hill KG, Abbott RD, Catalano RF, Hawkins JD. The contribution of gang membership to delinquency beyond delinquent friends. Criminology 1998; 36(1):93–115.
54. Olds DL, Henderson CR, Kitzman HJ, Eckenrode JJ, Cole RE, Tatelbaum RC. Prenatal and infancy home visitation by nurses: Recent findings. The Future of Children 1999; 9(1):44–65.
55. Schweinhart LJ, Weikart DP. Success by empowerment: The high/scope Perry preschool study through age 27. Young Children 1993.
56. Cunningham PB, Henggeler SW. Engaging multiproblem families in treatment: Lessons learned throughout the development of multisystemic therapy. Family Process 1999; 38:265–281.
57. Aos S, Barnoski R, Lee R. Preventive programs for young offenders: Effective and cost-effective. Overcrowded Times 1998; 9(2):1–11.
58. Bry BH, Catalano RF, Kumpfer K, Lochman JE, Szapocznik J. Scientific findings from family prevention intervention research. In: Ashery RS, Robertson EB, Kumpfer KL, eds. Drug abuse prevention through family interventions. Rockville, MD: US Department of Human Services, National Institute on Drug Abuse; 1998:103–129.
59. Dishion TJ, Andrews DW. Preventing escalation in problem behaviours with high-risk young adolescents: Immediate and 1 year outcomes. Journal of Consulting and Clinical Psychology 1995; 63:538–548.
60. Sanders MR, Markie-Dadds C, Tully L, Bor W. The Triple P-Positive Parenting Program: A comparison of enhanced standard, and self directed behavioral family intervention. Journal of Consulting and Clinical Psychology 2000; 68(4):624–640.
61. Webster-Stratton C, Hammond M. Treating children with early-onset conduct problems: A comparison of child and parent training interventions. Journal of Consulting and Clinical Psychology 1997; 65(1):93–109.
62. Long P, Forehand R, Wierson M, Morgan A. Does parent training with young noncompliant children have long-term effects? Behavior Research and Therapy 1994; 32(1):101–107.
63. Catalano RF, Gainey RR, Fleming CB, Haggerty KP, Johnson NO. An experimental intervention with families of substance abusers one-year follow-up of the focus on families project. Addiction 1999; 94:241–254.
64. DeMarsh J, Kumpfer KL. Family-oriented interventions for the prevention of chemical dependency in children and adolescents. In: Griswold-Ezekoye S, Kumpfer KL, Bukoski WJ, eds. Childhood and Chemical Abuse: Prevention and Intervention. New York: The Haworth Press; 1986:117–151.
65. Conduct Problems Prevention Research Group. Evaluation of the first three years of the Fast Track prevention trial with children at high-risk for adolescent conduct problems. Journal of Abnormal Child Psychology 2002; 30(1):19–35.
66. O'Donnell J, Hawkins JD, Catalano RF, Abbott RD, Day LE. Preventing school failure, drug use, and delinquency among low-income children long-term intervention in elementary schools. American Journal of Orthopsychiatry 1995; 65(1):87–100.
67. Hawkins JD, Guo J, Hill K, Battin-Pearson S, Abbott R. Long term effects of the Seattle social development intervention on school bonding trajectories. In: Maggs J, Schulenberg J, eds. Applied Developmental Science Special Issue: Prevention as Altering the Course of Development 2001:225–236.

68. Petterson P, Hawkins JD, Catalano R. Evaluating comprehensive community drug risk reduction interventions. Evaluation Review 1992; 16(6):579–602.

69. Toumbourou JW. Implementing Communities That Care in Australia: A community mobilization approach to crime prevention. Trends and Issues in Crime and Criminal Justice 1999; 122:1–6.

70. Joing Ma J, Truswell AS. Wernicke–Korsakoff syndrome in Sydney hospitals before and after thiamine enrichment of flour. Medical Journal of Australia 1995; 163:531–534.

71. Mattick RP, Oliphant D, Ward J. The Swiss scientific studies of medically prescribed narcotics. The effectiveness of other opioid replacement therapies: LAAM, heroin, buprenorphine and naltrexone. Sydney: Sydney National Drug and Alcohol Research Centre; 1997.

72. Smart RG, Mann RE. The impact of programs for high-risk drinkers on population levels of alcohol problems. Addiction 2000; 95(1):37–52.

73. Hawkins JD. Academic performance and school success: Sources and consequences. In: Weissberg RP, Gullotta TP, Hampton RL, Ryan BA, Adams GR, eds. Healthy children 2010: Enhancing children's wellness. CA: Sage Publications; 1997:278–305.

74. Dunn C, Deroo L, Rivara FP. The use of brief interventions adapted from motivational interviewing across behavioral domains: A systematic review. Addiction 2001; 96(12):1725–1742.

75. Brown JM. The effectiveness of treatment. In: Heather N, Peters TJ, Stockwell T, eds. International handbook of alcohol dependence and problems. Chichester: John Wiley; 2001:497–508.

76. Drug Policy Expert Committee. Drugs: meeting the challenge. Stage two report. Melbourne: Government of Victoria; 2000:1–215.

77. Hansen W. School-based substance abuse prevention: A review of the state of the art in curriculum, 1980–1990. Health Education Research 1992; 7(3):403–430.

78. McBride N, Midford R, Farringdon F, Phillips M. Early results from a school alcohol harm minimization study: The School Health and Alcohol Harm Reduction Project. Addiction 2000; 95(7):1021–1042.

79. Australian Institute of Health and Welfare. Heart, stroke and vascular diseases. National Centre for Monitoring Cardiovascular Disease. Canberra: Australian Institute of Health and Welfare; 2001.

80. Commonwealth Department of Health and Aged Care. Directions in injury prevention. Report 2: Injury prevention interventions – good buys for the next decade. Canberra: Commonwealth Department of Health and Aged Care; 1999.

81. National Mental Health Strategy. Promotion, prevention and early intervention for mental health. Canberra: Department of Health and Aged Care; 1999.

82. Victorian Health Promotion Foundation. Victorian Health Promotion Foundation mental health strategy. Melbourne: Victorian Health Promotion Foundation; 2000.

83. Normand J, Lempert RO, O'Brien CP. Under the influence? Drugs and the American Work Force. Washington: National Academy Press; 1994.

84. Baer JS, Kivlahan DR, Blume AW, McKnight P, Marlatt AG. Brief intervention for heavy-drinking college students 4-year follow-up and natural history. American Journal of Public Health 2001; 91(8):1310–1316.

85. Werch C, Anzalone D, Brokiewicz L, Felker J, Carlson J, Castellon-Vogel A. An intervention for preventing alcohol use among inner city middle-school students. Archives of Family Medicine 1996; 5(3):146–152.

86. Botvin GJ, Schinke S, Orlandi MA. School-based health promotion substance abuse and sexual behavior. Applied and Preventive Psychology 1995; 4:167–184.

87. White D, Pitts M. Educating young people about drugs: A systematic review. Addiction 1998; 93(10):1475–1487.
88. Tobler NS. Meta analysis of 143 adolescent drug prevention programs, quantitative outcome results of program participants compared to a control or comparison group. Journal of Drug Issues 1986; 16(4):537–567.
89. Wilhelmsen W, Laberg J, Klepp KI. Evaluation of two student and teacher involved alcohol prevention programs. Addiction 1994; 89:1157–1165.
90. Shope JT, Copeland LA, Marcoux BC, Kamp ME. Effectiveness of a school based substance abuse prevention program. Journal of Drug Education 1996; 26:323–337.
91. Hansen WB, Graham JW. Preventive alcohol, marijuana and cigarette use among adolescents: Peer pressure resistance training versus establishing conservative norms. Preventive Medicine 1991; 20(3):414–430.
92. Botvin G, Epstein J, Baker E, Diaz T, Ifill-Williams M. School based drug abuse prevention with inner-city minority youth. Journal of Child and Adolescent Substance Abuse 1997; 6:5–19.
93. Project MATCH Research Group. Matching alcoholism treatments to client heterogeneity treatment main effects and matching effects on drinking during treatment. Journal of Studies on Alcohol 1998; 59(6):631–639.
94. Toumbourou JW, Hamilton M, U'Ren A, Stevens-Jones P, Storey G. Narcotics Anonymous participation and changes in substance use and social support. Journal of Substance Abuse Treatment 2002; 23(1):61–66.
95. Lenton S, Heale P, Erickson P. The regulation of cannabis possession, use and supply. A discussion document prepared for the Drugs and Crime Prevention Committee of The Parliament of Victoria. Perth: National Drug Research Institute Monograph 2000; 3.
96. Weatherburn D, Jones C, Freeman K, Makkai T. The Australian heroin drought and its implications for drug policy. Bureau of Crime Statistics and Research Crime and Justice Bulletins 2001; B59:1–15.
97. Douglass RL. The legal drinking age and traffic casualties. A special case of changing alcohol availability in a public health context. In: Wechsler H, ed. Minimum drinking-age laws. An evaluation. Washington DC: Lexington Books, Health and Company; 1980:93–132.
98. Grube JW. Preventing sales of alcohol to minors results from a community trial. Addiction 1997; 92(S2):S251–S260.
99. Osterberg E. Effects of price and taxation. In: Heather N, Peters TJ, Stockwell T, eds. International handbook of alcohol dependence and problems. Chichester: John Wiley; 2001:685–698.
100. Chikritzhs T, Jonas H, Heale P, Stockwell T, Dietze P, Hanlin K, et al. Alcohol-caused deaths and hospitalizations in Australia, 1990–1997. Perth: National Drug Research Institute and Turning Point, Alcohol and Drug Centre Inc. National Alcohol Indicators Project 2000; 1:1–49.
101. Carroll T, Lum M, Taylor J, Travia J. Evaluation of the launch phase of the National Alcohol Campaign. Sydney: Commonwealth Department of Health and Aged Care; 2000.
102. DeJong W. College students' use of designated drivers: The data are in. Prevention Pipeline 1997; 25–27.
103. Johnson CA, Pentz MA, Weber MD, Dwyer JH, Baer N, MacKinnon DP, et al. Relative effectiveness of comprehensive community programming for drug abuse prevention with high-risk and low-risk adolescents. Journal of Consulting and Clinical Psychology 1990; 58(4):447–456.

104. Stevens MM, Freeman DH, Mott L, Youells F. Three-year results of prevention programs on marijuana use: The new Hampshire study. Journal of Drug Education 1996; 26(3):257–273.

105. Perry CL, Williams CL, Veblen-Mortenson S, Toomey TL, Komro KA, Anstine PS, et al. Project Northland: Outcomes of a communitywide alcohol use prevention program during early adolescence. American Journal of Public Health 1996; 86(7):956–965.

106. Holder HD, Saltz RF, Grube JW, Voas RB, Guenewald PJ, Treno AJ. A community prevention trial to reduce alcohol-involved accidental injury and death: Overview. Addiction 1997; 92(Suppl 2):S155–S171.

107. Holder HD, Saltz RF, Grube JW, Treno AJ, Reynolds RI, Voas RB, et al. Summing up: Lessons from a comprehensive community prevention trial. Addiction 1997; 92 (Suppl 2):S293–S301.

108. Tierney JP, Grossman JB, Resch NL. Making a difference. An impact study of Big Brothers/Big Sisters. Philadelphia: Public/Private Ventures; 1995.

109. Spoth R, Redmond C, Hockaday C, Yoo S. Protective factors and young adolescent tendency to abstain from alcohol use: A model using two waves of intervention study data. American Journal of Community Psychology 1996; 24(6):749–770.

110. Blyth A, Bamberg J, Toumbourou J. Behaviour exchange systems training: A program for parents stressed by adolescent substance abuse. Camberwell: Australian Council for Educational Research; 2000.

111. Toumbourou JW, Blyth A, Bamberg J, Forer D. Early impact of the BEST intervention for parents stressed by adolescent substance abuse. Journal of Community and Applied Social Psychology 2001; 11:291–304.

112. Spoth R, Redmond C, Shin C. Direct and indirect latent-variable parenting outcomes of two universal family-focussed preventive interventions: Extending a public health-oriented research base. Journal of Consulting and Clinical Psychology 1998; 66(2):385–399.

113. Spoth RL, Redmond C, Shin C. Reducing adolescents' aggressive and hostile behaviors: Randomized trial effects of a brief family intervention 4 years past baseline. Archives of Pediatrics and Adolescent Medicine 2000; 154(2):1248–1257.

114. Perry CL, Williams CL, Forster JL, Wolfson M, Wagenaar AC, Finnegan JR, et al. Background, conceptualization and design of a community-wide research program on adolescent alcohol use: Project Northland. Health Education Research Theory and Practice 1993; 8(1):125–136.

115. Stanton MD, Todd TC. The family therapy of drug abuse and addiction. New York: Guilford Press; 1982.

116. Liddle HA. Family-based treatment for adolescent problem behaviors: Overview of contemporary developments and introduction to the special section. Journal of Family Psychology 1996; 10(1):3–11.

117. Klein NC, Alexander JF, Parsons BV. Impact of family systems intervention on recidivism and sibling delinquency: A model of primary prevention and program evaluation. Journal of Consulting and Clinical Psychology 1977; 45(3):469–474.

118. Alexander JF, Parsons BV. Functional Family Therapy. Monterey, CA: Brooks/Cole; 2002.

119. Robbins MS, Alexander JF, Newell RM, Turner CW. The immediate effect of reframing on client attitude in family therapy. Journal of Family Psychology 1996; 10(1):28–34.

120. Black D, Tobler N, Sciacca J. Peer helping/involvement: An efficacious way to meet the challenge of reducing alcohol, tobacco, and other drug use among youth? Journal of School Health 1998; 68(3):87–93.

121. Dishion TJ, McCord J, Poulin F. When interventions harm – peer groups and problem behavior. American Psychologist 1999; 54(9):755–764.

122. Palinkas LA, Atkins CJ, Miller C, Ferreira D. Social skills training for drug prevention in high-risk female adolescents. Preventive Medicine 1996; 25(6):692–701.

123. Toumbourou J, Hamilton M, Fallon B. Treatment level progress and time spent in treatment in the prediction of outcomes following drug-free therapeutic community treatment. Addiction 1998; 93(7):1051–1064.

124. Thurman QC, Giacomazzi A, Bogen P. Cops, kids, and community policing: An assessment of a community policing demonstration project. Crime and Delinquency 1993; 39(4):554–564.

125. Anders J, Gye C. Early intervention through collaborative practices. Reducing Criminality: Partnership and Best Practice Conference, Perth. Canberra: Australian Institute of Criminology; 2000.

126. Toumbourou JW, Patton G, Sawyer S, Olsson C, Web-Pullman J, Catalano R, et al. Evidence-based interventions for promoting adolescent health. Melbourne, Centre for Adolescent Health; 2000: 1–150.

CHAPTER **7**

Changing physical activity and exercise patterns

Felicity Morris
Precilla Choi

INTRODUCTION

In Australia, UK, US, Canada, and other Westernized societies the range of problems associated with inactivity is vast and of great concern to local and global health bodies.[1,2] Physical activity is considered a vital factor in public health (expenditure and risk) and for wellbeing. It has also been considered to be a 'major modifiable risk factor'[2] (p. 3) in relation to mortality and morbidity. Thus, addressing the endemic problem of physical inactivity in the Western world is paramount.

The question of how to get people to increase their physical activity levels sufficiently in order to glean health benefits, and sustain them in the long term, has been the subject of a huge body of research. This has been conducted worldwide within a variety of disciplines across the health and medical sciences. The question remains unanswered, however, despite trials of a multiplicity of interventions at national and local levels, designed to encourage increases in physical activity and exercise. The assumption behind a large proportion of these was that increasing activity was a simple matter of giving people information about the need to do so, together with suggestions as to how changes may be made. This assumption appears to have been proved incorrect as research studies have shown that participation in physical activity has actually declined. For example, in an Australian study of over 3500 people, the percentage of adults who achieve sufficient levels of activity for health benefits (defined as at least 150 minutes of moderate activity per week) went from 62.2% in 1997 to 56.6% in 1999, remaining stable in 2000.[3] This is even though people's understanding of the importance of being active to health increased from 63.7% in 1997 and 63.9% in 1999 to 66.4% in 2000.[3]

Given that people know how important physical activity is in relation to morbidity and mortality, why is it that we find it so difficult when it comes to acting to change ourselves? Why can we not 'Just Do It ® ™' when we know we should? In this chapter we will present some answers to this question that have been gleaned from research, and then move on to look at the effectiveness of interventions that have been designed, and implemented, to change people's physical activity and exercise patterns within primary care, communities and target groups.

WHY ARE WE SO INACTIVE?

Throughout the Western world men and women continue to live lives that contrast greatly with their predecessors for whom life was hugely active, for example, in walking great distances to work, lifting or carrying objects from one place to another, and many other forms of physical work. Many of these types of activities are now automated or assisted by technological means. This growth of technology has led to a widespread decrease, on a daily basis, in what might be termed active living[4] with many work sites being places where sedentary (seated most of the time) behaviour is the norm. Workers will now more often use automated modes of travel from floor to floor, and spend extended periods of time seated while engaged in diverse mental tasks or waiting for machines to complete tasks. These are tasks that previously may have involved a fair amount of bending or stretching to complete – think of the now obsolete roneo graph machines where a handle needed to be turned to produce copies!

So, if we are not being active at work, what about during our non-work or leisure time? According to the 2002 US National Health Interview Survey[5] only 32% of US, adults (18+ years) participate in sufficient leisure time activity. The estimates also show significant age differences. In the 18 to 24 year age group, 45% males and 34% of females, participated in regular leisure time physical activity. Of the 24 to 64-year-olds, 36% of males participated compared with 31% of females. Men aged between 65 to 74 years comprised 29% and women 23% of those doing leisure time physical activity. Men 75 or older formed 35%, and women 29% of those participating in leisure time physical activity. This pattern appears to be consistent throughout the Western world.[6] Analysis showed Australian, Canadian, English, Finnish, and US citizens' participation in moderate-intensity activity levels to range from 29% to 51%. Differences have also been found between immigrants and non-immigrants in Sweden.[7] Their public health survey of 5600 people revealed Swedish immigrants born in Arabic-speaking and Eastern European countries to be more likely to be sedentary than Swedish born people. When age and educational status were taken into account, the findings remained consistent. Moreover, the physical activity levels of people born in other Western countries were more similar to the Swedish born.

How can this lack of leisure time physical activity be explained, especially when we understand how important physical activity is for our health and wellbeing? Differences in health behaviours (including physical activity and exercise) are often attributed to certain sociodemographic factors.[8] For example,[6] research showed physical activity patterns are generally highest for males, younger people, those with more education, and those who earn a good income. Studies also highlighted the sudden large-scale increase in the propensity to be sedentary with the onset of older age. Alongside these are the many reasons that the very large body of research into why people do not exercise has revealed. Termed barriers, some of these are external or environmental and relate to where the person lives. For example, research comparing people who lived in a coastal area with those living inland found the coastal residents to be 23% less likely to be sedentary, 27% more likely to participate in sufficient activity to accrue health benefits and 38% more likely to report involvement in vigorous levels of physical activity.[9] A US study found neighbourhood characteristics such as the presence of footpaths, having enjoyable scenery and hills and the presence of traffic to be highly related to physical activity.[10] Safe neighbourhoods are also important.[11] In their study the lower level of exercise participation among black Americans compared to non-black was partly explained by their greater likelihood of living in a less safe neighbourhood.

By far though, the research indicates that it is the personal barriers that are the greatest hindrance, and that a great number of these are perceived to exist. They deserve enormous attention as they are more amenable to change than other barriers and dealing with personal barriers may also enable a person to overcome other barriers. The most common personal barrier – and this is consistently found in different countries – is lack of time.[12] There are also statistically significant differences between groups. For example,[13] study of 5000 sedentary Australians found lack of time to be more frequently reported by younger people and those with children and less frequently by those with higher education levels. Other researchers have emphasized the time problem is particularly pertinent to women, especially to today's women who are likely to be employed outside the home as well as being primarily responsible for caring duties and work within the home. This may explain the consistent finding that men participate in more physical activity than women. Women's higher prioritization of caregiving activities compared to self-care activities (including exercise) has been attributed to their socialization into caregiving roles.[14] This can then continue in the later years post-retirement with available time being filled with caring tasks outside of the home (e.g. volunteer community work to help others such as working at a food bank) instead of a physical exercise program[15] because 'serving others is less selfish'.[16]

There are also additional barriers for many girls and women that are related to the body such as poor body image and misperceptions of physical ability.[17] Other commonly reported personal barriers across gender and age include discomfort, fear of injury, misconceptions about exercise, and other physical activities. Among older adults, injury and poor health are the main barriers.

The list of barriers is a very long one but overarching all of them is self-motivation.[12] This point is well-illustrated by the findings of a Canadian study of two groups of older people – active and inactive.[15] Both groups reported negative views about physical exercise (e.g. it can be uncomfortable) and both reported barriers (e.g. health problems) but the active group firmly believed in the value of physical exercise. As a result, they countered every negative thought with a positive one, and every barrier with a solution. Thus, they differed from the inactive group in their motivation to be active.[15] As there is no evidence to indicate that people who are active have more leisure time available to them than people who are not, how to motivate people to make time for this important health behaviour is an important question that needs to be answered if behaviour change is going to occur. This applies to both starting to be more physically active and remaining so as earlier research has found self-motivation to predict exercise adherence.[18] As we shall see later when discussing the results of interventions, difficult as it is to begin a physical activity program, it is even harder to stay motivated to continue with it.

What factors, then, influence motivation? A good starting point is health beliefs because these shape the beliefs about the barriers and benefits. Research by sociologists has shown health beliefs to be important in the motivational process in the context of physical activity. This process is very complex and a detailed discussion is beyond the scope of this chapter. However to illustrate, one example is that many people consider becoming ill to be a matter of 'luck' or 'chance' and therefore not within their control[19] which then reduces their belief in the benefit of participating in physical activity. Many people also do not see themselves as being at risk of becoming ill and this misperception means that there is a lack of congruence between public health messages and personal, subjective experiences. Another example is in how people define health which is done in a number of ways. One definition is a lack of illness symptoms and another is being physically fit enough to perform their every day tasks, whatever these may be.[19–21] If a person is not experiencing any symptoms of illness and can perform their everyday tasks without any difficulty (and remember that our every day tasks are increasingly sedentary), the person is more likely to believe they are healthy and therefore not in need of exercise. This was well-illustrated in the UK's Allied Dunbar National Fitness Survey in 1990.[22] The survey respondents acknowledged the importance of being physically active and agreed that most people were not active enough. However, most considered themselves to be sufficiently active although, as with the studies mentioned before, most were not. Thus, people seem to consider not exercising enough and not being fit and healthy to be issues for others and not for themselves. In addition, four out of five survey respondents believed themselves to be very or fairly fit but, when tested in the exercise physiology laboratory, many failed basic fitness tests with women doing far worse than men across all age levels. For example, one third of the men and two thirds of the women were found to be unable to sustain walking up a 1 in 20 slope at a reasonable pace without becoming over exerted. This begs the question of how often we walk up a 1 in 20 slope in the course of conducting our every day tasks and in the absence of the need to do so due to greater sedentariness in our lifestyles, we have become unaware of our decline in fitness.

In summary, to answer the question of why we are so inactive, the impact of technology and environmental developments both in the home and the workplace has undoubtedly severely affected what, and how much physical activity people do, on an hourly basis. Being physically active, therefore, has to be an active choice but this is not a simple matter due to the many barriers that are seen to exist. To overcome these, the benefits have to be seen to outweigh the costs but due to health beliefs such as perceiving oneself to already be fit and healthy and not at risk of becoming ill, the benefits are not seen to outweigh the costs. A recent study[23] which asked people to write down as many advantages and disadvantages of exercising that they could think of found that both active and inactive participants did not differ on the number of disadvantages or the time it took to think of them. However, the inactive participants were much slower to think of advantages and listed significantly fewer than the active participants. The authors concluded that one reason why sedentary people are not motivated to 'participate in regular exercise may be because they cannot think of reasons to exercise'.[23] How then can physical activity promotion programs overcome this and succeed in getting people to be more active? This is the question that we turn to next.

INCREASING PHYSICAL ACTIVITY

In preparing to write this chapter, our computer searches of interventions implemented over the past decade indicate that, worldwide, there have been some extremely innovative projects, designed to increase physical activity. In particular, a number of large scale recent projects have been implemented but the effectiveness of many of these have not been, or are still being, assessed so will not be discussed in this chapter. Neither will this chapter present a comprehensive or systematic review of all of the research because that would take up a whole book. Therefore, what is presented are firstly those interventions with adults that have been reported in scientific journals during the 1990s to July 2003 which have conformed to appropriate scientific standards such as randomized controlled designs or controlled quasi-experimental designs. We feel this is of primary importance in a book that aims to be evidence-based. Interventions that do not follow scientific standards – i.e. the interventions contained a number of 'conditions' where different participants receive different components of interventions (experimental condition) or no components (control or comparison condition) – do not add to the evidence base.

Secondly we report only those interventions that have shown some success at follow-up because the stated aim of the book is to provide evidence-based information to assist the design and delivery of behaviour change programs. In applying this criterion to determining which interventions to include in this chapter we decided to take an increase in physical activity levels as the simple definition of success (further discussion on appropriate measures of success for interventions takes place within the chapter). Follow-ups ranged from short-term (less than six months after receiving the intervention) across the medium-term (more than six months but less than 12 after the intervention) to the longer-term (at 12 months or more). We discuss studies from primary care and community settings that were specifically designed to increase physical activity levels, as this is the topic of the chapter. We do not, therefore, include those studies whose focus has been physical activity related changes in particular illness symptoms or mood.

Different terms are used to describe the types of interventions that have been implemented. In this chapter research on lifestyle, active lifestyle, and active living is that which concentrates on motivating individuals to change daily routines or increase physical activity with due consideration of the context (demands) and environment (locality) within which individuals live. This can include, for example, encouraging people to take the stairs instead of the escalator or to park their car farther away from their destination so that they will have to walk some distance. This approach contrasts with exercise prescription-based interventions because, in general, their primary focus is getting an individual with a particular condition or sedentary lifestyle to become active by following a prescription of exercise of a specified duration, intensity and frequency (e.g. a gym-based program at a certain level three times a week). Thus, exercise prescriptions concentrate on exercise advice whereas active living approaches first and foremost have a broader perspective encouraging movement throughout the activities of daily life.

PRIMARY CARE-BASED INTERVENTIONS

Primary care settings as platforms for key providers of encouragement to increase physical activity and exercise have attracted a lot of attention from researchers since the early 1990s leading to a number of trials of interventions with this focus. Primary care-based interventions vary in detail but are generally targeted at people with specific risk factors or health conditions. They are usually delivered by a general practitioner or other health professional and include components shown in Box 7.1.

A fictional example of a primary care-based intervention might be as follows. Margaret works at a telephone call centre for long shifts where she is seated; her short breaks are her cue to have another cigarette. She's been a heavy smoker for over 15 years and is now back to see her GP with yet another chest cold. Her GP recognizes that she is at risk of developing serious health problems and, as his previous attempts to get her to stop smoking failed, he decides to change focus. He asks if she would like to join a program

> **Box 7.1**   Components used in primary care interventions to increase physical activity
>
> Theory base: Transtheoretical Model, Health Belief Model, Theory of Planned Behaviour, Self-Efficacy Theory
> Counselling
> Phone contact
> Group education
> Written prescription
> Step counters
> Videos
> Assessment only
> Written materials
> Assessment/feedback
> GP/Health professional advice

to help her increase her activity levels to improve her general health. Margaret agrees, and the receptionist makes a time for her to come back and complete a number of computer-based questionnaires and an appointment for the first of six motivational counselling sessions over the next twelve weeks. She is also given some brochures on how to safely increase her activity levels and some information on local leisure centres. Margaret may also get some vouchers for free use of the leisure centres too!

Margaret is an example of someone with multiple risk factors – in her case they are smoking and physical inactivity.[24] Smith et al.'s 2002 Australian review of evidence-based research from the National Institute of Clinical Studies (NICS)[24] examined eight studies concerned with multiple risk factors published between 1988 and 1999, and 12 studies addressing the single risk factor of physical inactivity, published between 1996 and 2002. They found that, of the interventions for multiple risk factors, four out of the seven that had looked at long term (12 months or more) success, showed significant improvements in physical activity. No particular success indicators concerning the components of effective interventions emerged. That is, how many or what components were included in the intervention, (ranging from assessment and advice, assessment only, advice and further counselling, and telephone contacts) or who delivered the intervention, were not clear contributing factors to increased activity levels.

Turning now to interventions implemented for those with only one risk factor, mixed results were found but there were somewhat clearer implications for intervention design. At greater than six months but less than 12 months (short-term) three of the studies showed increases in physical activity. Two of only five studies that undertook long-term follow-up (12 months or more) found significant outcomes. Four of the five studies found short term increases in physical activity but these were not maintained at medium and long-term follow-up.

The findings of the single risk factor interventions indicated three elements that contribute to intervention effectiveness. These were firstly, the greater the number of intervention components (often greater numbers of 40-minute counselling sessions), in general the more effective was the intervention. Secondly, it did not matter which health professional (GP, nurse or other) delivered the intervention. Thirdly, it was primarily those participants who did no physical activity or were insufficiently active at recruitment who reported the most significant increases in physical activity.

The overall conclusion of the Smith et al.'s review was that interventions being delivered in primary care settings are effective in the short term. However, they emphasized the difficulty in comparing between studies due to the use of different outcome measures, and the use of a variety of benchmarks for success instead of standardized benchmarks like participants reaching sufficient activity levels to experience health benefits as stated by the US Surgeon General.[24]

Two studies are worth mentioning specifically here because of their research design and large sample size. The first is the UK-based Newcastle Exercise Project (NEP) which addressed the single risk factor of insufficient physical activity.[25] The NEP took place in a socioeconomically deprived part of Newcastle, England and consisted of 217 men and 306 women recruited while attending their local general practice surgery. The participants were divided into five groups, one receiving nothing (control group) and the other four receiving different combinations of a number of strategies. The most effective intervention group, in the short term (three months), was the one that received the greatest number of components. This group received a 75-minute assessment and feedback session, brochures, information about leisure centres, risk factor advice, six 40-minute motivational counselling interviews and 30 activity vouchers. In the long term (12 months) however, the initial reported increases in activity were not sustained. Long-term increases were also not observed for the other groups leading NEP researchers to conclude that although the number of components within the intervention may influence short-term increases, it makes no difference in the long term. These results illustrate Smith et al.'s[24] review conclusions concerning lack of success indicators with regard to components used in multiple risk factor studies.

The second study is the also UK-based Change of Heart study (TCHS) whose focus was the multiple risk factors of fat intake, physical activity, and smoking.[26] It was designed to assess the impact of behavioural counselling on change in activity levels and the other risk factors and was implemented with 883 patients from 20 British general practices. All participants received encouragement and suggestions on how to change and education about the benefits of changing their lifestyle. The experimental group also received either two or three 20-minute behavioural counselling sessions (depending on how many risk factors they had). When compared with the control group (those who received no counselling), the counselling group did initially (four months later) increase their activity levels but these increases had diminished over time when measured at 12 months.

One final intervention will be described here because it illustrates the extensive reach, and international popularity, of primary care-based interventions to increase activity. It is also an exemplary illustration of the processes of designing and implementing a primary care-based intervention. The Physician-based Assessment and Counselling for Exercise (PACE) program[27–30] began in the USA, was then taken up in Italy, and a pilot study to assess the feasibility of implementation in the Netherlands has also been completed.

The US (1996) PACE interventions were initially trialed with 255 inactive people. Using strategies based on the Health Belief Model, the Theory of Planned Behaviour, and Self-Efficacy Theory motivationally tailored information (based on what stage of change for physical activity the person was at) was given during an initial three to five minute counselling session and at subsequent contacts. The control group received no counselling sessions. The results showed that at four and six weeks after the intervention participants increased their walking activity by an average of 37 minutes per week while the control participants increased theirs by only 7 minutes.

The intervention was then extended to adolescents (PACE+) and the results published in 2001. It was set in four paediatric and adolescent medicine outpatient clinics and implemented with 117 adolescents of 11–18 years aimed to promote changes in moderate and vigorous physical activity. Participants received one of three combinations of components. These were (1) initial assessment, development of action plans, consultation with health professional and mail contact with the trained and supervised research staff; (2) occasional telephone and mail contact only from the trained and supervised research staff; or (3) frequent telephone and mail contact only from the trained and supervised research staff. Participants' moderate activity levels did increase for each condition over four months. It cannot be stated what components or mix of components were more successful than others, and whether the outcomes were due to the intervention or would have happened anyway. It was found, however, that more contact time with providers did not lead specifically to greater activity levels measured at four months. This finding has an implication for design of future interventions in terms of cost associated with providing interventions.

In Italy the PACE intervention[29] was implemented with 96 overweight participants. These participants received either PACE or usual care (control group). Those who received PACE showed, after five and six months, significantly increased belief in the ability to do more activity (self-efficacy), and shifts in stage of physical activity (from not being aware of a need to change, to thinking about change, to preparing to change, to becoming active and to maintaining the increased activity level). The study also found that the Italian women did not increase their activity levels as much as their US counterparts. This was attributed to demographic and cultural differences. Being married with children, and holding strong family and lifestyle orientations specific to their geographic location appeared to explain this difference between US and Italian women's PACE outcomes. This highlights the importance of understanding demographic and cultural differences when designing and implementing interventions.

In the Netherlands the feasibility pilot study[30] was undertaken with 29 general practices from city and rural areas to assess whether the program could be implemented within primary care. Assessment, therefore, was of the primary care practitioners' views of the program and not whether the participants became more active. Participants received two visits with a GP or Practice Nurse (PN), two telephone calls (one at the beginning and one at eight weeks after their second visit with the GP or PN) with a trained and supervised physical activity counsellor. Results have indicated that practitioners thought this was a program that stimulated patients to become physically active, and that it was suitable for wider implementation across the Netherlands.

Summary and comments on primary care-based physical activity interventions

Interventions to increase physical activity have been applied with large numbers of people, in primary care settings, using theoretical frameworks and models in the design of the interventions. While standardized benchmarks and outcome measures are needed to aid comparisons between studies and truly determine success,[24] in general, it would appear that people are prepared to attempt change when prompted to do so by a primary care provider like their GP, health visitor or dietician. It would also appear that different combinations of components are equally effective in initiating change. However, where long-term follow-up took place, the results indicated that even if people take up more physical activity, maintenance of the newly acquired level of activity is very difficult for the majority.

Of note is that some form of counselling is a major component of most short term successful interventions.[24,31] However, the US Preventive Task Force review[32] concluded that the evidence concerning its effectiveness is inconclusive. Assessment of counselling effectiveness in physical activity interventions is highly problematic for a number of reasons. Firstly the interventions vary hugely in the length of time of the sessions ranging from three to 45 minutes. This could be because there are different kinds of counselling such as motivational or behavioural, and each has a different focus and protocol as well as taking different lengths of times to deliver. We question, however, whether 'counselling' delivered in three minutes can legitimately be called counselling. Secondly, even if the kind of counselling (e.g. motivational or behavioural) is explicated in the published report of the study, the actual protocol is usually not. In general a behavioural change counselling session, might include discussion of the benefits of increased physical activity, what the participant perceives to be barriers and how they might overcome this followed by goal setting for the participant to make their desired changes. Subsequent sessions would then look at how progress is being made (or not as the case may be) and review goals. If the counselling does not contain the above it could be argued that it is inappropriate and possibly harmful to the participant. Intervention designers can attempt to minimize the type of harm that inappropriate counselling could do by ensuring it is health professionals who are trained and skilled in the necessary specific micro- and macro-skills employed routinely by professional counsellors.

In contrast to some of the community interventions, the primary care interventions generally have a basis in patient self-management, self-determination, and individual (though supported by their health professional) efforts and responsibility for their success. Less attention is given to issues of patients' environments and or the community demographics, facilities or support. They therefore tend to be of the exercise prescription genre, in that they focus on health risk, prevention and promotion, and encouraging individuals to change despite the demands upon them and contexts in which they live. Of equal value are those approaches that adopt a broader lifestyle context than the exercise prescription or referral approach and it is these that we turn our attention to next.

COMMUNITY AND LIFESTYLE/ACTIVE LIVING-BASED INTERVENTIONS

Community interventions

Community intervention focus has undergone a shift since the 1980s where promotion of vigorous activity to increase physical fitness was the aim. However, the realization of how inactive and/or unfit people are changed the focus to that of promoting moderate physical activity in order to reduce sedentariness.[33] Box 7.2 illustrates the components now used in these community interventions. A range of interventions have been implemented that focus on specific groups within the community such as inactive older people,[34] people with illnesses like diabetes,[35,36] workgroups,[37] those with low cardiorespiratory fitness,[38] newly partnered couples,[39] those living in a socially and economically deprived area,[40] young adults,[41] and children.[42] Details of those studies that were well designed can be found in Table 7.1. Three will be described here to illustrate three research designs: having a true control condition, a comparison condition and neither a control nor comparison. We will then move on to discuss lifestyle/active living interventions that are generally aimed at the whole community as opposed to specific groups within.

The first study we describe is the Netherlands community intervention known as 'Aging Well and Healthily'. This study did have a true control condition and was conducted in eight municipalities and involved 21 groups (full data collected from 269 participants). Some groups began the program right away (experimental condition) and received health education from a peer educator and an exercise program from a physical activity instructor. The remainder of the groups served as the waiting control condition, not receiving the intervention until nine months later when post-tests had been conducted. Results showed significant increases in physical activity for both the experimental and control participants. Before the start of the program 48% of

Box 7.2   Components used in community interventions to increase physical activity

Theory base: Social Learning, Transtheoretical Model, Self–Efficacy Theory, Social Cognitive Theory
Advice
Assessment
Written material
Coordinator/kit
Gym membership/exercise vouchers
Support person
Group education/exercise/activities
Group activities
Telephone contact
Competition participation
Website access
Motivational video cassette tape
Marketing, e.g. T-shirts/magnets
Guided activities
Choice
Collaboration with stake holders

participants reported that they were not physically active but at follow-up (4–6 months later) 82% reported being active and this was more significant for women participants. There was no longer-term follow-up in this study.

The second study that we describe did not have a true control group but did have a comparison group and was aimed at people with diabetes.[36] In this study participants took part in one of two conditions (again no true control condition was used in this intervention). In the first condition participants received personalized support through a helping relationship, group teaching, face-to-face follow-up contact, mailed brochures and exercise classes (power walking, water aerobics or low-impact aerobics). In the second condition, which was the comparison condition, participants received group-teaching sessions, telephone contact, a brochure and six months of exercise classes only. Those benefiting the most in both intervention groups were those who were in the pre-action stages of change (contemplation, preparation). This indicated that both conditions were effective in creating significant improvements in physical activity levels and were equally effective for participants in pre-action stages of change. For those who were more active prior to the start of the intervention, the condition providing personalized support was most effective in increasing their physical activity levels.

The study that did not have either a control or a comparison group that we wish to describe is Australia's most recently published study, the two-year community intervention, known as 'Concord: A great place to live'.[43] This

Table 7.1 Community-based interventions

Year and authors	Title and country	Participants and demographics	Methods		Main findings
2002 Burke et al.[39]	Physical activity interventions for new couples AUSTRALIA	137 newly partnered couples	**Theory base** Health Beliefs Model Social Cognitive Theory		Self-efficacy for physical activity, and positive health behaviours increased for both high and low conditions in comparison to usual care condition at time 2 (16 weeks) and in the high condition at time 3 (1 year).
			Between groups conditions[+] *High level* Receive information modules every 2 weeks Half by mail Half by contact sessions (demonstration of exercise techniques, answered questions and reviewed progress)	*Low level* Main contact to deliver first information module Other modules mailed every second week (self-directed change and overcoming barriers to change)	**Usual care** No information or contact	Exercising at moderate intensity increased for all groups at time 2 and time 3, but differences not significant between groups.
			Within groups conditions Time 1: Baseline (pre-test) Time 2: Post-test after 16-week intervention Time 3: Follow-up 1 year after commencing program		Fitness levels significantly increased for high condition at time 2 and 3 relative to control and low conditions. (suggesting that self report was an overestimate for control and low conditions)

Continued

Table 7.1 Community-based interventions—cont'd

Year and authors	Title and country	Participants and demographics	Methods	Main findings
2002 Burke et al. (cont'd)			**Dependent variables** Dietary intake (3-day diet records) 7-day recall of physical activity Blood pressure Perceived barriers to physical activity and positive health behaviours Health beliefs Self-efficacy	
2002 Hopman-Rock & Westhoff[52]	AWH (Aging Well and Healthy) NETHERLANDS	269 adult participants 65 years + Independent community living Physically inactive Across 8 municipality	**Theory base** Theory of planned behaviour (specifically attitude and self-efficacy/behavioural control) **Between groups conditions** *AWH Intervention* Health education by a peer educator Low intensity exercises taught by fitness instructor *A small payment was required by participants* *Control* No treatment (treatment offered after study) **Within groups conditions** Time1: Baseline (pre-test)	**Results** Participants in the AWH condition reported being more physical active at time 2 (4–6 months after) than control condition. (activity increased from 48% to 82%). This was more significant for women participants *Comments* The long-term impact of this intervention is unknown

Table 7.1 Community-based interventions—cont'd

2002 Hopman–Rock & Westhoff (cont'd)			Time 2: Post-test 4–6 months after intervention **Dependent variables** Measures on a pedometer Physical activity questionnaire for use with older adults including questions on household activities, sports activities, leisure time activities	
2002 Lowther & Mutrie[53]	Physical activity for economically deprived UNITED KINGDOM	370 adult participants Scottish housing estates 65% female	**Theory base** Social Cognitive Theory	Physical activity increased for both fitness assessment and exercise consultation groups from baseline to time 2 (4 weeks) and time 3 (3 months) in comparison to controls
				Physical activity was maintained for the intervention groups at time 4 (6 months) attributed to the intervention re-test at 3 months
			Between groups conditions Fitness assessment Exercise vouchers Computerized fitness assessment flexibility Peak flow (VO_2 submax) on cycle exercise prescription	Physical activity declined for these groups at time 4 (1 year)
			Exercise consultation Exercise vouchers Exercise consultation for 30 minutes	No effect of type of intervention (exercise consultation or fitness assessment) on physical activity for sedentary participants at time 3 (3 months), but exercise consultation intervention was more effective in promoting physical activity in sedentary participants at time 5 (1 year)
			Control Exercise vouchers	

Continued

Table 7.1 Community-based interventions—cont'd

Year and authors	Title and country	Participants and demographics	Methods	Main findings
2002 Lowther & Mutrie (cont'd)			**Within groups conditions** Time 1: Baseline (pre-test) Time 2: Post-test 4 weeks after intervention Time 3: Follow-up 3 months after intervention Time 4: Follow-up 6 months after intervention Time 5: Follow-up 1 year after intervention **Dependent variables** Scottish Physical Activity Questionnaire	Sedentary participants tended to select the exercise consultation over the fitness assessment intervention
2002 Woods et al.[41]	Helping sedentary young adults become active UNITED KINGDOM	459 participants Sedentary students 14–23 years	*Theory base* Transtheoretical Model **Between groups conditions** *Self-instructional Intervention* 2 personally addressed packages on active living delivered by exercise psychology experts *Control* Usual care (access to student facilities at university)	Significantly more participants in the self-instructional intervention improved their stages of change than the control at time 2

Table 7.1 Community-based interventions—cont'd

2002 Woods et al. (cont'd)		**Within groups conditions** Time 1: Baseline (pre-test) Time 2: Post-test after 6-month intervention period **Dependent variables** Habitual exercise behaviour Stages of change questionnaire (short)		**Results** Decline in Internet usage over 8 weeks for both conditions although less so for Active Lives condition.
2001 McKay et al.[35] UNITED STATES	D-Net Active Lives PA Intervention	78 adult participants Type 2 diabetic patients 53% female 40 + years (average = 52 years) Sedentary	**Theory base** Social Cognitive Theory	
			Between groups conditions *Active Lives Intervention* 8 week personalized PA program via Internet Planning process (5 steps to action) with online coach Online coach question and answer facility Identify benefits and barriers Goal setting Assisted scheduling	Information only Information of diabetes via Internet Real time blood glucose tracking with graphic feedback	Those who used the personal online coach in the Active Lives condition reported greater change in moderate to vigorous activity at time 2 (post-test) that those who didn't No significant differences between control and Active Lives conditions in physical activity and depression scores

Continued

Table 7.1 Community-based interventions—cont'd

Year and authors	Title and country	Participants and demographics	Methods	Main findings
2001 McKay et al. (cont'd)			Personal database to track pnformation resource + motivational stories Communication to other Active Lives participants online **Within groups conditions** Time 1: Baseline (pre-test) Time 2: Post-test after 8-week intervention **Dependent variables** Physical activity (assess whether respondents meet CDC PA recommendations) Total PA score for previous week in minutes of vigorous, moderate activity and walking Depression scales	
2001 Mau et al.[36]	Women with diabetes HAWAII	147 adult participants Women Diabetes	**Theory base** Transtheoretical Model **Between groups conditions** *Family Support Intervention* Culturally *Standard Intervention* Culturally competent program for 6 months	Participants in the family support intervention condition were more likely to advance from pre-action to action/ maintenance stage at time 2 (post-test) than participants in the standard intervention Participants in the family support intervention condition who advanced to the action/ maintenance stage showed

Table 7.1 Community-based interventions—cont'd

2001 Mau et al. (cont'd)		competent program for 6 months (role play, peer educators) Exercise classes and follow-up Designated Ohana (family) Support (OS) person Instructed on how to ask OS for assistance in making lifestyle changes **Within groups conditions** Time 1: Baseline (pre-test) Time 2: Post-test after 6-month intervention **Dependent variables** Food frequency questionnaire (total calories consumed per day) Modified activity questionnaire (estimates of calories expended) Stages of change inventory	(role play, peer educators) Exercise classes and follow-up	more improvement in fat intake and physical activity than those at the same stage in the standard intervention condition
2001 Stewart et al.[34]	CHAMPS II UNITED STATES	173 adult participants 66% female 65–90 years physically under-active	**Theory base** Social Cognitive Theory Transtheoretical Model	*Results* At Time 1 (pre-test), there was no difference between the control and CHAMPS condition. Participants were not exercising at all

Continued

Table 7.1 Community-based interventions—*cont'd*

Year and authors	Title and country	Participants and demographics	Methods	Main findings
2001 Stewart et al. (cont'd)			**Between groups conditions** *CHAMPS Intervention* Self-efficacy enhancement Development of balanced activity program based on stage of change Motivational (goal setting) techniques Educational Counselling via phone Newsletters *Control* Waitlisted (for participation at end of program) **Within groups conditions** Time 1: Baseline (pre-test) Time 2: Post-test after 1-year intervention **Dependent variables** Estimated calories expended per week in moderate intensity physical activity Self-report CHAMPS physical activity questionnaire for older adults	Calorific expenditure for the CHAMPS condition increased more at time 2 (1 year later) than the control condition. (487 per week in moderate intensity activity and 687 in activity of any intensity) CHAMPS particularly effective for women over 75 years and overweight participants **Comments** Long-term outcomes are unknown

Table 7.1   Community-based interventions—cont'd

2001 Titze et al.[37]	Office in Motion SWITZERLAND	379 adult participants Office workers 8 offices in Switzerland	**Theory base** Transtheoretical Model	Significant progression in stages of change for intervention offices at time 2 (post-test) than control offices
				The level of physical activity at baseline influenced the effect of the intervention
			Between groups conditions *Intervention Program* Information Action for daily life activities Fitness lessons Counselling	*Control* No intervention
				Proportion of physically active people for intervention condition at time 2 increased to 21%
			Within groups conditions Time1: Baseline (pre-test) Time 2: Post-test after 4-month intervention period	
			Dependent variables 7-day recall questionnaire on physical activities (daily life, leisure and sport) stages of change questionnaire	
1999 Dunn et al.[38]	Project Active (Lifestyle vs. Structured Exercise) UNITED STATES	235 adult participants (116 women, 119 men) Sedentary	**Theory base** Social Cognitive Theory Transtheoretical Model	**Results** Both lifestyle and structured activity conditions had significant and comparable improvements in physical activity, cardiovascular fitness, blood pressure, percentage of body fat at time 2 (24 months)

Continued

Table 7.1 Community-based interventions—cont'd

Year and authors	Title and country	Participants and demographics	Methods	Main findings
1999 Dunn et al. (cont'd)			**Between groups conditions** *Lifestyle Physical Activity* Advised to accumulate 30 minutes of moderate intensity physical activity on most days of the week (suited to lifestyle) Group meetings teaching cognitive and behavioural strategies related to physical activity (1 per week for 16 weeks, 1 per fortnight until week 24 Completed stages of change each month and given intervention manual tailored to individual readiness Assignments During 18 month follow-up meetings were decreased from 1 per month, (1 per three months, 1 per 6 months)	*Structured Exercise* Individual supervised sessions 5 days per week for 6 months at fitness center Group leader assisted goal setting and reinforcement Individualization of programs Participants who missed sessions were followed up and encouraged to return During 18 month follow-up, group met every 3 months for group activities Monthly activities calendar	**Conclusion** Lifestyle Physical Activity intervention is just as effective as a Structured Exercise program in improving physical activity, cardiovascular fitness and blood pressure

Table 7.1 Community-based interventions—cont'd

1999 Dunn et al (cont'd)		**Within groups conditions** Time 1: Baseline (pre–test) Time 2: Post–test after 24-month intervention **Dependent variables** 7-day physical activity recall VO_2 peak by treadmill Plasma lipid and lipoprotein cholesterol concentrations Blood pressure Body composition	Newsletter on benefits of activity and research findings
1996 Calfas et al.[27]	225 adult participants	**Theory base** Health Belief Model Theory of Planned Behavior (behavioural control/self-efficacy variable) Transtheoretical Model **Between Group Conditions** *PACE* Counselling and booster phone call on: Increasing social support Increasing self-efficacy Reducing barriers to activity Increasing knowledge of benefits of activity	Physician-based counselling condition showed larger increase in activity from baseline at time 2 and time 3 than the control condition (37 mins increase in walking compared to 7 mins increase).
	PACE (Physician-based Assessment and Counseling for Exercise). UNITED STATES		
		Control Usual care	

Continued

Table 7.1   Community-based interventions—*cont'd*

Year and authors	Title and country	Participants and demographics	Methods	Main findings
1996 Calfas et al. (cont'd)			Note: Counselling sessions were tailored based on the stage of change of the patient (via a stages of change questionnaire) **Within groups conditions** Time 1: Baseline (pre-test) Time 2: Post-test 4 weeks after intervention Time 3: Follow-up 6 weeks after intervention **Dependent variable** Readiness to adopt physical activity Self-reported physical activity levels	

study was developed in partnership with the Concord Local Government area and the Central Sydney Health Promotion unit and is noteworthy for its innovation because of the range of components and strategies adopted and the level of collaboration with different community organizations and the residents themselves. It ran between 1997 and 1999, across an inner Western region of Sydney and aimed to assist women in becoming more physically active by increasing the opportunities to participate. This was done in a variety of ways such as organizing community walking events, setting up walking groups and conducting a range of different kinds of physical activity classes. In addition, walking maps were produced and made available and signage put up to indicate walking routes. A range of barriers to physical activity was addressed from the environmental to the personal with the program being promoted through regular newsletters, T-shirts, fridge magnets and banners. Although there was no control group, the program was assessed using a pre-(May–June 1997) and post-(May–June 1999) intervention survey design. Women aged between 20 and 50 years took part. Pre-intervention surveys were completed by 1762 women and post-interventions surveys by 1801.

The results showed that at post-intervention there were significantly fewer (15.2%) sedentary women than there had been at pre-intervention (21.6%). This could be seen in the significant increase in the proportion of women who took part in a low level of physical activity at post-intervention (47.9%) compared to pre-intervention (41.6%). No changes to moderate or high physical activity levels were found. The conclusion that this intervention was somewhat successful must be made with caution however as there was no control or comparison group and this is a point worthy of some further consideration. Of those studies that have incorporated a control group, some differed and some did not in their effectiveness. Moreover, the findings of studies that used not a true control but a comparison group are also equivocal. It would appear that some form of intervention, even when it is just being in a waiting list control group, can often be sufficient to heighten awareness and subsequently initiate some behaviour change.

The Concord study illustrates the practical difficulties large-scale community interventions have in incorporating a control or comparison group. The lifestyle and active living type interventions that have been conducted to date also have this issue as they tend to be aimed at the general community and not specific groups within the community per se. It is these that we turn to next.

Lifestyle/active living–based interventions

Traditionally community interventions have often been designed using structured physical activity programs but more recently, considerable variations have taken place with the advent of lifestyle-based interventions. These have come about as a result of the recommendations that adults should undertake at least 30 minutes of accumulated moderate physical activity on most and preferably all days of the week. Since many people state lack of time as a factor that prevents them from being more physically active, strategies that promote the incorporation of physical activity into daily tasks may facilitate the attainment of the advocated 30-minute target. Consequently people should be encouraged to opt for the active rather than passive alternative when presented with a choice such as taking the stairs instead of the escalator/lift or getting on or off buses a stop earlier than usual in order to incorporate some walking into their day. Thus, active living approaches focus on incorporating activity into daily lifestyles with due regard to context and locality.

Following the publication of Blamey et al.'s[44] seminal study in the UK, a number of similar studies examining the examining the effects of advertising campaigns to encourage people to use the stairs have been conducted in the USA[45,46], the UK[47] and Australia.[48] Details of these studies can be found in Table 7.2. Collectively, a range of settings have been used such as shopping malls, university/hospital buildings and train stations. In all of these studies posters or signs were placed at decision points for taking the stairs or the elevator and the decisions that people made were recorded by observers. All of the studies found that stair use increased significantly compared to baseline and, in the above mentioned UK and USA studies that included a post-intervention assessment (8–12 weeks), stair use remained higher than baseline after the posters had been taken down.

It should be apparent that research designs such as these cannot incorporate a control or comparison condition. In addition, observers discreetly record the numbers of people who take the stairs and elevators at specific times of the day and make comparisons between the number of observations at baseline, following intervention and post intervention. They will not necessarily be observing the same people at the different phases of the study. The reliability of the observations can also be questioned due to the difficult job the observers have – i.e. counting huge numbers of people rushing to/from work in a train station. In an attempt to address this, an Australian study[48] used an infra-red motion sensor device to do the counting. Unlike the other studies, theirs found that stair use returned to baseline post-intervention and remained there at reintroduction of the intervention. It was also noted that the difference between baseline and intervention was smaller than that found in the other studies. However, a likely reason for the different results of the Australian study may be the use of the motion sensor device. The authors acknowledge that this meant that those who should have been excluded due to, for example, physical challenges, were not.

Another innovative, but again methodologically challenging study is the UK Project 'Walk Stop'.[49] The intervention consisted of placing posters at bus stops for a two-week period that encouraged people to 'walk a stop' by either walking to the next stop or getting off the bus a stop earlier than their destination. One week before the posters were displayed people waiting at bus stops were interviewed ($n = 131$) to assess their intention to either walk to the next stop or get off a stop early. The posters were displayed for one week and the week after that people waiting at the same bus stops ($n = 115$) were interviewed again. The results were that people were more likely to walk a stop before getting on the bus rather than get off a stop early. Also, the percentage

Table 7.2 Community/active living interventions

Year and authors	Title and country	Participants and demographics	Methods	Main findings
2003 Mutrie et al.[49]	Project Walk Stop UNITED KINGDOM	246 adult participants Bus commuters at 9 bus stops in Glasgow	**Theory base** Theory of Planned Behavior (intention and self-efficacy/behavioural control) Transtheoretical Model **Intervention** Adverts at bus stops encouraging bus commuters to walk a stop (walk to the next stop or alight early) **Within groups conditions** Time 1: Baseline (pre-test) Time 2: Post-test after 2-week intervention **Dependent variables** Intention to walk a stop Self-efficacy for walking a stop Stage of exercise change	Percentage of participants intending to walk a stop at least once a week increased at time 2 (12% to 26%). Higher levels of self-efficacy at time 2.
2002 Marshall et al.[54]	Motivational signs and incidental physical activity AUSTRALIA	People using a health care facility	**Theory base** Social Cognitive Theory (self-efficacy) **12-week observation study** Motivational messages about using the stairs in a hospital posted during weeks 4–5 then removed, posted again during weeks 8–9 then removed.	Stair use significantly increased after motivational messages were posted at time 1 (4–6 weeks), then dropped, when posters were removed. Stair use did not significantly change from baseline after motivational messages were posted at time 2 (8–9 weeks).

Continued

Table 7.2 Community/active living interventions—cont'd

Year and authors	Title and country	Participants and demographics	Methods	Main findings
2002 Marshall et al. (cont'd)			**Within groups conditions** Time 1: Baseline (observation for 4 weeks – prior to signage) Time 2: Post-test after first intervention phase at 4–5 weeks Time 3: Post-test after second intervention phase at 8–9 weeks **Dependent variables** Anonymous counts of use of stairs vs. elevators using a motion sensing device over 12-week period	Stair use decrease below baseline in final weeks of observational study.
2001 Boutelle et al.[46]	Signs Artwork Music to promote stair climbing UNITED STATES	Employees at a school of public health building (approx 700 part-time and full-time employees)	**Theory base** Social Cognitive Theory (self-efficacy) **Observation study** *Phase 1:* Signs instructing people to 'Take the stairs for your health' adjacent to the elevators at a school of public health building, stickers above the elevator buttons and on the stairwell doors for 3 weeks. *Phase 2:* Signs plus artwork (changed weekly) and music (changed daily) in stairwell.	Signage significantly increased stair use from baseline to time 1. Artwork and music made a significant additional contribution to stair use from time 2 to time 3 Neither phase differentially affected men or women.

Table 7.2   Community/active living interventions—cont'd

| 2001 Bontelle et al. (con'd) | | **Within groups conditions**
Time 1: Baseline (observation prior to signage)
Time 2: Post-test immediately after phase 1
Time 3: Post-test immediately after phase 2

Dependent variables
Observer counts of use of stairs vs. escalators 3 days a week for 3 hours each. | |
| 2001 Bock et al.[55] | Individual motivation tailored intervention | 150 adult participants
Sedentary
Average age 44 years | **Theory base**
Social Cognitive Theory
Transtheoretical Model

Between groups conditions
Motivation matched intervention
Self-help manuals
Individually tailored feedback reports matched to stage of change including motivational information, overcoming barriers and increasing self-efficacy | *Standard print-based intervention*
American heart self-help books addressing walking, swimming and cycling for heart health | Significantly more participants in the Motivation matched intervention condition exceeded exercise participation goals at the end of the intervention period (time 4) and maintained then 6 months after the intervention (time 5) than in the Standard print-based intervention. |

Continued

Table 7.2 Community/active living interventions—*cont'd*

Year and authors	Title and country	Participants and demographics	Methods	Main findings
2001 Bock et al. (cont'd)			**Within groups conditions** Time 1: Baseline (pre-test) Time 2: 1 month into the intervention Time 3: 3 months into the intervention Time 4: 6 months into the intervention Time 5: Follow-up 6 months after the intervention (month 12) **Dependent variables** 7 day recall of physical activity Motivational readiness for physical activity (stages of change) Self-efficacy Affect	
2001 Kerr et al.[56]	Observation of prompted stair climbing UNITED KINGDOM	Shoppers at shopping mall in Midlands region of United Kingdom	**Theory base** Social Cognitive Theory (self-efficacy) **12-week observation study** Motivational messages on stair risers in shopping mall over 12 weeks **Within groups conditions** Time 1: Baseline (observation for 2 weeks prior to signage) Time 2: Post-test after 12 week intervention	Stair use was significantly increased from time 1 to time 2. When motivational messages were removed, stair usage remained higher than baseline.

Table 7.2 Community/active living interventions—cont'd

Year/Author	Intervention	Population	Methods	Results
1995 Blamey et al.[44]	Stay healthy, save time, use the stairs UNITED KINGDOM	Commuters at a train station in city centre	**Dependent variables** Observed stair choices **Theory base** Social Cognitive Theory (self-efficacy) **Observation study** Motivational messages about using the stairs adjacent to the escalators at a train station posted for 3 weeks. **Within groups conditions** Time 1: Baseline (observation for 1 week prior to signage) Time 2: Monitor during 3 weeks signs were present Time 3: Post-test immediately after signs removed Time 4: Follow-up 4 and 12 weeks after signage intervention. **Dependent variables** Observer counts of use of stairs vs. escalators on Monday, Wednesday and Friday from 8.30 am–10 am (those carrying luggage or pushing prams were excluded)	Stair use increased from baseline during the 3 weeks of signage (from 8% to 17%). Stair use decreased during the weeks immediately after signage was removed, but remained higher than baseline even 12 weeks after the intervention. Stair choices were more significant from men than women
2001 Coleman et al.[45]	Stair use in US–Mexico border community		**Theory base** Social Cognitive Theory (self-efficacy)	Women's stair use increased at all intervention sites, while men's increased at only 2 sites (airport and bank)

Continued

Table 7.2   Community/active living interventions—*cont'd*

Year and authors	Title and country	Participants and demographics	Methods	Main findings
2001 Coleman et al. (cont'd)	UNITED STATES		**Intervention** 2 × 2ft signs encouraging stair use in both English and Spanish placed between stairs and elevators at 4 sites (airport, bank, office building and university of Texas campus) **Between groups conditions** *Individual promotion sign* Stair promotion for individuals in English and Spanish (depicting an individual climbing the stairs) *Family promotion sign* Stair promotion for family in English and Spanish (depicting family climbing the stairs) **Within groups conditions** Time 1: Baseline (pre-test) Time 2: Intervention phase (1 month) Time 3: Post-intervention phase **Dependent variables** Observer counts of use of stairs vs. escalators (those carrying luggage or pushing prams were excluded)	No difference in individual and family promotion message to stair climbing in the Hispanic community

of participants intending to walk a stop before getting the bus at least once a week changed from 12%, to 26% after the intervention.

As with the stair walking studies, the people interviewed were not necessarily the same both times. This study was also only able to measure intention to walk a stop and not whether people's behaviour actually changed although this is still a positive finding, as we know from the Theory of Planned Behaviour (see Chapter 2) that intention is highly predictive of behaviour.

With the growth of active living/lifestyle interventions, the question of which is more effective at increasing physical activity levels – either this or the exercise prescription type of intervention – is very pertinent. This question was addressed in a study of 315 sedentary men and women (average age 46 years) who took part in either an exercise prescription condition or a lifestyle condition.[38] The exercise prescription group received a structured exercise program with prescribed intensities, frequencies and durations. The lifestyle group, however, received encouragement to incorporate 30 minutes of moderate physical activity into their day together with assistance in small groups for varying amounts of time across the duration of the intervention.

At six months (short-term) both groups had very similar increases in moderate intensity physical activity. At 24 months only 20% in both groups had maintained the initial increase. These results strongly suggest that both types of intervention were equally successful in increasing moderate intensity physical activity and that neither was more successful in maintaining the increases.

The final study that we would like to mention is one that used pedometers as a motivational tool because these are becoming popular in physical activity interventions. In Minnesota, USA, pedometers were used in the efforts of a large health-care and health insurance organization (with over 660 000 members) to help people become more active.[50] In the eight-month long study, 92 participants were provided with a pedometer, an action planner, an exercise log, biweekly motivational cards, and the opportunity to enter draws with prizes. As with the Concord program there was no control or comparison group. Evaluations were conducted by phone with 42 participants eight weeks after the intervention was completed. They reported that the program had helped them to increase their activity levels. Further evaluation took place at eight months after the study began using a mailed questionnaire with 30 of these being returned for analysis. These indicated increased steps per day, continued use of the pedometer at least twice a week and that the program was 'somewhat' to 'very' motivating for increasing physical activity. Following this successful program more partnerships with workplaces have been formed and more than 10 000 people have enrolled in the program.

Summary and comments on community-based physical activity interventions

Two different kinds of community interventions have been outlined in this section and both have been somewhat successful in promoting the uptake of greater amounts of physical activity. Targeting particular interventions to particular groups has produced good short- to medium-term results but whether these approaches are effective long-term is often not known. Larger scale targeted intervention studies require greater funds and longer-term commitment of both the deliverers and the instigating researchers. What also comes out very strongly is that in setting up community interventions, a lot of time and effort into building partnerships with community, council or other organizations is required and the success of the program is dependent on the level of collaboration and cooperation. The benefits of this however can be seen in the Concord project with the wide range of strategies put in place that addressed so many barriers to physical activity.

Another issue for community interventions is that they tend to recruit participants who are already active and some have noted the difficulty in recruiting participants who were sufficiently inactive. It appears that people who are already active are open to becoming more active, whereas those who are least active are not willing or able to explore the possibilities of being more active. Can it be said, therefore, that community interventions are successful when they do not recruit sufficient numbers of inactive people? Moreover, when for example in the Concord study, so many different kinds of barriers were addressed but more sedentary people did not participate, does this not illustrate that addressing barriers is not enough? Somehow people's lack of will and motivation needs to be addressed too. Within the primary care setting counselling may be effective in this regard but counselling is not normally a component of community interventions.

CONCLUSIONS

From the research into interventions to increase physical activity a number of clear conclusions have emerged. Firstly, no particular kind of intervention (primary care or community) is more or less effective than another. Secondly, the evidence concerning strategies used (e.g. counselling, education materials, exercise prescriptions) is equivocal. We do not know which are more or less effective than others although there is some suggestion that all strategies have some value. Thirdly, any success is short-term only. We might be able to start but maintaining the increased physical activity level is another matter altogether. Future interventions, therefore, must focus on maintenance strategies. To enable interventions to be evaluated, future research studies must conform to scientific standards. They must use standardized measures of success based on clear definitions that incorporate a range of physical activities and not just participation in the program recommended/provided by the intervention. They must also include long-term follow-up, which goes beyond the end of the intervention. This sounds expensive, and indeed it is, but not only has research clearly identified the preventive and therapeutic aspects of physical activity, it has also documented the higher medical costs associated with inactivity.[51]

It is noteworthy that it is often older adults who have and are taking part in community interventions. Is it the case that their health beliefs have changed because as they have grown older they have come to perceive themselves as less healthy and at risk of becoming ill? Have they, therefore, now got reasons to be active and consequently come to consider the benefits of increasing physical activity to outweigh the costs? Maybe so but people need to be active throughout the lifespan and not just when they get older and more likely to be at risk. How then can people be motivated to incorporate regular physical activity into their lives and maintain it?

It must be borne in mind that any behaviour is the result of a complex interaction between internal (physical and psychological) and external (social and environmental) factors. Therefore, where possible a holistic approach should be adopted which encompasses all possible determinants (physical – limitations of illness or body shape, psychological – low self-efficacy for physical activity and environmental – safety/access to facilities) of physical activity. Thus, to be truly effective, the application of a really broad perspective (the big picture) of activity that encompasses every aspect of an individual's life, (contexts and environments) is required which spans the whole of life (age and lifestyle) but with due consideration that people are individual in terms of experience and their capacity to act in particular ways at specific times in their life. We need, therefore, interventions within primary care, within the community and interventions that are both prescribed and lifestyle oriented.

While there is far less research on the effectiveness of maintenance strategies for physical activity, information from the general area of motivation can be helpful. For example, we know that choice is a powerful motivator to act, whereas feeling that one has no choice, or that something is being imposed, is far less likely to result in lasting change. Maintenance is also influenced by individual preferences relating to group or individual involvement in the activity (physical or otherwise), as well as choice of the kind of activity and, having positive thoughts about the ability to increase one's activity. Thus, veering away from the imposition of programs or prescriptions and moving towards giving people ways to rethink and reassess their desired changes after adopting physical activity could be effective for maintenance. This would also assist in finding ways of countering monotony of activity experienced by those who prefer variety in their choice of activity. In addition, social reasons are very often reported as strong motivators to exercise therefore opportunities to be physically active while being socially engaged should also be considered.

The holistic approach means that the agenda for increasing physical activity levels and maintaining them is a big one. It is, however, very necessary. While empowering people to act to reduce health risk specifically, or more generally to increase quality and enjoyment of life, is good, it is not enough because, as the evidence shows, endeavouring to get and stay active is truly not a matter of just doing it.

References

1. Services USDoHaH. Physical activity and health: A report of the Surgeon General. Atlanta: Centres for Disease Control and Prevention, National Centre for Chronic Disease Prevention and Health Promotion; 1996.

2. Armstrong T, Bauman A, Davies J. Physical activity patterns of Australian adults: Results of the 1999 National Physical Activity Survey. Canberra: Australian Institute of Health and Welfare; 2000.

3. Bauman A, Ford I, Armstrong T. Trends in population levels of reported physical activity in Australia 1997, 1999, and 2000. Canberra: Australian Sports Commission; 2001.

4. McElroy M. Resistance to exercise: A social analysis to inactivity, 1st edn. Champaign: Human Kinetics; 2002.

5. CDC. http://www.cdcgov/nchs/nhis.htm//2000_NHS.; 2002.

6. Biddle SJH, Mutrie N. Psychology of physical activity, 1st edn. London: Routledge; 2001.

7. Lindstrom M, Sundquist J. Immigration and leisure-time physical inactivity: A population based study. Ethnicity and Health 2001; 6(2):77–85.

8. Armitage CJ, Conner M. Social cognitive models and health behaviour: A structured review. Psychology and Health 2000; 15(2):173–190.

9. Bauman A, Smith B, Stoker L, Booth M. Geographical influences upon physical activity participation: Evidence of a 'coastal effect'. Australian and New Zealand Journal of Public Health 1999; 2(3):322–324.

10. Brownson RC, Baker EA, Houseman RA, Brennan LK, Bacak SJ. Environmental and policy determinants of physical activity in the United States. Americal Journal of Public Health 2001; 91(12):1995–2003.

11. Grzywacz JG, Marks NF. Social inequities and exercise during adulthood: Toward an ecological perspective. Journal of Health and Social Behaviour 2001; 42(2):202–220.

12. Biddle SJH, Mutrie N. Psychology of physical activity: determinants, well-being and interventions. London: Routledge; 2002.

13. Owen N, Bauman A. The descriptive epidemiology of a sedentary lifestyle in adult Australians. International Journal of Epidemiology 1992; 21:305–310.

14. Mutrie N, Choi PYL. Is 'fit' a feminist issue? Dilemmas for exercise psychology. Feminism and Psychology 2000; 10(4):544–551.

15. O'Brien CS. Grounding theory in self-referent thinking: Conceptualizing motivation for older adult physical activity. Psychology of Sport and Exercise 2003; 4:81–100.

16. O'Brien Cousins S. Thinking out loud: What older adults say about triggers for physical activity. Journal of Aging and Physical Activity 2001; 9(347–363).

17. Choi PYL. Femininity and the physically active woman. London: Routlege; 2000.

18. Dishman RK. Compliance/adherence in health-related exercise. Health Psychology 1982; 1:237–267.

19. Blaxter M. Health and lifestyles. London: Tavistock/Routledge; 1990.

20. Bauman A. Diversities in conceptions of health and physical fitness. Journal of Health and Human Behaviour 1961; 2:39–46.

21. Watson J. Males bodies: Health, culture, and identity. Buckingham: Open University Press; 2000.

22. Allied Dunbar National Fitness Survey. London: Sports Council and Health Education Authority; 1992.

23. Cropley M, Ayers S, Nokes L. People don't exercise because they can't think of reasons to exercise: An examination of causal reasoning within the transtheoretical model. Psychology, Health and Medicine 2003; 8(4):409–414.

24. Smith BJ, Merom D, Harris P, Bauman AE. Do primary care interventions to promote physical activity work?: Systematic review of the literature. The New South Wales Centre for Physical Activity and Health Report No. CPAH 03-0002. Melbourne: The National Institute of Clinical Studies; 2002.

25. Harland J, White M, Drinkwater C, Chinn D, Farr L, Howel D. The Newcastle exercise project: A randomised controlled trial of methods to promote physical activity in primary care. British Medical Journal 1999; 39:828–832.

26. Steptoe A, Kerry S, Rink E, Hilton S. The impact of behavioral counselling on stage of change in fat intake, physical activity and cigarette smoking in adults at increased risk of coronary heart disease. American Journal of Public Health 2001; 91(2):265–270.

27. Calfas KJ, Long BJ, Sallis JF, Wooten WJ, Pratt M, Patrick K. A controlled trial of physical counselling to promote the adoption of physical activity. Preventive Medicine 1996; 25:225–233.

28. Patrick K, Sallis JF, Prochaska JJ, Lydston DD, Calfas KJ, Zabinski MF, et al. A multicomponent program for nutrition and physical activity change in primary care: PACE+ for adolescents. Archives of Pediatrics and Adolescent Medicine 2001; 155(8):940–946.

29. Nigg CR, Bolognesi M, Massarini M. A transtheoretical model-based physical activity intervention targeting overweight/obese primary care patients: PACE results from Italy. In: Stelter R, ed. FEPSAC XIth European Congress of Sport Psychology Proceedings: University of Copenhagen; 2003:121.

30. Van Poppel MNM, Van Sluijs EMF, Van Mechelen W. A PACE intervention in Dutch general practice: Feasibility and short term results. In: Stelter R, ed. FEPSAC XIth European Congress of Sport Psychology Proceedings: University of Copenhagen; 2003:135.

31. Eakin EG, Glasgow RE, Riley KM. Review of primary care-based physical activity intervention studies. Journal of Family Practice 2000; 49(2):158.

32. Eden KB, Orleans CT, Mulrow CD. Does counselling by clinicians improve physical activity?: A summary of evidence for the US Preventive Services Task Force. Annals of Internal Medicine 2002; 137(3):208–215.

33. Levin S, Gans KM, Carleton RA, Bucknam L. The evolutions of a physical activity campaign. Family of Community Health 1998; 21(1):65–79.

34. Stewart AL, Verboncoer CJ, McLellan BY, Gillis DE, Rush S, Mills CM, et al. Physical activity outcomes of CHAMPS II: A physical activity promotion program. Journal of Gerontology: Biomedical Sciences and Medical Sciences 2001; 56: M465–M470.

35. McKay HG, Seeley JR, King D, Glasgow RE, Eakin EG. The diabetes network Internet-based physical activity intervention. Diabetes Care 2001; 24(8):1328.

36. Mau MK, Grove JS, Glanz K, Johnson B, Severino R, Curb JD. Mediators of lifestyle behavior change in native Hawaiians. Diabetes Care 2001; 24(10):1770–1775.

37. Titze S, Martin BW, Seiler R, Stronegger W, Marti B. Effects of a lifestyle physical activity intervention on stages of change and energy expenditure in sedentary employees. Psychology of Sport and Exercise 2001; 2(2):103–116.

38. Dunn AL, Marcus BH, Kampert JB, Garcia ME, Kohl HW, Blair S. Comparison of lifestyle and structured interventions to increase physical activity and cardiorespiratory fitness: A randomised trial. Journal of the American Medical Association 1999; 281(4):327.

39. Burke V, Mori GN, Gillam HF, Beilin LJ, Houghton S, Cutt HE, et al. An innovative program for changing health behaviours. Asia Pacific Journal of Clinical Nutrition 2002; 11(Suppl.):S586–S597.

40. Lowther M. Promoting physical activity in a socially and economically deprived community: A twelve month randomised control trial of fitness assessment and exercise consultation. Journal of Sports Sciences 2001; 20(7):577–588.

41. Woods C, Mutrie N, Scott M. Physical activity intervention: A transtheoretical model-based intervention designed to help sedentary young adults become active. Health Education Research: Theory and Practice 2002; 17(4):451–460.

42. Sherman N. Increasing children's physical activity levels. JOPERD 2000; 71(4):8.

43. Wen L, Thomas M, Jones H, Orr N, Moreton R, King L, et al. Promoting physical activity in women: Evaluation of a 2 year community-based intervention in Sydney, Australia. Health Promotion International 2002; 17(2):127–137.

44. Blamey A, Muttrie N, Aitchison T. Health promotion by encouraged use of stairs. British Medical Journal 1995; 311:289–290.

45. Coleman KJ, Gonzalez EC. Promoting stair use in a US–Mexico border community. Americal Journal of Public Health 2001; 91(12).

46. Boutelle KN, Jeffery RW, Murray DM, Schmitz MKH. Using signs, artwork and music to promote stair use in a public building. American Journal of Public Health 2001; 91(12).

47. Kerr J, Eves F, Carroll D. Six month observational study of prompted stair climbing. Preventive Medicine 2001; 33(5):422–427.

48. Marshall AL, Bauman AE, Patch C, Wilson J, Chen J. Can motivational signs prompt increases in incidental physical activity in an Australian health-care facility? Health Education Research 2002; 17:743–749.

49. Mutrie N, Comrie M, Crawford F, McMahon R, Noble A, Sutherland R. Project 'Walk Stop': Promoting walking to bus commuters. In: Stelter R, ed. FEPSAC XIth European Congress of Sport Psychology Proceedings: University of Copenhagen; 2003:118.

50. Lindberg R. Active living: On the road with the 10,000 steps program. Journal of the American Dietetic Association 2000; 100(8):878–879.

51. Pratt M, Macera CA, Wang G. Higher direct medical costs associated with physical inactivity. Physician and Sports Medicine 2000; 28(10).

52. Hopman-Rock M, Westhoff MH. Health education and exercise stimulation for older people: Development and evaluation of the program 'Healthy and Vital'. Tijdschr Gerontol Geriatric 2002; 33(2):56–63.

53. Lowther M, Mutrie N, Scott EM. Promoting physical activity in a socially and economically deprived community: A twelve month randomised control trial of fitness assessment and exercise consultation. Journal of Sports Sciences 2002; 20(7):577–588.

54. Marshall AL, Bauman AE, Patch C, Wilson J, Chen J. Can motivational signs prompt increases in incidental physical activity in an Australian health-care facility? Health Education Research 2002; 17:743–749.

55. Bock BC, Marcus BH, Pinto BM, Forsyth LH. Maintenance of physical activity following an individualized motivationally tailored intervention. Ann Behav Med 2001; 23(2):79–87.

56. Kerr J, Eves F, Carroll D. Six-month observational study of prompted stair climbing. Preventive Medicine 2001; 33(5):422–427.

CHAPTER **8**

Tobacco dependence, smoking prevention and cessation

Renee Bittoun
Colette Browning

INTRODUCTION

Tobacco smoking has been recognized as a significant behavioural risk factor for many diseases word-wide including heart disease, stroke and lung diseases. The World Health Organization estimates that smoking-related diseases kill one in 10 adults globally.[1] Tobacco smoking is known to cause almost 20 000 deaths per annum in Australia and leads the cause of mortality and morbidity of all drugs of dependency combined.[2] In the UK 114 000 people per annum die from smoking-related diseases equating to 20% of the deaths in the UK per annum.[3] In the US over the period 1995–1999, 440 000 people died per annum from smoking-related causes and expenditure on smoking-related diseases is estimated to be in the order of $157 billion per year.[4] In Australia it is estimated that the social cost of smoking to the Australian community is $12.7 billion annually.[2]

Historically the behaviour of smoking was seen by some as 'dirty, obsessive, lazy and self-indulgent' and at best was considered a bad habit that could be arrested with will power, behavioural changes and some perseverance.[5] In the latter half of the 20th century an inordinate amount of scientific research has shone light on this addictive behaviour but the term 'habit' is unlikely to be used in the lexicon of researchers of tobacco use today.[6] Their discoveries regarding tobacco use and nicotine dependence are an exemplary study of the nature of addictions. Thus in order to aid smokers in quitting a better understanding of the current evidence regarding tobacco use and the advances that have been made is essential.

In countries where there have been concerted efforts by governments to reduce smoking rates through public education and legislative interventions, it is pleasing to note that smoking rates have decreased. Reported daily tobacco use has diminished in Australia from approximately 45% of males smoking in the 1950s to 19.5% in 2001. This reduction is one of the best in the Western world[7] and is mainly due to the implementation of the vigorous public anti-smoking campaigns that began in the 1980s as a result of the overwhelming medical evidence linking smoking and ill health. From 1955 programs were developed in Australia to help smokers quit. Many private organizations used hypnotherapy and acupuncture (although neither have been shown to be particularly efficacious[8]) and the Five Day Plan of group counselling conducted by the Seventh Day Adventist Organization was widely available. Few studies were conducted to assess the success of these programs. Clinics and programs devoted to smoking cessation began in the 1970s. The 'Quit For Life' media campaigns commenced in Sydney in 1983 and were followed in Melbourne in 1986. Surveys showed responses to anti-smoking advertising resulted in 2.8% quit rates in the general smoking population.[9]

Since the mid-1990s in Australia there has been a systematic approach to tobacco control through the National Tobacco Campaign (NTC). A special issue of Tobacco Control in 2003 describes the various components and outcomes of the campaign.[10] The NTC involved collaboration between the Federal and State governments as well as the Cancer Council, involved media campaigns and Quitline, a telephone advice/counselling service provided by the Cancer Council.[11] The focus of the campaign was on the harmful effects of tobacco use and included mass media advertising. The campaign was aimed at adults between 18 and 40 years of age and also targeted those from lower socioeconomic groups and culturally and linguistically diverse backgrounds. By 2001 smoking rates hade reduced to 25% for men and 21% for women.[12] Internationally these results were regarded as highly successful. Though small percentage reductions these results however translate to many thousands of annual quitters.[10] However over the campaign period the price of cigarettes also increased significantly, smoke free environments were legislated and nicotine replacement therapies were marketed by pharmaceutical companies.[10]

There is evidence that the steady drop in smoking prevalence has begun to plateau in Australia. This may be due to the target becoming harder to treat.[13] Increasingly a role has developed for pharmacological interventions to aid this harder target group. Today tobacco use in Australia has become an age and socioeconomic related phenomenon. Younger people and those of lower socioeconomic status are more likely to be smokers. For example 18.7% of males from white-collar occupations smoke compared to 40.9% of blue-collar workers. There is, as elsewhere in the world, a high incidence of smoking in those with mental health concerns and in indigenous populations.[13] In Australia 51% of indigenous people currently smoke.

In the UK smoking rates have been falling since the mid-seventies but have plateaued since 1990. In 2002, 27% of women and 25% of men smoked.[14] The prevalence of smoking in young teenagers has remained at 9 to 11% since 1998. There has been a reduction in smoking rates for boys aged 15 years from 24% in 1982 to 18% in 2003 but smoking rates in girls over this period have remained stable at around 25–26%.[15] In the US, 25% of men and 21% of women smoke. Of those living in poverty 33% smoke. Education level impacts on smoking rates. Of those with 9–11 years education 35% smoke while only 12% of those with more than 16 years of education smoke.[16]

While smoking rates in countries such as the UK, US and Australia have dropped other countries show alarming rates of smoking. For example in China, the Republic of Korea and Cambodia 67% of men smoke while in Japan and Malaysia 51% of men smoke.[1]

Nicotine action, addiction and withdrawal

Nicotine is a fast-acting drug with a short activity (half-life). The most effective means of delivering nicotine to the brain is through smoking. It encourages the expression in the brain of a wide array of neurotransmitter substances that all have very positive neurological effects in some people. There is growing evidence for the heritability of tobacco dependence.[17] With as little as one inhalation from a cigarette, addicted smokers immediately feel less anxious, less moody, are able to concentrate more effectively, feel less distressed, less hungry, less aggressive and are relieved of strong urges to smoke. These positively reinforcing effects that occur very quickly are the bases for nicotine dependence.[18]

Dependent smokers finely titrate (or adjust) their nicotine blood levels by inhaling deeper or longer to effect a higher nicotine level, or inhaling lighter and puffing quicker to lower levels. Many smokers 'self-medicate' by smoking tobacco to counteract anxiety or a depressed mood. Smokers smoke both for these positive rewards gained and the relief of reduced withdrawal symptoms.

The brain areas affected by nicotine, by implication, influence their respective roles in human behaviour. There are potential nicotine receptor sites on every neuron (nerve cell) in the brain, and therefore every receptor in the brain could be affected. However, there is evidence that individuals have different numbers of accessible receptor sites and that these may be genetically predetermined.[17]

Most smokers show at least some symptoms of tobacco withdrawal. It is a well-documented syndrome comprising a combination of anxiety, distress, aggressiveness, urges to smoke, inability to concentrate, increase in appetite and general moodiness.[19] These acute symptoms occur in some smokers even between cigarettes as nicotine blood levels quickly fall and may certainly manifest to some degree in many smokers within hours of their last intake when nicotine plasma levels have fallen to very low levels. Acute withdrawals can persist for days or weeks but are generally finite within a timeframe of two weeks. Longer-term symptoms of withdrawal can include depression and infrequent but irritating urges to smoke linked to situations of psychological distress and other strong, often negative triggers. Smokers have learned that these trigger events can be 'cured' by smoking.[20] Other physical symptoms of withdrawal that may occur within weeks of quitting include mouth ulcers and a cough which, ironically, may appear for the first time or increase when having quit smoking.

Smokers have also learned the beneficial neurological effects of smoking that can occur in combination with other substances such as alcohol, caffeine and cannabis. There are potent cue-conditioned responses resulting in strong urges to smoke that accompany the use of these substances.[21] Smokers are known to consume at least twice the amount of alcohol and caffeine as non-smokers and to suffer alcohol or caffeine toxicity on quitting smoking.[19]

Individual differences in smokers

Smokers are not a homogeneous group. In the 1970s Fagerstrom was one of the first scientists to show that smokers ranged in dependency from mild to moderate to severe levels of tobacco dependency and that response to smoking cessation initiatives was related to levels of dependency. Fagerstrom developed the first of many smoking questionnaires that correlated active smoking to levels of dependency. Ability to quit was shown to be directly related to measurable levels of addiction.[22,23] Multiple attempts to quit unsuccessfully have also been shown to correlate with higher levels of dependency.[24] There is substantial evidence both in Australia and overseas that most smokers want to quit.[25] However relapse is endemic in smokers who make an unaided quit attempt with 50% to 75% relapsing within one week of a concerted quit attempt, and more than 62% within the first two weeks with an ever reducing likelihood of relapsing after three months. At best, between 5 to15% of smokers committed to quitting on their own are still not smoking one year later.[24]

It is evident that some smokers have few symptoms of withdrawal when nicotine deprived; many spontaneously cease smoking without aid and do not relapse, while others self-report formidable and overwhelming symptoms, and though persistently attempt to quit, always consistently relapse.[24] There is now growing evidence that the fundamental nature of the addiction to nicotine may be dependent on an individual's sensitivity to nicotine in the brain and ability to metabolize nicotine in the liver, much of which seems to be genetically determined.[26,27] There is growing evidence of differences in liver metabolism of nicotine. Poor metabolizers are reported to smoke less and find quitting easier than fast metabolizers. Racial origin can also impact on nicotine metabolism.[28]

Initiation into smoking, that is, the first cigarettes ever smoked, is ruled by a multiplicity of factors including peer pressure, bravado, rebellion, advertising, weight control and curiosity. To date there is no evidence that adolescents who continue to smoke (the vast majority of smokers commence before age 18) are of a particular character trait, personality type, gender (as many boys as girls smoke) or socioeconomic status. Social context and attitudes however play an important role in influencing smoking uptake. A study of children aged 11 to 15 years found that children who had smoked or were current smokers were more likely to live in social contexts where smoking was part of their everyday life. They also held positive attitudes to smoking.[29]

Some researchers believe that the reactions to the very first cigarettes smoked are a clue as to whether a person will go on to smoke continuously. Pomerleau believes that pre-existing sensitivities to nicotine determine long-term use. The more sensitive (or reactive) the first-time smoker is to nicotine the more likely he or she is to go on to become a regular, daily smoker.[30] Nick Martin and his colleagues at the Queensland Institute of Medical Research have contributed considerably to the debate on the genetic predisposition to smoking in their large twin studies.[31] These studies showed that identical twins separated at birth from their parents and each other are likely to be dependent smokers irrespective of personal histories of exposure or non-exposure or environmental and cultural circumstances if their biological parents were dependent smokers.[31] There is now substantial evidence in the scientific literature on the genetic predisposition or heritability of nicotine dependency.

Smoking as a compulsive addictive behaviour

It is inevitable that many smokers, having received such overwhelming chemical joy from smoking and concomitant displeasure from not smoking, should seek to continue to use tobacco regularly, if not simply to allay withdrawals between cigarettes and remain 'normal'. The mood alteration that commonly occurs in other drug dependencies, the 'highs', seem not to occur in smoking. Rather it is the avoidance of the 'lows' that typifies the dependent smoker. The overall emotional effects on the smoker can now be almost directly linked with the increase and then decrease of nicotine in the brain areas directly affected.[32] For example there have been reports of individuals demonstrating an acute lack of concentration or an inability to perform tasks requiring short-term memory during nicotine deprivation which may be directly attributed to the deprivation of nicotine in the area of the brain involved.[33]

In general, smokers report distinct cognitive and behavioural effects from smoking including perceptions of relaxation, euphoria, stimulation, as well as anxiolytic and dysphoric effects. Having successfully initiated into smoking (almost always in adolescence) dependent smokers have thus launched into a cycle of pleasure and displeasure, learning along the way that smoking relieves much of this displeasure almost instantaneously. Relief from symptoms usually occurs within the first few puffs of a cigarette. The learning of the 'relief' factor of smoking becomes an insidious component of a smoker's behaviour. The experience of relief is used in all types of anxiety states or negative situations and events. The brain responds not only chemically to nicotine but also electrically. Profound electroencephalogram (EEG) changes can take place in smokers with and without a cigarette. For example, alpha wave frequency, an index of relaxation, is enhanced within seconds of smoking and then is reduced as the nicotine blood levels abate.

Many smokers in our society are now aware of the impact that smoking has on health and wellbeing, however many persist with it despite this awareness. According to the DSM 1V, one of the criteria for dependency (on any substance) is that the drug is used in the face of the full knowledge of the detrimental effects, both medical and social. Studies have shown that some smokers are not only continuing to smoke in the face of their illnesses but are particularly prone to lying about it.[34] Ultimately this behaviour should not grossly violate the principle of bounded rationality but the evidence of contradictions between desire (not to smoke) and behaviour (smoking) in smokers is very strong. Smoking shows a convincing argument for compulsive addictive behaviour as:

- 96% of smokers smoke daily.
- Few smoke less than 5/day.
- 50% smoke within 30 minutes of waking.
- 48% have not abstained for more than 1 week in the past 5 years.
- 70% of smokers in UK say they wish to quit.
- Heavier smokers wish to quit.
- 79% of smokers have tried to quit, 58% more than once.
- 75% of self-quitting attempts fail in the first week and poignantly, smokers who attempt to quit many times still want to quit.[35]

Smoking prevention and cessation interventions

As previously indicated most smokers would like to give up smoking.[25] A report based on the UK Office of National Statistics Omnibus Survey[36] found that 70% of smokers wished to quit, 79% had tried to quit in the past and 51% said they intended to quit in the next year. Almost all wanted to quit for health-related reasons.

In many countries around the world there have been dramatic spontaneous reductions in smoking when governments have committed to strong anti-smoking campaigns. Educating smokers about the health consequences of smoking through the media, health warnings on tobacco products, the banning of all tobacco advertising, increasing the cost of tobacco through taxation and strong laws prohibiting environmental tobacco smoke exposure have played the most important roles in changing the smoking behaviour of smokers and discouraging its uptake. As well as broad mass-media campaigns and legislative approaches smoking cessation interventions include pharmacological interventions including nicotine replacement and fading, psychological approaches such as group behaviour therapy, hypnotherapy, telephone counselling, and inter-

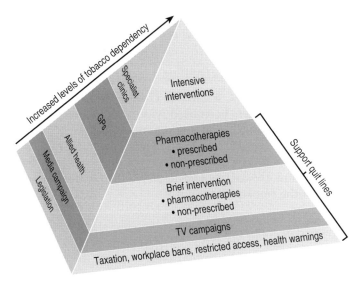

Fig. 8.1 Smoking cessation pyramid. Bittoun, 2005.

ventions incorporating behavioural change models, and health professional advice approaches. Figure 8.1 shows a hierarchy of these smoking cessation approaches. At the bottom of the pyramid are the broader strategies that may help smokers quit spontaneously, while at the top are the more intensive approaches that may be required for the heavily dependent smoker. Settings for interventions have included primary care settings, schools, families and work places. The Cochrane Tobacco Addiction Group provides an excellent range of systematic reviews of these various interventions available online at: http://www.update-software.com/Abstracts/TOBACCOAbstractIndex.htm.

Below we summarize the outcomes of some of the various approaches to smoking cessation. We have limited the scope of the summary to interventions aimed at adult populations. For a review of smoking prevention and control for young people the reader is referred to a number of reviews in the area.[29,37–40]

Individual approaches

Cold-turkey quitting

When questioned, quitting alone, unaided or 'cold turkey' has been shown as the commonest method used by smokers to stop smoking. A tempting assumption from this evidence is that all smokers are therefore best left to quit 'cold turkey' on their own. Unfortunately closer attention reveals that most smokers relapse who attempt cold turkey and that multiple attempts over many years are necessary to achieve a permanent abstinence.[24] In the many studies carried out in the general population of smokers few were stratified into levels of dependency, thus a good assessment of spontaneous (i.e. unaided) quitting by dependency level is as yet unavailable.

Individual telephone counselling: Quitline

In Australia as part of the NTC a national *Quitline* service was established in 1997. Smokers help lines have been used widely as an integrated component of mass media campaigns and smoking cessation programs.[41,42] *Quitline* provides counselling and access to information about quitting smoking. Evaluations of the effectiveness of the approach have been positive. For example over a one year period 3.6% of smokers accessed the *Quitline* and at 12-month follow-up, 28% of the smokers had quit.[43]

Hypnotherapy and acupuncture

There is much anecdotal evidence that both of these therapies have helped many smokers quit smoking (reports of up to 95% abstinence). There is no reported evidence that either hypnotherapy or acupuncture has any effect on withdrawals or relapse prevention.[8] A Cochrane Review of acupuncture for smoking cessation conducted in 2002 concluded 'There is no clear evidence that acupuncture, acupressure, laser therapy or electrostimulation are effective for smoking cessation'[44] (p. 2). Similar conclusions were reached based on a Cochrane review of hypnotherapy for smoking cessation conducted in 1998.[45]

Individual behaviour change approaches: The stages of change model in smoking cessation

Prochaska and his colleagues described smoking cessation as a process rather than an all-or-none phenomenon. Smokers in this model move through different motivational stages from 'no motivation to quit' to 'maintaining the new behaviour'.[46] They describe five stages of change and define the first three stages as measuring levels of intention to quit and the last two stages by (non-smoking) behaviour.[47] This approach has widespread acceptance by health services providing smoking cessation programs. For example a survey of health authorities in England reported in Riemsma et al.[47] found that training courses mainly focused on the stages of change model to explain smoking behaviour change. However, a recent review of stage-based interventions to promote smoking cessation concluded that that there was limited evidence for their effectiveness when compared to non-staged interventions or no intervention.[47] Riemsma and his colleagues examined 23 randomized controlled trials aimed at assessing the effectiveness of stage-based interventions in smoking behaviour change. Of these, eight trials showed evidence in favour of the effectiveness of the approach, 12 trials showed no effects and three trials were inconclusive. Trials that were more likely to confirm the effectiveness of stage-based interventions were more likely to be large or use self-report to assess smoking status. Despite the need to be able to accurately identify an individual's stage of change only two trials provided validation information about the method used to assess the stage of change. The authors also point out that most trials included limited information about the intervention design.

Nicotine replacement therapy (NRT)

Nicotine replacement therapy involves obtaining controlled and reducing doses of nicotine through gum, patches, lozenges or sprays. Efficacy of treatment is determined by continued biochemically proven abstinence of at least six months from commencement of treatment. A recent Cochrane review on the effectiveness of different forms of nicotine replacement therapy for smoking cessation[48] found that NRT significantly increased the odds of quitting. Odds ratio in therapies is the effectiveness of the active treatment versus a placebo. Odds of 1 implies no effect, odds of 2 implies twice as effective and so on. Table 8.1 shows the odds ratios for the various nicotine delivery methods.[48]

NRT is often combined with advice or counselling. Education on the nature of tobacco dependency, withdrawal symptoms and the time-course of withdrawals, encouragement and evidence-based tips, frequent follow-ups and adjustment or changes in pharmacotherapy when needed have all shown to be important components of counselling. However studies of the efficacy of NRT interventions that included advice or counselling have found that less than half of the participants continue not to smoke after one year (see Table 8.2). While odds ratios seem impressive, at best with any single pharmacotherapy, from 30% to 40% of smokers were shown to still not smoke one year after treatment depending on the

Table 8.1   Odds ratios for nicotine replacement therapy for smoking cessation

Type of NRT	Odds ratio
Nicotine gum	1.66
Nicotine patches	1.81
Nasal spray	2.35
Inhaled nicotine	2.14
Nicotine lozenges	2.05

As cited in Silagy et al.[48]

Table 8.2   Efficacy of NRT when combined with advice or counselling

Cessation advice/counselling	Percentage who were non–smokers at 12 months
No action	1
Brief advice in primary care	5
Brief advice plus NRT in primary care	10
Intensive professional counselling alone	15–20
Intensive professional counselling plus NRT	30–40

Based on Fagestrom,[49] Silagy et al[50] and Baillie et al.[51]

intensity of the adjuvant advice or counseling.[8,49–51] Hence the majority of smokers do not quit smoking despite formal medical or counselling interventions.

The nicotine delivered by NRT is often inadequate for some smokers and they may continue to need to smoke, and/or have withdrawals despite commencing on these therapies. Many clinicians have felt it appropriate to supplement nicotine patch therapy with nicotine gum. Unpublished data from a trial conducted at St Vincent's Clinic in Australia has shown greatly increased long-term efficacy when smokers, who were stratified into levels of dependency, were given a combination of nicotine patch and a nicotine gum. Fagerstrom et al have shown distinct advantages in a combination therapy trial that was double-blind and placebo controlled.[52] There is scope for the combination of patches, wearing several at once, and the combination of patch and other, perhaps inhaled forms of nicotine.[53]

Nicotine fading by reduction of numbers of cigarettes or nicotine content

Many smokers have felt comforted by the notion that by reducing the so-called nicotine intake by reducing the number of cigarettes they smoke per day or reducing the intake of nicotine by smoking the so-called milder cigarettes would assist them in quitting smoking. A smoker is most likely to titrate the nicotine content required so that either more cigarettes are smoked when the concentration of nicotine is lowered or deeper inhalations are made as compensation for reducing the number of daily cigarettes smoked. However if strict smoking criteria are adhered to, that is a regimented daily reduction, this method may have some positive outcome. If numbers of cigarettes are strictly allocated and reduction of nicotine content is persistently towards an outcome of no smoking/nicotine altogether, then some reports have shown 25% confirmed abstinence at one year.

Other, similar, methods have been recommended to smokers to help them quit. For example, delaying a cigarette by one hour per day over several days with the aim to delay further into the day until no more cigarettes are smoked. Ultimately every cigarette that is smoked in this procedure becomes increasingly more rewarding and reinforcing, thus paradoxically enhancing the dependency as smokers lurch towards the next cigarette. Inevitably the likelihood of success using this tactic is very small and does not rule out or even reduce smokers of the symptoms of withdrawal once they are nicotine free. Using nicotine-free cigarettes is another method commonly used by smokers in nicotine fading. No study has ever shown this as an acceptable technique to quit smoking. Unfortunately for the smoker, in a vain attempt to derive some physical pleasure from inhaling this type of cigarette, the tendency is to inhale deeply and extract more carbon monoxide and particulate matter than ever before.

Other pharmacological interventions

Bupropion, traded as Zyban and Wellbutrin, increases the release of dopamine and noradrenaline, and it is these activities that are believed to be the cause of the positive effects it has in smoking cessation. In the US this treatment is the only aid in smoking cessation (apart from NRT) cleared for marketing by the Food and Drug Administration. The safety and efficacy of bupropion has been well-studied,[54] however there is some debate as to the long-term efficacy above placebo effect using this treatment.[55] There is currently no indicator that best predicts efficacy in smoking cessation pharmacotherapy for any given smoking patient. Suitability for nicotine replacement therapy (NRT) and bupropion (Zyban) is contingent on medical status, however patients may find one type of treatment more practical than another.

Clonidine (clonidine hydrochloride) is a post-synaptic agonist reducing sympathetic activity, mimicking a nicotine effect. Clonidine, an anti-hypertensive medication, has been used in the treatment of opiate withdrawals and has shown some efficacy in the treatment of nicotine withdrawal. In tablet form however there are considerable side effects, particularly the lowering of blood pressure and constipation. Transdermal clonidine patch has shown some benefit in acute nicotine withdrawals with fewer side effects and considerable relief of cravings, anxiety and irritability, though it continues to be disfavoured as a treatment in smoking cessation.[56]

Buspirone is a serotonergic agonist that acts as an anxiolytic. In patients whose major symptom of withdrawal may be anxiety, this agonist has shown some positive effects. However a Cochrane review of the effectiveness of anxiolytics for smoking cessation conducted in 2000 concluded that the evidence was weak.[57]

Antidepressants are increasingly popular in smoking cessation for the treatment of dysphoria so commonly a symptom of withdrawal and the cause of relapse. As these medications may have delayed onset of effects, it has been recommended that treatment should commence several weeks prior to a quit date. Combination therapy, the combination of antidepressants and nicotine replacement is currently undergoing trial and evaluation. A Cochrane review conducted in 2003 found that nortriptyline and bupropion increased the odds of cessation.[57]

Naltrexone, has been considered appropriate in smoking cessation, as its opioid antagonistic effects may be helpful in reducing the positive effects of smoking. Trials are underway in respect of these effects. Mecamylamine is also another blocker of the positive effects of nicotine. This antagonist has also shown poor efficacy due mainly to side effects. Particularly severe constipation is known to deter the user.[58] Silver nitrate and silver acetate have been used as aversive substances to produce a 'bad taste' while smoking. Not only does lack of compliance interfere with successful abstinence but also continuation to smoke despite the bad taste is proof of the lack of efficacy of these products. Glucose or dextrose as a treatment for smoking cessation is a recent promising innovation based on the increased demand for sweet substances that smokers manifest during the withdrawal phase. It is hypothesized that either the satiation effects of glucose dampen a desire to smoke or that glucose directly affects the neuronal systems involved with nicotine. A few trials to date have shown encouraging outcomes.[59]

Small group interventions

Interventions such as group behaviour therapy and family-based approaches have been used to facilitate smoking cessation. A Cochrane review of 52 trials where group therapy was compared to self-help, individual counselling, other intervention types or no intervention, found that group therapy was more effective than no intervention controls but no more effective than individual counselling. Support and skills training normally provided by group approaches were not enhanced by the inclusion of specific cognitive or behavioural skills.[60]

Community-based interventions

Community-based interventions provide a vehicle for incorporating individual and social factors to reduce smoking rates and such approaches are gaining widespread appeal. However the success of such approaches for smoking cessation has been limited. The US Community Intervention Trial for Smoking Cessation (COMMIT), a large randomized trial involving 11 communities over five years, is an example of such an approach.[61–63] The intervention was targeted to adults and used community organization and participation as the theoretical basis of the intervention. Teachers, health professionals and volunteers delivered the intervention through worksites, churches businesses and schools. Mass media, advertising and resource guides were incorporated in the intervention. While follow-up analyses found a reduction in the prevalence of smoking in all communities there was no difference in reduction in overall prevalence between the intervention and comparison communities. However in those smoking less than 25 cigarettes per day the intervention group showed a higher quit rate. In Australia The Cancer Action in Rural Towns project (CART), a randomized trial,[64] targeted several health risk and preventive behaviours including smoking, and breast, skin and cervical cancer screening in 10 pairs of rural towns. Community organizations, worksites, schools, health services and the media were used to deliver the intervention. Analyses conducted at 3 to 3.5 years from the start of the intervention found no differences in quit rates for women between the intervention and comparison towns. However men in the intervention towns showed higher quit rates than men in the comparison towns. A Cochrane review of 32 community based-studies of smoking cessation (including COMMIT and CART) found that reduction in smoking prevalence was modest.[65]

CONCLUSION

While population smoking rates have decreased in many Western countries there is evidence that this trend has plateaued and that we need to target certain groups in the community such as those from low socioeconomic backgrounds, those with mental illnesses, young women and indigenous groups. Worldwide many countries still exhibit alarming smoking rates. Countries where success is most evident, such as in Australia, have employed national strategies to address smoking prevention and cessation using multiple channels including mass media, smoke-free legislation, high tobacco taxes, and coordinated and systematic advice and interventions for smokers.

Most of the interventions reviewed in this chapter have targeted the individual. Nicotine replacement therapy has demonstrated success at six months follow-up but the long-term efficacy of such approaches have been questioned. Other pharmacological treatments have shown mixed effects with antidepressants showing some promise to address depression as a withdrawal symptom. Telephone counselling and telephone advice lines appear useful as part of combined strategies for smoking cessation. Group intervention approaches appear to provide no added benefit above individual counselling but may be more cost effective. Individual behaviour change approaches using models such as the Stages of Change Model have also shown mixed results. Community-based interventions have demonstrated reductions in smoking rates within specific cohorts such as moderate smokers and men but overall outcomes from such approaches are modest.

There is increasing evidence that integrated approaches are needed that recognize the role of the social environment in smoking cessation. A survey of Australians aged 14 years and over found that independent of education level smoking cessation was strongly associated with knowing that tobacco smoke was harmful, living in households where smoking was restricted and having few friends who smoke.[66] Despite the great strides taken in most countries to reduce smoking rates more work needs to be done in targeting specific hard to reach (or change) groups. To do this we need to better understand the social factors and psychological that influence smoking uptake. Toumbourou's analysis of motivational influences on drug use (see Chapter 6) could well be applied in the smoking arena.

References

1. WHO. The World Health Report. Geneva: WHO; 2003.
2. Collins DJ, Lapsley HM. The social costs of smoking in Australia. NSW Public Health Bulletin 2002; 15:92–94.
3. Peto R, Lopez AD, Boreham J, Thun M, Heath C. Mortality from smoking in developed countries 1950–2000. Oxford: Oxford University Press; 1994.
4. Center for Disease Control. Annual smoking – attributable mortality, years of potential life lost, and economic costs – United States, 1995–1999. Morbidity and Mortality Weekly Report 2002; 51(14):300–303.
5. Larson P, Haag H, Silvette H. Tobacco experimental and clinical studies. Baltimore: Williams & Wilkins; 1961.
6. Perkins K. Tobacco smoking is dependence, not a 'habit'. Nicotine and Tobacco Research 1999; 1(2):127–128.
7. Mackay J, Eriksen M. The tobacco atlas. Brighton: World Health Organisation 2002.
8. US Department of Health and Human Services. Treating tobacco use and dependence. Clinical Practice Guideline. In: Online. Available: www.surgeongeneral.gov/tobacco/default.htm.; June 2000.

9. Dwyer T, Pierce J, et al. Evaluation of the Sydney 'Quit for Life' anti-smoking campaign. Part 2. Changes in smoking prevalence. Medical Journal of Australia 1985; 144(7):344–347.

10. Woodward K. Tobacco control on Australia. Tobacco Control 2003; 12(Suppl II):ii1–ii2.

11. Hill D, Carroll T. Australia's national tobacco campaign. Tobacco Control 2003; 12(Suppl II):ii9–ii14.

12. White V, Hill D, Siahpush M, et al. How has the prevalence of cigarette smoking changed among Australian adults? Trends in smoking prevalence between 1980 and 2001. Tobacco Control 2003; 12(Suppl II):ii23–29.

13. Dengenhardt L, Hall W. The relationship between tobacco use, substance-use disorders and mental health; results from the National Survey of Mental Health and Well-being. Nicotine and Tobacco Research 2001; 3(3):225–234.

14. Jarvis M. Monitoring cigarette smoking prevalence in Britain in a timely fashion. Addiction 2003; 98:1569–1574.

15. Department of Health. Drug use, smoking and drinking among young people in England 2004.

16. National Center for Health Statistics. Smoking. http://www.cdc.gov/nchs/fastats/smoking.htm; 2004.

17. Rosecrans J, Karan L. Neurobehavioural mechanisms of nicotine action: Role in the initiation and maintenance of tobacco dependence. Journal of Substance Abuse Treatment 1993; 10:161–170.

18. Benowitz C. Pharmacologic aspects of cigarette smoking and nicotine addiction. New England Journal of Medicine 1988; 319(20):1318–1330.

19. Bittoun R. The management of nicotine addiction. A guide for counselling in smoking cessation. Sydney: University of Sydney Press; 1998.

20. Glassman A, Covey L, et al. Smoking cessation and the course of major depression: A follow-up study. Lancet 2001; 357:1929–1932.

21. Shiffman S, Murray E. Situational determinants of coping in smoking relapse crises. Journal of Applied Social Psychology 1987; 17(1):3–15.

22. Fagerstrom K. Measuring degree of physical dependence to tobacco smoking with reference to individualization of treatment. Addictive Behaviours 1978; 17:367–377.

23. Hajek P. Individual differences in quitting smoking. British Journal of Addiction 1991; 86(5):555–558.

24. Garvey A, Bliss R, Hitchcock J, et al. Predictors of smoking relapse among self-quitters: A report of the normative aging study. Addictive Behaviors 1992; 17:367–377.

25. Hill D, White V, Scollo M. Smoking behaviours of Australian adults in 1995: Trends and concerns. Medical Journal of Australia 1998; 168(5):209–213.

26. Pomerleau O, Collins A, Shiffman S, et al. Why some people smoke and others do not: New perspectives. Journal of Consulting and Clinical Psychology 1993; 61(5):723–731.

27. Picciotto M, Zoli M, Rimondini R, et al. Acetylcholine receptors containing the beta 2 subunit are involved in the reinforcing properties of nicotine. Nature 1998; 391(8):173–177.

28. Tyndal R, Sellers E. Genetic variations in CYP2A6-mediated nicotine metabolism alters smoking behaviour. Therapeutic Drug Monitoring 2002; 24(1):163–171.

29. Buller D, Borland R, Woodall W, Hall J, Burris-Woodall P, Voeks J. Understanding factors that influence smoking uptake. Tobacco Control 2003; 12(Suppl 4): iv16–iv 25.

30. Pomerleau O, Kardia S. Genetic research on smoking. Health Psychology 1999; 18(1):3–6.

31. Heath A, Martin N. Genetic models for the natural history of smoking: evidence for a genetic influence on smoking persistence. Addictive Behaviors 1993; 18:19–34.

32. Wonnacott S, Russell M, Stolerman IP. Nicotine psychopharmacology: Molecular, cellular, and behavioural aspects. Oxford: Oxford University Press; 1990.

33. Warburton D, Rusted J, Fowler J. Comparison of the attentional and consolidation hypotheses for the facilitation of memory by nicotine. Psychopharmacology 1992; 108(4):443–447.

34. Bittoun R, McMahon M, Bryant D. Smoking in hospitalised patients. Addictive Behaviours 1991; 16:79–81.

35. Stolerman P. Evidence that nicotine is addictive. The effects of nicotine on biological systems II. Montreal, Canada; 1994.

36. Lader D, Meltzer H. Smoking related behaviour and attitudes. London: Office of National Statistics; 2002.

37. Lantz PM, Jacobsson PD, Warner KE, Wasserman J, Pollacj HA, Berson J, et al. Investing in youth tobacco control: A review of smoking prevention and control strategies. Tobacco Control 2000; 9:47–63.

38. Stead L, Lancaster T. A systematic review of interventions for preventing tobacco sales to minors. Tobacco Control 2000; 9:1169–1176.

39. Wakefield M, Chaloupka F. Effectiveness of comprehensive tobacco control programmes in reducing teenage smoking in the USA. Tobacco Control 2000; 9:177–186.

40. Sowden A, Arblaster L, Stead L. Community interventions for preventing smoking in young people (Cochrane review). Chichester: John Wiley; 2004.

41. Zhu S-H, Anderson C, Johnson C. A centralised telephone service for tobacco cessation: the Californian experience. Tobacco Control 2000; 9(Suppl II):ii48–55.

42. Platt S, Tannahill A, Watson J, et al. Effectiveness of antismoking telephone helpline: Follow-up survey. British Medical Journal 1997; 314:1371.

43. Miller C, Wakefield M, Roberts L. Uptake and effectiveness of the Australian telephone Quitline service in the context of a mass media campaign. Tobacco Control 2003; 12(Suppl II):ii53–ii58.

44. White A, Rampes H, Ernst E. Acupuncture for smoking cessation Cochrane Review Issue 3. Chichester: John Wiley; 2004.

45. Abbott N, Stead L, White A, Barnes J. Hypnotherapy for smoking cessation Cochrane Review Issue 3. Chichester: John Wiley; 2004.

46. Prochaska JO, DiClemente CC. The Transtheoretical Approach: Crossing traditional boundaries of therapy. Homewood, Ill: Dow Jones-Irwin; 1984.

47. Riemsma R, Pattenden J, Bridle C, Sowden A, Mather L, Watt I, et al. Systematic review of the effectiveness of stage based interventions to promote smoking cessation. British Medical Journal 2003; 326:1175–1177.

48. Silagy C, Lancaster T, Stead L, Mant D, Fowler G. Nicotine replacement therapy for smoking cessation Cochrane Review Issue 3. Chichester: John Wiley; 2004.

49. Fagerstrom K. Review of nicotine gum and tailoring treatment to types of smokers. Journal of Smoking Related Diseases 1994; 5(Suppl 1):179–148.

50. Silagy C, Mant D, Godfrey F. Meta-analysis on efficacy of nicotine replacement therapies in smoking cessation. Lancet 1994; 343:139–142.

51. Baillie A, Mattick R, Hall W, et al. Meta-analytic review of the efficacy of smoking cessation interventions. Drug and Alcohol Review 1994; 13:157–170.

52. Fagerstrom K, Schneider N, Lunell E. Effectiveness of nicotine patch and nicotine gum as individual versus combined treatments for tobacco withdrawal symptoms. Psychopharmacology 1993; 111:271–277.

53. Bittoun R. Combination therapy in the hard-to-treat smoker. In: 2nd National Conference on Tobacco Control, Adelaide; 2002.

54. Fiore M, Smith S, Gorenby D, et al. The effectiveness of the nicotine patch for smoking cessation. A meta-analysis. JAMA 1994; 27(24):1940–1947.

55. Simon J, Duncan C, Carmody T, et al. Bupropion for smoking cessation. A randomized trial. Arch Intern Med 2004; 164(16):1797–1803.

56. Gourlay S, Stead L, Benowitz N. Clonidine for smoking cessation. Cochrane Database of Systematic Reviews 2000; (CD000058).

57. Hughes J, Stead L, Lancaster T. Anxiolytics for smoking cessation Cochrane Review Issue 3. Chichester: John Wiley; 2004.

58. Clarke P. Tobacco smoking, genes and dopamine. Lancet 1998; 352(9122):84–85.

59. West R. Glucose for smoking cessation. Does it have a role? CNS Drugs 2001; 15:261–265.

60. Stead L, Lancaster T. Group behaviour therapy programmes for smoking cessation Cochrane Review Issue 3. Chichester: John Wiley; 2004.

61. The Commit Research Group Community intervention trial for smoking cessation (COMMIT). Summary of design and intervention. Journal of the national Cancer Institute 1991(83):1620–1628.

62. The COMMIT Research Group Community intervention trial for smoking cessation (COMMIT). II Changes in adult cigarette smoking and prevalence. American Journal of Public Health 1995; 85:193–200.

63. Taylor S, Ross N, Cummings M, Glasgow R, Goldsmith C, Zanna P, et al. Community Intervention Trial for Smoking Cessation (COMMIT): Changes in community attitudes to smoking health. Education Research 1998; 13:109–122.

64. Hancock L, Sanson-Fisher R, Perkins J, McClintock A, Howley P, Gibberd R. The effect of a community action program on adult quit smoking rates in rural Australian towns: The CART project. Preventive Medicine 2001; 32:118–127.

65. Secker-Walker R, Gnich W, Platt S, Lancaster T. Community interventions for reducing smoking among adults Cochrane Review Issue 3. Chichester: John Wiley; 2004.

66. Siahpush M, Borland R, Scollo M. Factors associated with smoking cessation in a national sample of Australians. Nicotine and Tobacco Research 2003; 5:597–602.

CHAPTER **9**

Management of depression

Helen Lindner

INTRODUCTION

Depression is a condition that affects an individual in terms of behavioural, motivational, affective, cognitive, and somatic functioning.[1] The range of depression can be from a low or mild level of negative mood through to severe depression or major depressive disorder (MDD). Depression is not just a 'state of mind', but is related to chemical changes in the brain, and the development of negative thoughts and behaviours.[1] Typical symptoms of depression include constant feelings of sadness, irritability, or tension; decreased interest or pleasure in the individual's usual activities or hobbies; loss of energy, or feeling tired even when not engaging in activity; a change in appetite, with significant weight loss or weight gain; a change in sleeping patterns, such as a difficulty with sleep onset, awakening earlier than usual, or sleeping too much; restlessness or feeling slowed down; decreased ability to make decisions or concentrate; feelings of worthlessness, hopelessness, or guilt; or thoughts of suicide or death.

World Health Organization's[2] International Classification of Disease (ICD-10) states that depression includes the following symptoms:

- Two weeks of abnormal depressed mood.
- Loss of interest and decreased energy.

- Loss of confidence.
- Excessive guilt.
- Recurrent thoughts of death.
- Poor concentration.
- Agitation or retardation.
- Sleep disturbances.
- Change in appetite.

WHO proposes that a diagnosis of mild depression would include the first two symptoms and at least one other symptom, whereas severe depression would be diagnosed when the first two symptoms, and at least five other symptoms, had been reported by an individual.

Another classification system for the diagnosis of depression comes from the Diagnostic and Statistical Manual of Mental Disorders, Fourth Edition (DSM-IV).[3] The DSM-IV presents a classification for major depressive disorder (MDD). This disorder is diagnosed when there has been one or more major depressive episodes of '...at least two weeks of depressed mood or loss of interest accompanied by at least four additional symptoms of depression' (DSM-IV[3] p. 345). The additional four symptoms of depression are to be selected from significant weightloss or gain when not dieting, insomnia or hypersomnia nearly every day, psychomotor agitation, fatigue or loss of energy, feelings of worthlessness or excessive or inappropriate guilt, diminished ability to think or concentrate, and recurrent thoughts of death.[3]

The term dysthymia is used to describe a milder state of depression, where depressed mood is evident '... for more days than not, accompanied by additional depressive symptoms that do not meet criteria for a major depressive episode' (DSM-IV[3] p. 345), and for at least two years. This condition resembles major depression, but is characterized by a lesser degree of symptom-severity. Other mood disorders, such as seasonal affective disorder, postpartum depression, premenstrual dysphoric disorder (PDD), and bipolar disorder, can display similar symptomatology. Seasonal affective disorder has a recurrence of the symptoms during certain seasons of the year, but involves symptoms that are seen with any major depressive episode. Postpartum depression can occur in women following the recent birth of a baby. It typically occurs in the first few months after delivery, but can happen within the first year following birth. Postpartum depression is different from the 'baby blues', which tend to occur the first few days after delivery and resolve within a short period of time. The symptoms of postpartum depression are typical of those seen with any major depressive episode. Premenstrual dysphoric disorder (PDD) is the experience of negative mood during the premenstrual or late luteal phase of the menstrual cycle. Women who experience this type of depressive symptomatology report a remission of these feelings once the menstrual flow has commenced. Due to the short-term cyclical nature of PDD, this type of depression does not respond well to pharmacology. However, coping skills-focused interventions, such as cognitive behaviour therapy, has been shown to be efficacious in reducing premenstrual symptomatology, including depressed mood.[4]

A severe mood disorder that is different from MDD, is bipolar disorder. These two types of depression require quite different pharmacological treatments. This chapter will not include any further discussion of bipolar disorder.

CAUSES OF DEPRESSION

No single cause has been identified for the onset of depression. However, a number of risk factors, or a combination of risk factors, have been identified as associated with the experience of depressive symptoms. Genetics has been found to play an important part in the onset of depression, where individuals who have a family history of depression can be more prone to depression themselves. Life stressors and traumas, such as financial problems, a relationship breakup, or the death of a loved one can precede depression. Additionally, depression can be experienced following changes in life-situations, like starting a new job, leaving school, or getting married. Another factor related to depression has been found to be low self-esteem and a negative outlook on life situations. However, the causal link between these factors and depression are unclear, as these traits may actually be caused by low-level depression, such as dysthymia. Serious medical conditions like heart disease, diabetes, cancer, and HIV have consistently been found to be associated with depression. It is worthwhile noting that the diagnosis criteria of the DSM-IV[3] (p. 356) included a note: 'Do not include symptoms that are clearly due to a general medical condition'. This comment emphasizes the need to be thorough in the assessment procedure of depression when there is a co-morbidity of a physical illness that could include depressive-type symptoms related to pain or medication. Depression can cause medical conditions to worsen, as the physical and cognitive symptoms of depression can weaken the immune system and influence the effective management of conditions, such as chronic pain. Furthermore, depression can be caused by medications used to treat medical conditions.

Co-morbidity of other disorders has been found to be common with depression. For example, anxiety disorders, eating disorders, schizophrenia, and substance abuse are often reported concurrently with depression. The causal link between the co-morbidity of conditions has not been resolved, but there has definitely been an indication of a strong risk association.

THE EPIDEMIOLOGY OF DEPRESSION

Depression has been identified as one of the most prevalent forms of mental illness,[5] and has been reported to be the most common single reason for attending a general practitioner.[6]

The burden of depression on society and individuals is represented to be substantial.[7] Thomas and Morris investigated the cost of depression in a UK sample, and estimated that the cost of depression was in excess of £9 billion with £370 million of this cost being associated with direct treatment costs.

They also reported that 2615 lives, and 1097 million working days were lost due to depression in 2000. Furthermore, the substantial burden of depression has been documented in Australia.[8]

Ustun et al.[9] estimated the burden of depression for 2000 in terms of disability adjusted life years (DALYs). They reported that depression was the fourth leading cause of disease burden (4.4% of total DALYs), and that depression accounts for approximately 12% of all total years lived with disability worldwide.

Dewa et al.[10] identified that depression-related workplace disability was a major problem in Canada, with 1521 employees from financial and insurance companies reporting depression-related absences from work for at least ten consecutive work days (2% of workforce), with approximately 12% of these individuals reporting more than one short-term disability episode in the prior 12 months.

Gender differences in the experience of depression have been widely reported. For example, Hunt and Yanke[11] reported that females were approximately 1.5 times more likely to suffer from depressive symptoms than males, with odds ratio of 1.58 (95% CI, 1.06–2.37). A number of sources of statistics associated with the prevalence of depression are presented in Table 9.1. These data indicate a higher rate of depression in the European samples, compared to the North American samples. However, the assessment of depression in the Chisholm et al.[12] paper was specifically for those patients who met the DSM-IV criteria for a diagnosis of major depressive disorder, and therefore could reflect a restricted assessment of a broader range of depression, as measured in the other studies.

It has been noted by numerous investigators that the co-morbidity of depression with physical illness, particularly chronic illnesses, tends to add to the burden and financial cost of depression (e.g. Chisholm et al.[12]). Chisholm et al.[12] reported that the economic consequences of depression were more highly related to the presence of medical co-morbidity than by the severity of depression symptomatology.

Table 9.1 Statistics on the prevalence of depression in European and North American samples

Researchers	Sample–age	Males	Females
Pelkonen et al. (2003)	Finnish 22 years	9 %	13 %
Ayuso-Mateos et al. (2001)	European 8–65 years	6.61 %	10.05 %
Chisholm et al. (2004)	North America		
	15–29 years	3.10 %	6.02 %
	30–44 years	3.01 %	4.65 %
	45–59 years	2.23 %	3.78 %
	60–69 years	2.20 %	3.53 %

Additionally, a study undertaken by Surtees et al.[13] of functional health status, chronic medical conditions, and depression in a sample of 20 921 UK residents, reported that depression had an independent impact on functional health, which was equivalent in magnitude to that associated with chronic physical illness.

Two papers quantified the increase in costs for those with both diabetes and depression compared with those with diabetes alone. Ciechanowski et al.[14] relied on a sample of several hundred individuals with diabetes in a single health plan and showed that those with greater depressive symptoms had between 51% and 86% higher costs. Egede et al.[15] used data from 825 individuals with diabetes who participated in the Medical Expenditure Panel Survey (MEPS), and showed that those with both major depression (85 patients) and diabetes had 4.5 times greater annual health care expenditures than those with diabetes alone. It is noted that the number of patients who reported major depression represented 10.3% of the sample. This percentage reinforces other research findings that depression is a major health concern for our communities.

The presence of co-morbid depressive symptoms has been reported to have a significant impact on health outcomes, health-care utilization, and overall functioning in patients with chronic illness. Depression has additional importance in the chronic illness condition of diabetes because of its association with poor adherence with diabetes treatment, poor glycaemic control, and an increased risk of micro- and macrovascular disease complications.[16] Research has found that depression in individuals with diabetes has been associated with poor adherence to dietary recommendation, and hyperglycaemia,[16,17] poor metabolic control disorder,[18] complications of diabetes, decreased quality of life, and increased health-care use and expenditure.[14] To investigate the association of depression and adherence, DiMatteo et al.[17] conducted a meta-analysis. The relationship between depression and non-compliance was substantial and significant, with an odds ratio of 3.03 (95% CI, 1.96–4.89). That is, compared with non-depressed patients, the odds were three times greater that depressed patients would be non-compliant with medical treatment recommendations.

TREATMENT OF DEPRESSION

The treatment of depression on an individual, group or community level, all have common factors, such as pharmacological therapies, psychological therapies, and education and awareness-based components. Therefore, an overview of these approaches will be presented, followed by a specific review of the empirical literature in each of the targeted areas of the individual, group, and community settings.

Evidence for efficacious treatment of depression has included both psychological and drug therapies.[19,20] Although both drug and non-drug interventions have been shown to be beneficial for the treatment of depression, the most common form of treatment worldwide is antidepressant medication.[21]

However, as highlighted by WHO,[22] patient adherence to drug medication is problematic. In fact, non-adherence to antidepressant medication has been reported to be 40% of patients within 12 weeks of treatment,[23] 43% patients within six months,[24] and 32–42% patients had not even filled their prescription.[25] Therefore, it could appear that the role of psychological intervention for the depression could not only be to address the symptoms of depression, but could also be to address adherence to prescribed antidepressant medication. Factors related to adherence of medication have been identified as influencing treatment-seeking behaviour including 'personal control'.[26] Halter assessed a sample of student nurses on their attitudes toward depression, and reported that the nurses would be more likely to seek help for depression if they perceived that the depression was not under personal control. Furthermore, Parker and Parker[27] found that patients, who attributed somatic cues of depression to psychological factors, reported greater treatment-seeking behaviour than patients who perceived the somatic cues as 'normal'. Specifically, analyses of responses from 900 'routine' general practice patients revealed a significant association between a non-treatment seeking response from patients and an interpretation of depressive symptomatology as 'normal' experiences.

Pharmacological treatment of depression

Eccles et al.[28] presented a report on the guidelines for the choice of antidepressants for depression in primary care. Their report stated: 'There is a substantial range of toxicity associated with different antidepressants as currently used in primary care. The SSRIs and lofepramine are associated with the smallest risk of fatal poisoning (III)' (p. 107). However, the report also made the statement: 'A general policy of switching from tricyclics to SSRIs does not appear cost-effective. Where the toxic effects of tricyclic antidepressants give cause for concern, substitution with lofepramine appears relatively cost-effective (III)' (p. 107). These statements on the recommendations for 'older' types of antidepressants compared to the 'newer' strains of antidepressants were based on the category of evidence III. It is noted that this level of evidence is based on 'non-experimental descriptive studies, such as comparative studies, correlation studies and case–control studies' (p. 104). The lack of category of evidence from levels I or II is a problem with accepting these recommendations. Further research, based on meta-analysis of randomized controlled trials or quasi-experimental studies needs to be presented for a clear understanding of the effectiveness, side effects, and drop-out rates associated with antidepressants.

Claxtan et al.[29] compared the two types of antidepressants of tricyclic antidepressants and selective serotonin reuptake inhibitors (SSRIs) on work absenteeism. They reported that drug treatment using the newer antidepressants, SSRIs, was related to a lower mean number of days absent, compared to treatment using the older types of tricyclic antidepressants.

Psychological treatments of depression

Psychological treatment of depression has predominantly been in the form of cognitive behaviour therapy (CBT).[30] CBT has been described as 'a family of treatments which includes cognitive therapy' (King[31] p. 83). Beck et al.[30] (p. 3) claimed that the general characteristics of CBT for depression is 'an active, directive, time-limited, structured approach ... based on an underlying theoretical rationale that an individual's affect and behaviour are largely determined by the way in which he structures the world'. Numerous empirical investigations have demonstrated the effectiveness of CBT (see reviews by Evans et al.,[32] Hollon et al.[33] and Jacobson & Hollon[34]). Beck's work on treatment for depression has pivoted around the basic premise that an individual's emotions, behaviours, and motivations are largely determined by their views or thoughts about 'the world'. According to Beck et al.,[30] an individual who develops maladaptive schemas or cognitive distortions could be vulnerable to depression. Specifically, for depression, an individual's thoughts tend to be a hopelessness or worthlessness about themselves, their present world, and their future. Investigations by Jacobson et al.[34] and Gortner et al.[35] found that individuals, who underwent an intervention that incorporated identification and modification of maladaptive thought patterns, revealed a clinical improvement in depressive symptomatology. Furthermore, these improvements were maintained at six-month and two-year follow-up assessment times. Therefore, a component of CBT for the treatment of depression should include interventions focused on cognitive restructuring through the identification and disputation of negative thoughts. A typical procedure for verbal challenging of negative thoughts could be to work through the following questions with the patient: What is the evidence for these negative thoughts? What alterative views are there? What are the advantages and disadvantages of this way of thinking? What logical errors are you making?

Additionally, Fennell[1] proposed that CBT therapy for depression should include cognitive strategies (e.g. challenge cognitive distortions, such as catastrophizing, demanding expectations, and self-downing types of thinking, distraction techniques, counting thoughts); behavioural strategies (e.g. monitoring activities, pleasure, and mastery activities, scheduling activities, graded task assignment, increase social contacts); and preventive strategies (e.g. identifying assumptions, challenging assumptions). A behavioural experiment has been proposed as another effective component of a CBT intervention for depression. Behavioural experiments follow a procedure where by the patient makes a prediction, reviews existing evidence for and against the prediction, devises a specific experiment to test the validity of the prediction, notes the results of the experiment, and then draws conclusions from the experiment.

The validity of CBT, as an evidence-based practice for the treatment of depression, was questioned by King.[31] He described the criteria by which any claim for evidence-based practice should be considered. Specifically, King identified the concept of efficacy of treatment, the patient's initial treatment response, the duration of treatment effects, the issues of treatment specificity versus person specificity, and consumer acceptance of the treatment modality, as areas that need to be presented and evaluated with a controlled investigation before an acceptance of CBT as an effective therapy for depression can be made. King proposed that much of the reported evidence of the efficacy of CBT falls short of meeting these criteria. Furthermore, there has been a dearth of empirical literature on the individual components of CBT.

Individual interventions for depression

Individual-based depression interventions tend to include drug and psychotherapy interventions through a face-to-face interaction. In contrast, recent investigations of depression treatment have included computerized psychotherapy programs and telephone intervention modalities.

Proudfoot et al.[36] undertook an investigation with 274 patients, who were suffering from depression, mixed anxiety and depression, or anxiety disorders, on the effectiveness of a computerized cognitive-behavioural therapy for anxiety and depression. The participants in this study were allocated to a computerized CBT, or 'treatment as usual' conditions, with or without medication. The computer-based therapy, called 'Beating the Blues', consisted of a 15-minute introductory videotape, and eight 50-minute therapy sessions. The sessions included cognitive components (automatic thoughts, thinking errors and distraction, challenging unhealthful thinking, core beliefs, and attributional style), and behavioural components (activity scheduling or problem-solving, and graded exposure, task breakdown, or sleep management). Proudfoot et al. reported a significant treatment effect for the computerized CBT in terms of depression. However, drug therapy was also reported as a significant variable in depression scores across the six-month assessment period. In a cost-effectiveness analysis of these data, McCrone et al.[37] reported that computers-delivered CBT had 81% change of being cost-effective, and impacted positively on cost per quality-adjusted life years.

The effectiveness of a CBT intervention delivered by telephone was investigated by Simon et al.[20] A total of 600 patients, who were beginning antidepressant treatment for depression, were allocated to either a usual primary care ($n = 195$), usual care plus a minimum of three telephone 'outreach' calls ($n = 207$), or usual care plus a structured 8-session CBT program ($n = 198$) delivered by telephone. All treatment modalities impacted positively on depression across a six-month period. However, the greatest improvement in depression was for patients in the telephone CBT group; intermediate improvements were reported for the patients in the 'outreach' group; and the least improvement was with patients in the usual care group. Specifically, analyses revealed significant statistical and clinical changes in depression from the plus-CBT therapy group, compared with the usual drug care therapy group. No significant changes in depression scores were found between the 'plus-outreach' and the usual care groups at the six-month assessment period.

These examples, together with the previous review of one-to-one psychological interventions, indicate a continuing development of evidence-based psychological interventions that aim to adapt to a variety of patient and environmental needs.

Group interventions for depression

The availability of group-based programs for depression appears to be limited. However, support for group-based interpersonal psychotherapy was found from research in rural Uganda.[38] Bolton et al.[38] assigned 108 men and 116 women to either the depression intervention or a 'usual treatment only' group. They reported a significant change in diagnosis for major depression for the 16-week group psychotherapy intervention (86% to 6.5%), compared to the control group (94% to 54.7%), although both groups significantly reduced over the study period.

In the area of maternal depression, a study by Verduyn et al.[39] investigated the effect of a group cognitive–behavioural therapy (CBT) on maternal depression and child behaviour problems. Women recruited from the general population were assigned to either a CBT for depression and parenting skills enhancement group; a mothers' support group; or a no intervention group. Analysis revealed no significant differences between the groups, but within-group comparison at the end of treatment, at six-month, and 12-month follow-up, revealed maternal depression (and child problems) had improved significantly in the CBT group. These findings supported a tentative indication that group interventions seemed to provide some benefits to mothers with depression, with a possibly improved outcome resulting from CBT for children with behavioural problems.

As with the above research, many of the investigations of group interventions for depression appear to have a co-morbid condition, such as pain,[40] conduct disorder,[41] stroke,[42] breast cancer[43] and HIV-infected gay men.[44]

A study that focused on a sample with major depression was one undertaken by Araya et al.[45] Specifically, Araya et al. recruited 240 adult female primary-care patients with major depression, who were from low-income environments in Santiago, Chile. The research aimed to compare the effectiveness of a stepped-care program with usual care, using a randomized controlled trial methodology. The stepped care was a three-month, multi- component and psycho-educational group intervention. Analyses revealed a significant decrease in depression scores for the stepped-care program compared to the usual care group of women. It is noteworthy that at the six-month follow-up assessment point 70% of the stepped-care group, compared with 30% of the usual-care group, had recovered from the major depression episode.

Additionally, Peden et al.[46] investigated the effectiveness of a six-week cognitive–behavioural group intervention in reducing depressive symptoms, and decreasing negative thinking in a sample of 92 college women who were at risk for major depression. The women were randomly assigned to either a CBT intervention or a no-treatment control group. The cognitive–behavioural intervention specifically identified and reduced negative thinking, using the techniques of thought stopping and affirmations. Analyses revealed that the women in the intervention group experienced a greater decrease in depressive symptoms and negative thinking than those in the control group at post-intervention, with these effects continuing at the 18-month follow-up.

The paucity of research into group interventions for depression could reflect that the depression symptoms experienced by the patient could make attendance at group sessions too difficult for their range of functioning or the severity of the depression symptoms.[47] Furthermore, the appropriateness of group interventions could be questionable when treatment includes pharmacology that would require individual monitoring of the effectiveness of the drug to ensure accurate dosage routines. However, the effectiveness of interventions, in which the patient had the concurrent availability of individual-based drug treatment and group-based psychological interventions, needs to be further investigated.

Large group and community interventions for depression

The area of depression management in large groups or community settings has tended to be focused on education, acceptance of depression, and increasing help-seeking opportunities. Hegerl et al. undertook a telephone survey in two German cities on the beliefs and attitudes of the public towards depression and its treatment. Additionally, the study evaluated the effectiveness of a community-based program that was implemented in one of the cities. This program aimed to improve intervention opportunities and community acceptance for people suffering from depression. Hegerl et al. reported that, across a ten-month period, slight to moderate changes in perceived causes and treatment options for depression were observed in both cities, and that no change was found from an initial level of misconception about pharmacological therapy for depression.

In terms of interventions based in community settings, a depression intervention was undertaken by Ciechanowski et al.[49] These researchers investigated the effectiveness of a home-based program of detecting and managing minor depression or dysthymia among older adults. Ciechanowski et al. used a randomized controlled trial where 138 patients, aged 60 years or older with minor depression or dysthymia were assigned to the Program Encourage Active, Rewarding Lives for Seniors (PEARLS) intervention ($n = 72$) or usual care ($n = 66$). The PEARLS intervention involved a problem-solving approach to increasing social and physical activities, and discussed the potential treatment of depression using antidepressants. At the 12-months assessment time, the intervention group, compared to the control group of patients, were more likely to report a 50% reduction in depressive symptoms (43% vs 15%; OR = 5.21), and to achieve complete remission form depression (36% vs 12%; OR = 4.96). That is, the PEARLS intervention group of older people was approximately five times more likely to report an improvement or remission from depression than the non-PEARLS patients.

SUMMARY AND CONCLUSIONS

Depression has been identified as a major health issue in our society, both in developed and developing countries. Depressive symptomatologies, from major depressive disorders to mild and moderate levels of depression, have been identified as important health target areas. The skills for early diagnosis, treatment, and relapse prevention of the range of depression symptomatology need to be developed, and evidence-based practice for the treatment of depression needs to be carried out for both pharmacological and psychological interventions. Furthermore, the factors associated with the high non-adherence rate for medical treatments and lifestyle interventions for depression need to be explored.[22] However, the current research indicates a role for drug, behavioural, and cognitive therapies in the treatment of depression.

A growing area of concern is the role of depression in chronic physical illnesses, such as diabetes and heart disease. Frasure-Smith et al.[50] proposed that depression was a major prognostic factor for heart disease, equal to other factors such as coronary atherosclerosis. Depression has been found to be common in patients following acute myocardial infarction (AMI), and other coronary syndromes,[51] and has been reported to be three times higher than in the general population.[52,53] Strik et al.[54] found an incidence of 31% of major and minor depression in 'first-time' AMI patients at one-year post the cardiac incident. Furthermore, it has been reported that patients with heart disease and depression have increased morbidity (e.g. Carney et al.[55]), health-care costs (e.g. Shiotani et al.[56]), and a decreased quality of life,[57] compared to heart disease patients without depression. Therefore, the role of the health practitioner and allied health professions in the identification, support, and treatment of depression appears to be a growing field in the current aging population, where chronic illness is rapidly becoming more prevalent.

References

1. Fennell MJ. Depression. In: Hawton K, Salkavoskis PM, Kirk J, Clark D, eds. Cognitive behavioural therapy for psychiatric problems: a practical guide. Oxford: Oxford University Press; 1989.
2. World Health Organization. The ICD-10 Classification of Mental and Behavioural Disorders. Clinical Descriptions and Diagnostic Guidelines. Geneva: WHO; 1992.
3. American Psychiatric Association. Diagnostic and Statistical Manual of Mental Disorders, 4th edn. Washington, DC: American Psychiatric Association; 2000.
4. Kirkby RJ. Changes in premenstrual symptoms and irrational thinking following cognitive–behavioral coping skills training. Journal of Consulting and Clinical Psychology 1994; 62:1026–1032.
5. Murray C, Lopez A. The global burden of disease: A comprehensive assessment of mortality and disability from diseases, injuries and risk factors in 1990. Cambridge: Harvard University Press; 1996.
6. Goldberg DP, Huxley P. Common mental disorders. London: Routledge; 1992.
7. Thomas CM, Morris S. Cost of depression among adults in England in 2000. British Journal of Psychiatry 2003; 183:514–519.

8. Andrews G, Sanderson K, Corry J, Lapsley HM. Using epidemiological data to model efficiency in reducing the burden of depression. Journal of Mental Health Policy Economics 2000; 3:175–186.

9. Üstün TB, Ayuso-Mateos JL, Chatterji S, Mathers C, Murray CJL. Global burden of depressive disorders: methods and data sources. British Journal of Psychiatry 2004; 184:386–392.

10. Dewa CS, Hoch JS, Lin E, Paterson M, Goering P. Pattern of antidepressant use and duration of depression-related absence from work. British Journal of Psychiatry 2003; 183:507–513.

11. Hunt DC, Yonke CT. Use of a behavioural risk survey by employers to identify leading health problems among employees and their dependents. Journal of Public Health Management Practice 2002; 8:26–32.

12. Chisholm D, Sanderson K, Ayuso-Mateos JL, Saxena S. Reducing the global burden of depression: Population-level analysis of intervention cost-effectiveness in 14 world regions. British Journal of Psychiatry 2004; 184:393–403.

13. Surtees PG, Wainwright NWJ, Khaw K, Day N. Functional health status, chronic medical conditions and disorders of mood. British Journal of Psychiatry 2003; 183:299–303.

14. Ciechanowski PS, Katon WJ, Russo JE. Depression and diabetes: Impact of depressive symptoms on adherence, function and costs. Archives of Internal Medicine 2000; 160:3278–3285.

15. Egede LE, Zheng D, Simpson K. Comorbid depression is associated with increased health care use and expenditures in individuals with diabetes. Diabetes Care 2002;25(3):464–470.

16. Lustman PJ, Anderson RJ, Freedland KE, de Groot M, Carney RM, Clouse RE. Depression and poor glycemic control: A meta-analytic review of the literature. Diabetes Care 2000; 23:934–929.

17. DiMatteo MR, Lepper HS, Croghan TW. Depression is a risk factor for noncompliance with medical treatment; meta-analysis of the effects of anxiety and depression on patient adherence. Archives of Internal Medicine 2000; 160(14):2101–2107.

18. de Groot M, Anderson R, Greedland KE, Clouse RE, Lustman PJ. Association of depression and diabetes complications: A meta-analysis. Psychosomatic Medicine 2001; 63:619–630.

19. Dowrick C, Dunn G, Ayuso-Mateos JL, Dalgard OS, Page H, Lehtinen V, et al. Problem solving treatment and group psychoeducation for depression: Multicentre randomised controlled trial. Outcomes of Depression International Network (ODIN) Group. British Medical Journal 2000; 321(7274):1450–1454.

20. Simon GE, Ludman EJ, Tutty S, Operskalski B, Von Korff M. Telephone psychotherapy and telephone care management for primary care patients starting antidepressant treatment. JAMA 2004; 292:935–942.

21. Peveler R, Kendrick A. Treatment delivery and guidelines in primary care. British Medical Bulletin 2001; 57:193–206.

22. World Health Organization. Adherence to long-term therapies: Towards Policies for Action. Geneva: WHO; 2003.

23. Peveler R, George C, Kinmonth AL, Campbell M, Thompson C. Effect of antidepressant drug counselling and information leaflets on adherence to drug treatment in primary care: Randomised controlled trial. British Medical Journal 1999; 319:612–615.

24. Schumann C, Lenz G, Berghofer A, Muller-Oerlinghausen B. Nonadherence with long-term prophylaxis: A 6-year naturalistic follow-up study of affectively ill patients. Psychiatry Research 1999; 89(3):247–257.

25. Lin EH, Katon WJ, Simon GE, Von Korff M, Bush TM, Walker EA, et al. Low-intensity treatment of depression in primary care: Is it problematic? General Hospital Psychiatry 2000; 22(2):78–83.

26. Halter MJ. Stigma and help seeking related to depression: A study of nursing students. Journal of Psychosocial Nursing and Mental Health Services 2004; 42:42–51.

27. Parker G, Parker K. Influence of symptom attribution on reporting depression and recourse to treatment. Australian and New Zealand Journal of Psychiatry 2003; 37:469–474.

28. Eccles M, Freemantle N, Mason J. North of England evidence-based guideline development project: Summary version of guidelines for the choice of antidepressants for depression in primary care. Family Practice 1999; 16(2):103–111.

29. Claxton AJ, Chawla AJ, Kennedy S. Absenteeism among employees treated for depression. Journal of Occupational and Environmental Medicine 1999; 41:605–611.

30. Beck AT, Rush AJ, Shaw BF, Emery G. Cognitive therapy pf depression. New York: Guilford; 1979.

31. King R. Evidence-based practice: Where is the evidence? The case of cognitive behaviour therapy and depression. Australian Journal of Psychology 1998; 33:83–88.

32. Evans MD, Hollon SD, DeRubeis RJ, Piasecki JM, Grove WM, Garvey MJ, et al. Differential relapse following cognitive therapy and pharmacotherapy for depression. Archives of General Psychiatry 1992; 49(10):802–808.

33. Hollon SD, Evans MD, DeRubeis RJ. Cognitive mediation of relapse prevention following treatment for depression: Implications of differential risk. In: Ingram RE, ed. Contemporary psychological approaches to depression. New York: Guilford Press; 1990:117–136.

34. Jacobson NS, Hollon SD. Cognitive behaviour therapy vs. pharmacotherapy: Now that jury's returned its verdict, it's time to present the rest of the evidence. Journal of Consulting and Clinical Psychology 1996; 64(1):74–80.

35. Gortner ET, Gollan JK, Dobson KS, Jacobson NS. Cognitive–behavioral treatment for depression: Relapse prevention. Journal of Consulting and Clinical Psychology 1998; 66:377–384.

36. Proudfoot J, Ryden C, Everitt B, Shapiro DA, Goldberg D, Mann A, et al. Clinical efficiacy of computerised cognitive–behavioural therapy for anxiety and depression in primary care: Randomised controlled trial. British Journal of Psychiatry 2004; 185:46–54.

37. McCrone P, Knapp M, Proudfoot J, Ryden C, Cavanagh K, Shapiro DA, et al. Cost-effectiveness of computerised cognitive–behavioural therapy for anxiety and depression in primary care: Randomised controlled trial. British Journal of Psychiatry 2004; 185:55–62.

38. Bolton P, Bass J, Neugebauer R, Verdeli H, Clougherty KF, Wickramaratne P, et al. Group interpersonal psychotherapy for depression in rural Uganda. JAMA 2003; 289:3117–3124.

39. Verduyn C, Barrowclough C, Roberts J, Tarrier T, Harrington R. Maternal depression and child behaviour problems. Randomised placebo-controlled trial of a cognitive–behavioural group intervention. British Journal of Psychiatry 2003; 183:342–348.

40. Ersek M, Turner JA, McCurry SM, Gibbons L, Kraybill BM. Efficacy of a self-management group intervention for elderly persons with chronic pain. Clinical Journal of Pain 2003; 19(3):156–167.

41. Rohde P, Clarke GN, Mace DE, Jorgensen JS, Seeley JR. An efficacy/effectiveness study of cognitive–behavioral treatment for adolescents with comorbid major

depression and conduct disorder. Journal of the American Academy of Child and Adolescent Psychiatry 2004; 43(6):660–668.

42. Clark MS, Rubenach S, Winsor A. A randomized controlled trial of an education and counselling intervention for families after stroke. Clinical Rehabilitation 2003; 17:703–712.

43. Kissane DW, Bloch S, Smith GC, Miach P, Clarke DM, Ikin J, et al. Cognitive–existential group psychotherapy for women with primary breast cancer: A randomised controlled trial. Psycho-Oncology 2003; 12(6):532–546.

44. Weiss JL, Mulder CL, Antoni MH, de Vroome EM, Garssen B, Goodkin K. Effects of a supportive-expressive group intervention on long-term psychosocial adjustment in HIV-infected gay men. Psychotherapy and Psychosomatics 2003; 72:132–140.

45. Araya R, Rojas G, Fritsch R, Gaete J, Rojas M, Simon G, et al. Treating depression in primary care in low-income women in Santiago, Chile: A randomised controlled trial. Lancet 2003; 361:995–1000.

46. Peden AR, Rayens MK, Hall LA, Beebe LH. Preventing depression in high-risk college women: A report of an 18-month follow-up. Journal of American College Health 2001; 49:299–306.

47. Sanford M, Byrne C, Williams S, Atley S, Miller J, Allin H. A pilot study of a parent-education group for families affected by depression. Canadian Journal Psychiatry 2003; 48(2):78–86.

48. Hegerl U, Althaus D, Stefanek J. Public attitudes towards treatment of depression: Effects of an information campaign. Pharmacopsychiatry 2003; 36:288–291.

49. Ciechanowski P, Wagner E, Schmaling K, Scwartz S, Williams B, Diehr P, et al. Community-integrated home-based depression treatment in older adults: A randomised controlled trial. JAMA 2004; 291:1569–1577.

50. Frasure-Smith N, Lespérance F, Talajic M. Depression and 18-month prognosis after myocardial infarct. Circulation 1995; 91(4):999–1005.

51. DeVon H, Zerzic J. Symptoms of acute coronary syndromes: Are there gender differences? A review of the literature. Heart and Lung 2002; 31:235–245.

52. Fontana A, Kerns R, Rosenberg R, Colonese K. Support, stress, and recovery from coronary heart disease: A longitudinal causal model. Health Psychology 1989; 8(2):175–193.

53. Ladwig KH, Kieser M, Konig J, Breithardt G, Borggrefe M. Affective disorders and survival after acute myocardial infarction. Results from the post-infarction late potential study. European Heart Journal 1991; 12:959–964.

54. Strik JMH, Lousberg R, Cheriex EC, Honig A. One year cumulative incidence of depression following myocardial infarction and impact on cardiac outcome. Journal of Psychosomatic Research 2004; 56(1):59–66.

55. Carney R, Rich M, Freedland K, Saini J, teVelde A, Simeone C, et al. Major depressive disorders predicts cardiac events in patients with coronary artery disease. Psychosomatic Medicine 1988; 50:627–633.

56. Shiotani I, Sato H, Kinjo K, Nakatani D, Mizuno H, Ohnishi Y, et al. Depressive symptoms predict 12-month prognosis in elderly patients with acute myocardial infarction. Journal of Cardiovascular Risk 2002; 9(3):153–160.

57. Lane D, Carroll D, Ring C, Beevers DG, Lip GY. Mortality and quality of life 12 months after myocardial infarction: Effects of depression and anxiety. Psychosomatic Medicine 2001; 63(2):221–230.

CHAPTER 10

Interventions for insomnia

Kenneth Mark Greenwood

INTRODUCTION

Sleep disorders have serious social and public health consequences[1–3] and are widespread.[4] The consequences of disturbed sleep are serious and include loss of work productivity, increased incidence of road and work accidents, reduced income, poor health and increased use of the health-care system, tiredness during the day, increased irritability, loss of motivation, poor memory, decreased concentration, and muscle aches.[2,3,5–7] Obtaining too little sleep and too much sleep have both been associated with reduced longevity.[8] At the outset, it is important to understand that, while sleep disorders clearly have serious public health consequences, there has been little public health focus on sleep disorders to date.

Many types of sleep disorder are recognized in the various nosological schemes.[9,10] Of these, the most common is insomnia, which can be defined as 'a complaint of difficulty initiating or maintaining sleep or of non-restorative sleep that lasts for at least one month . . . and causes clinically significant distress or impairment in social, occupational, or other important areas of functioning'[9]

(p. 599) which cannot be attributed to other medical or psychiatric complaints. Several types of insomnia can be identified. This chapter is concerned with the most common, known as primary insomnia or psychophysiological insomnia.

THE EPIDEMIOLOGY OF INSOMNIA

Sateia et al.[4] suggested that the prevalence of insomnia in the general population may be 35%, with between 10% and 15% who may be assessed as having moderate to severe sleeping disorders. Similar figures are found in numerous studies, with variability due to the exact definition of insomnia used.

With such a high prevalence, lifetime incidence is also extremely high. Most people will have some period during their lives when obtaining adequate sleep is problematic.

Despite the consequences described above, insomnia is said to go unrecognized and untreated, with only one out of twenty people who complain of suffering from insomnia actually visiting a medical practitioner to discuss it specifically.[2]

Treatment approaches

Insomnia and other sleep problems are commonly treated with hypnotic medications, such as benzodiazepines. Kripke[11] concluded that drug-based therapies for the majority of sleep disorders are ineffective and dangerous. He also questioned their effectiveness in treating sleeping problems even in the short-term. Drug therapy is also expensive, as it is continuing.

A preferred therapy for insomnia involves a psychological approach, which is non-pharmacological and has a good evidence base. The current behavioural interventions for insomnia include a number of components including sleep hygiene, stimulus control therapy, sleep restriction therapy, and cognitive therapy.[12]

Individual interventions for insomnia

Several meta-analyses,[13,14] and systematic reviews[15,16] document the evidence base and have led to published practice parameters for the non-pharmacological treatment of insomnia by the American Academy of Sleep Medicine.[17] A number of published and evaluated treatment manuals exist.[18] While the current cognitive behavioural therapy (CBT) approaches to the treatment of insomnia are effective and result in clinically meaningful change for most individuals, it is clear that there is room for improvement.[19]

Group interventions for insomnia

The current CBT approaches have also been shown to be effective when delivered to small groups, and it has also been claimed by some that the group process can result in improvements in treatment outcome.[18]

Limitations of individual and group therapist directed intervention

Given the extensive literature on the efficacy of current CBT approaches to insomnia, this chapter does not concentrate on documenting the evidence for these approaches. Instead, attention is directed to less common approaches which may prove to be more effective in addressing the problem in larger numbers of individuals.

As stated earlier, the majority of those with sleep problems do not access psychological treatments.[20,21] One reason for this may be the expense in terms of the cost and time required to attend multiple (usually around six) sessions delivered in either an individual or small group format. It may also be that treatment in a group setting and/or public admission of having a 'psychological' problem act as a disincentive to seeking treatment. It is also the case that access to such treatments is limited geographically and that those in more remote areas are unlikely to have easy access to a qualified therapist. It may even be that the public and other health professionals are unaware of the existence and efficacy of such treatments. Whatever the case, it is clear that the majority of those with sleeping problems do not receive adequate treatment for their problem.[2]

It is clear that, while efficacious treatments are available, these are not commonly used and that sleep problems remain a serious problem in the community. A better treatment strategy is required that addresses the barriers to seeking treatment described above. One approach that is likely to be of value, and more acceptable and available to individuals with sleep problems, is the use of bibliotherapy or self-help treatment.

THE LITERATURE ON SELF-HELP FOR SLEEP PROBLEMS

Many self-help manuals for sleep problems are available commercially.[22,23] However, surprisingly little systematic research has been conducted on the efficacy of these in addressing sleep problems. Searches of both PsycINFO (from 1974 to Week 2, March, 2004) and MEDLINE (From 1966 to Week 2 March, 2004) were conducted using the keywords of self-help or bibliotherapy combined with keywords of insomnia or sleep. Only seven published reports containing empirical data relevant to the evaluation of self-help approaches for sleep problems were found in the scientific literature, and, of these, two were dissertation abstracts that have not subsequently been published and one reported on a mass-media intervention. Subsequent searches of the references cited by these reports yielded an additional three reports, one of which is a dissertation abstract. In addition, an unpublished report by the author was available for review.

Alperson and Biglan[24] evaluated the effectiveness of a brief 'self-help' intervention (two weeks only) consisting of stimulus control instructions and relaxation ($n = 14$: $n = 7$ young < 55 years and $n = 7$ old > 55 years) against a control intervention involving back exercises and instructions to engage in activity in bed ($n = 8$) and a self-monitoring only group ($n = 7$). Analyses compared baseline measures with those obtained 12 weeks later. Significantly larger changes in SOL (latency to sleep onset) were found in the young intervention group, but also in the control intervention group, compared to the self-monitoring only group. However, the change in the intervention group did not differ from that in the control intervention. No change was found in the older intervention group. While both the intervention group and the control intervention group increased total sleep time, this change was only significant in the control intervention group. No differences were found in the number of night awakenings. While quality of sleep ratings were most improved in the young intervention group, these changes were not significantly better than those found in the control intervention group. Thus, while positive changes were found in the young intervention groups, these did not differ from the control intervention. Moreover, change was not found in the older intervention group. The intervention investigated in this study was brief (two weeks only), the follow-up period short, and the number of participants small. The intervention did not include many of the components considered crucial in insomnia treatment (e.g. sleep hygiene recommendations, cognitive restructuring etc.). The intervention was also not strictly self-help as participants attended to be provided with their instructions, read these during a session, and were allowed to ask questions of the therapist. Importantly, no comparison with a 'standard' therapist-delivered intervention was conducted.

Bailey[25] employed a commercially available self-help manual, which was described as including general knowledge about sleep and instructions for a variety of behavioural self-control techniques. No other details were provided. Thirty adult complainers about SOL were randomly assigned to three conditions: (1) group contact, weekly; (2) brief contact via weekly telephone call; and (3) self-directed for a two-month period. The program was reported to be effective for those with some therapist contact. No reductions in SOL were found in the self-directed group, whereas the other two groups were reported to have decreased SOL and increased TST. No details of the magnitude of change were reported. As this report is the abstract of a dissertation, which has not been subsequently published, it is difficult to evaluate. However, the finding of no change in the self-directed group is of interest, suggesting the value of minimal therapist contact.

Morawetz[26] compared the results of 141 individuals randomly assigned to waitlist, therapist-led, and a self-help condition provided with a commercially available self-help tape containing stimulus control and relaxation instructions. Results were presented separately for those using sleep medication at pretest and those who were not. For those not using sleep medications, significant improvements in sleep diary and self-assessments, of similar magnitude to the therapist-led group, were achieved by the group using the self-help tape if their major problem was with sleep onset or early morning waking. Those presenting with sleep maintenance problems did not improve significantly, but showed changes in the direction of improvement. However, the self-help tape program was not effective for those using sleep medications compared to the waitlist group, although improvements were found in the therapist-led group. These results persisted at the four-month follow-up. The magnitude of the improvements seen was similar to those reported in the literature for therapist-led intervention. This study provides good data from a relatively large sample of the efficacy of self-help treatment in those not using sleeping medication. For those using sleep medication therapist contact was found to be important. However, whether the weekly group sessions are required, or a more minimal level of therapist contact would suffice was not assessed.

Gustafson[27] reported on the effects of a self-administered muscle relaxation training program provided to 22 participants. No comparison groups were involved. The effects observed were small, possibly because relaxation training is only a small part of the package of components normally included in insomnia treatment.

Riedel et al.[28] studied 50 insomniacs 60 years or older. Participants were randomly allocated into a group that viewed educational videotape and received a printed brochure and a group who also received weekly sessions of therapist guidance. An additional 25 insomniacs served in a waitlist condition. The intervention consisted of educational material about sleep in older individuals and instructions for sleep compression. While significant improvement was found in the videotape group, these changes were similar to those seen in the waitlist group and significantly less than those found in the therapist guidance group. These results point to the importance of therapist contact in this group. However, the changes found in the waitlist group suggest the possibility of reactivity to self-monitoring and indicate the need for a control group who are not required to self-monitor. The nature of the intervention and the particular nature of sleep problems in the elderly make it difficult to generalize from this study self-help interventions for younger individuals.

Iler[29] used the SleepBetter Without Drugs™ program developed by Morawetz (see web site: http://www.sleepbetter.com.au). Forty-eight individuals aged 19–81 years old took part, with 24 in the intervention group and 24 in a waitlist control group. After one week of monitoring, the intervention group received the program and continued daily monitoring for six weeks. It was reported that the intervention group significantly improved sleep on most subjective measures and that significant improvements were found on SOL, WASO (minutes awake after sleep onset), TST (total sleep time). However, no other details of means, effect size etc. are reported. As this report is the abstract of a dissertation, which has not been subsequently published, it is difficult to evaluate. No effect sizes are reported and no comparison with a therapist-led program was conducted.

Mimeault and Morin[20] randomly assigned 54 individuals with insomnia to a self-help treatment, self-help with brief weekly telephone consultation or a waitlist control group. Treatment individuals were mailed a booklet each week for six weeks. Telephone consultations were brief (<15 minutes). The intervention involved a number of components, but surprisingly omitted relaxation training. Individuals in both treated groups improved in a fashion similar to other reports of group or individual-based therapy, and, while the addition of telephone consultations slightly improved outcome at post-test, no difference was found between the two self-help groups at three-month follow-up. The authors admit that the power for detecting differences between the treatment groups was low. Unlike the results of Morawetz,[26] no differential response was found between those using sleeping medications and those who were not. No other analyses were conducted to determine predictors of response to self-help treatment.

Knuth,[30] in a dissertation abstract, described a multi-method approach for the treatment of insomnia, delivered using audiotapes, a videotape and a workbook. No details of the participants in the study or the results obtained are provided. The work has not subsequently been published.

Greenwood et al.[31] recently completed a study in which the SleepBetter Without Drugs™ program of Morawetz was provided to 17 volunteer male prisoners and a control group of seven were also assessed. While group changes in the direction of improved sleep were found in the treatment group, these were not statistically significant. Of the 17 individuals, 11 showed improvement, but only four individuals improved their sleep to a level where it was no longer considered a problem. Little change was observed in the control group. It was concluded that that simple provision of a self-help program, while of value, was not sufficient in its own right to alleviate sleep problems in this group.

Limitations of the self-help literature

The literature reviewed above does not provide quality evidence about the efficacy of self-help approaches for insomnia. It is important to know not only whether self-help treatment is efficacious relative to no treatment, but also to know its efficacy relative to therapist-led interventions of known potency. Given this, a self-help treatment containing the components thought to be important, and commonly included, in therapist-led interventions (stimulus control, sleep restriction, sleep hygiene education, relaxation training and cognitive restructuring) needs to be compared in a randomized controlled trial against a standard therapist-led intervention and the participants need to be representative of the group eligible for such treatment. The literature reviewed does not contain such a trial.

Evaluation of self-help insomnia treatment should include a treatment package that is comprehensive and contains similar components to the packages found to be effective when delivered in individual or group-based treatment modes. Of the studies reviewed above, only five of the nine could be considered to have utilized comprehensive treatment packages, and the omission of relaxation from the study of Mimeault and Morin[20] makes this study a questionable inclusion in this list.

Evaluation should include appropriate comparison groups. Only six of the nine studies reviewed above included a no-treatment group. Given that the efficacy of psychological treatment for insomnia has been established and the existence in the literature of many demonstrations of lack of change in untreated waitlist groups, it is considered that a no-treatment comparison group is not essential. A more important comparison group, however, is a therapist-led intervention, which would allow determination of the efficacy of self-help relative to the therapist-led approach that has been demonstrated to be effective in the literature. Only three of the nine studies included such a group.

The relative benefits of the presence or absence of some minimal therapist contact in self-help approaches has not been addressed in the literature. A few studies have included brief telephone contact from the therapist, with some reporting a benefit[25] and some not.[20] Minimal therapist contact is cost-effective and has been argued by some as necessary to engender the necessary degree of motivation for change.[28] Others have argued that any degree of therapist contact may decrease the client's ownership of change and undermine the persistence of treatment effects.[20] Morin et al.[13] reported that self-help improvement rates are slightly inferior to those obtained with treatment protocols implemented by therapists and that the addition of therapist guidance may help. However, the studies on which these conclusions were based are limited as shown above.

In summary, the reports of Bailey,[25] Iler[29] and Knuth[30] do not contain sufficient detail for proper evaluation.

Greenwood et al.[31] report on a very small and specialized group of prisoners and Riedel et al.[28] report on elderly individuals exposed to a treatment packages specific to that age group. The generalizability of both studies is questionable.

Gustafson[27] reports on a package including relaxation alone and the package used by Alperson & Biglan[24] cannot be considered to be comprehensive.

Only the studies of Morawetz[26] and Mimeault & Morin[20] can be considered to have designs sufficient to address the questions of interest. However, Mimeault & Morin[20] did not include a therapist-led comparison group and, thus, cannot properly address the issue of the efficacy of self-help relative to therapist-led intervention. Morawetz found that those on sleeping medication did not respond to the self-help package, but did not assess a self-help treatment with minimal therapist contact, which was found to be effective by Mimeault & Morin for this group.

In summary, the existing literature does not provide good quality information about the relative efficacy of self-help treatment for insomnia, how this should be delivered and the client characteristics predictive of success. Self-help approaches, however, do show promise. Of course, should good evidence of the efficacy of these interventions be obtained, a remaining challenge will be to encourage widespread access to, and use of, these approaches.

MASS MEDIA AND INTERNET INTERVENTIONS FOR INSOMNIA

Given the public health implications of poor sleep it is surprising that few attempts have been made to use mass media approaches to intervention.

Use of the mass media has been made in related areas. For instance, fatigue, particularly in drivers, has been addressed in various road safety programs (e.g. the Arrive Alive program in the state of Victoria, Australia http://www.arrivealive.vic.gov.au/about.html). This fatigue may be a consequence of poor sleep. The focus in these campaigns has been on fatigue while driving, the consequences of this, and the use of particular countermeasures such as the use of power naps. As such programs target only one symptom of sleep disturbance, and that the symptom may not be related to insomnia, they are not discussed further in this chapter.

Only two papers could be found in the literature relating to mass media interventions to insomnia. Oosterhuis and Klip[32] reported on a mass media self-help insomnia intervention conducted in the Netherlands involving eight-weekly, 15-minute television programs, nine radio lessons, a book and an audiotape. The program included many components typically found in modern therapeutic approaches to insomnia. Of the more than 200 000 people who watched the program, 23 000 ordered the additional material. Of these, a random selection of 400 volunteers was made and of these 105 people completed the evaluation. Changes similar to those reported in other sleep studies were reported, suggesting good efficacy for the self-help, mass media intervention. However, no comparison groups were used and the authors admit the possibility of selection bias in those who took part in the evaluation.

There is a great deal of information about sleep problems available on the Internet. While the quality of this information varies, there is no evidence in the literature of who makes use of this information and the extent to which they benefit from it.

Strom et al.[33] reported on an evaluation of a five-week, Internet-based treatment for insomnia. A total of 109 eligible participants were randomly allocated to Internet-based treatment or to a waitlist control group. However, the attrition rate was high (24%) with only 30 of 54 in the treatment group and 51 or 54 in the waitlist group providing post-test data. Weekly material was provided on websites for participants and e-mail contact with the therapists was allowed. The program content reflected a standard self-help program.[18,22] While significant improvements in sleep were found in the treatment group, these were also found in the control group. These changes tended to have quite modest effect sizes, and were much smaller than those reported in therapist-led interventions. For example, sleep onset latency decreased from 38.3 to 27.3 minutes in the treatment group and from 40.8 to 35.9 minutes in the waitlist group. As such, and despite the authors' positive evaluation, no specific benefit of the Internet-based treatment could be claimed.

In summary, the evidence for the efficacy of mass media interventions is limited. However, these have rarely been employed and, given the success of these approaches in others areas, further investigation of these approaches is warranted.

An intervention targeted at a community

The only community-based intervention for sleep problems appears to be the Walla Walla project described by William Dement.[34] Walla Walla in Washington State is the hometown of Dement. He returned there in 1988 as an eminent sleep researcher to give a public lecture on sleep. Dement, with colleague Nino-Murcia, reviewed the records of 750 local patients and found that sleep disorder diagnoses were absent. He then educated primary care physicians in that town in the diagnosis and treatment of sleep disorders and provided weekly telephone conferences for the physicians. As a consequence the number of diagnoses increased. A sleep curriculum has been prepared for local schools. A sleep disorders clinic has been established. As a consequence more than 2000 people have been diagnosed and treated for sleep disorders. While only sketchy details of the project are presented, the description clearly provides a model for what could be the future for community-based interventions in the field of sleep disorders.

SUMMARY AND CONCLUSIONS

This chapter has shown that, while therapist-led interventions for individuals and small groups are well developed, public health interventions in this area are in their infancy. Given the public health consequences of poor sleep and the prevalence of the problem, it is clear that such interventions are sorely needed.

Future directions in the study of insomnia and other sleep disorders

Much work remains to be done. The problem is not that we do not know how to intervene. The problem appears to be in convincing people with sleep problems to seek appropriate help. There appears to be a number of issues that need to be addressed in achieving this goal. The first is to convince people that sleep problems are serious, rather than an inconvenience that must be endured. The second problem is to convince people that effective, non-drug treatments exist. Preliminary data[35] indicate that people with sleep problems do seek help more often than previously thought, but that the sources of their help are rarely appropriately qualified health professionals. As a consequence they receive advice of dubious quality and become demoralized in their attempts to solve their sleep problem. A major impediment to seeking appropriate help is the common belief that all that will be offered to them is hypnotic drugs, which a large proportion of people wish to avoid. There is a clear role for public health practitioners to modify the beliefs that sleep problems are not serious and that effective treatments do not exist. Techniques that have been used successfully for other health problems would seem eminently suitable for adoption in achieving these aims.

A second area that needs to be addressed is to continue to work to develop cost-effective methods of treatment that will be affordable and available to the large numbers of people needing help. In this endeavor, approaches using self-help would seem to hold particular promise, as well as approaches involving the use of the Internet.

Little is known about the categories of individuals most likely to benefit from self-help approaches. Work is required to identify characteristics of individuals or their sleep problem that predict self-help treatment success.

Finally, research is required to expand the work done in the insomnia field into other less common, but often more serious, sleep disorders such as sleep apnoea, restless legs syndrome, periodic leg movement disorder, and the various circadian rhythms sleep disorders.

The field of sleep disorders is ripe for an injection of public health methodology. It is hoped that some readers of this chapter will take up this challenge.

References

1. Lamberg L. Promoting adequate sleep finds a place on the public health. JAMA 2004; 291:2415–2417.
2. Leger D. Public health and insomnia: Economic impact. Sleep 2000; 23(Suppl. 3): S69–76.
3. Leger D, Guilleminault C, Bader G, Levy E, Paillard M. Medical and socio-professional impact of insomnia. Sleep 2002; 25:621–625.
4. Sateia MJ, Doghramji K, Hauri PJ, Morin CM. Evaluation of chronic insomnia. Sleep 2000; 23:243–308.
5. Culebras A. Clinical handbook of sleep disorders. Boston, MA: Butterworth-Heinemann; 1996.
6. Kapur VK, Redline S, Nieto FJ, Young T, Newman AB, Henderson JA. The relationship between chronically disrupted sleep and health care use. Sleep 2002; 25:289–296.
7. Gallup. Sleep in America. Princeton, NJ: Gallup; 1991.
8. Grandner MA, Kripke DF. Self-reported sleep complaints with long and short sleep: A nationally representative sample. Psychosomatic Medicine 2004; 66:239–241.
9. American Psychiatric Association. Diagnostic and Statistical Manual of Mental Disorders, 4th edn. Washington, DC: American Psychiatric Association; 2000.
10. American Sleep Disorders Association. International classification of sleep disorders, revised: Diagnostic and coding manual. Rochester, MN; 1997.
11. Kripke DF. Chronic hypnotic use: Deadly risks, doubtful benefit. Sleep Medicine Reviews 2000;4.
12. Stepanski EJ, Perlis ML. A historical perspective and commentary on practice issues. In: Perlis ML, Lichstein KL, eds. Treating sleep disorders: Principles and practice of behavioral sleep medicine. Hoboken, NJ: John Wiley; 2003:3–26.
13. Morin CM, Culbert JP, Schwartz SM. Nonpharmacological interventions for insomnia: A meta–analysis of treatment efficacy. American Journal of Psychiatry 1994; 151:1172–1180.
14. Murtagh DRR, Greenwood KM. Identifying effective treatments for insomnia: A meta-analysis. Journal of Consulting and Clinical Psychology 1995; 63:79–89.
15. Edinger JD, Wohlgemuth WK. The significance and management of persistent primary insomnia. Sleep Medicine Reviews 1999; 3:101–118.
16. Morin CM, Hauri PJ, Espie CA, Spielman AJ, Buysse DJ, Bootzin RR. Nonpharmacologic treatment of chronic insomnia. Sleep 1999; 22:1–23.
17. Chesson ALJ, Anderson WM, Littner M, Davila D, Hartse K, Johnson S, et al. Practice parameters for the nonpharmacologic treatment of chronic insomnia: An American Academy of Sleep Medicine report: Standards of Practice Committee of the American Academy of Sleep Medicine. Sleep 1999; 22:1128–1133.
18. Morin CM. Insomnia: Psychological assessment and management. New York, NY: Guilford Press; 1993.

19. Harvey AG, Tang NKY. Cognitive behaviour therapy for primary insomnia: Can we rest yet? Sleep Medicine Reviews 2003; 7:237–262.
20. Mimeault V, Morin CM. Self-help treatment for insomnia: Bibliotherapy with and without professional guidance. Journal of Consulting and Clinical Psychology 1999; 67:511–519.
21. National Institute of Health. NIH releases statement on behavioral and relaxation approaches for chronic pain and insomnia. American Family Physician 1996; 53:1877–1880.
22. Morin CM. Relief from insomnia: Getting the sleep of your dreams. New York, NY: Doubleday; 1996.
23. Sharp TJ. The good sleep guide. Victoria: Penguin Book Australia; 2001.
24. Alperson J, Biglan A. Self-administered treatment of sleep onset insomnia and the importance of age. Behavior Therapy 1979; 10:347–356.
25. Bailey CA. Effects of therapist contact and a self-help manual in the treatment of sleep-onset insomnia. Dissertation Abstracts International 1983; 43:3724B.
26. Morawetz D. Behavioral self-help treatment for insomnia: A controlled evaluation. Behavior Therapy 1989; 20:365–379.
27. Gustafson R. Treating insomnia with a self-administered muscle relaxation training program: A follow-up. Psychological Reports 1992; 70:124–126.
28. Riedel BW, Lichstein KL, Dwyer WO. Sleep compression and sleep education for older insomniacs: Self-help versus therapist guidance. Psychology and Aging 1995; 10:54–63.
29. Iler JA. Efficacy of a nonpharmacological intervention for insomnia: An empirical investigation. Dissertion Abstracts International 1997; 58:2680B.
30. Knuth KM. A self-management treatment program for insomnia. Dissertation Abstracts International 2000; 61:2767B.
31. Greenwood K, Greaves J, Morawetz D. Self-help for sleep problems in male prisoners. In: Inaugural Conference of the Australasian Society for Behavioural Health and Medicine, Brisbane; 13–15 February 2003.
32. Oosterhuis A, Klip EC. The treatment of insomnia through mass media: The results of a televised behavioural training programme. Social Science and Medicine 1997; 45:1223–1229.
33. Strom L, Pettersson R, Andersson G. Internet-based treatment for insomnia: a controlled evaluation. Journal of Consulting and Clinical Psychology 2004; 72(1):113–120.
34. Dement WC. The promise of sleep: The scientific connection between health, happiness, and a good night's sleep. London: Pan; 1999.
35. Ong M, Greenwood KM. Treatment-seeking for sleep problems: The role of illness perceptions. In: Paper presented at the 2nd Annual Conference of the Australasian Society for Behavioural Health and Medicine, Christchurch; February, 2004.

CHAPTER **11**

Problematic gambling behaviour

Alun C. Jackson

INTRODUCTION

The push for evidence-based practice in the health and human services means that there is now little tolerance for 'implicit' and 'unsystematic' program theory.[1-3] The exception, of course, is where there are many knowledge gaps or contention about the underlying behavioural mechanisms which give rise to the behaviours targeted for change or the effectiveness of new interventions. Problem gambling is one such area, typified by debates on aetiology and measurement[4-8] as well as what constitutes best practice in individual, group and community level interventions.[9-11]

In addition to these broad issues of definition and measurement, Blaszczynski,[12] in developing a typology of pathological gambling, proposed that, while people experiencing problematic gambling behaviours shared many characteristics, there were clear 'types' of problem gamblers with varying pathways into problem gambling. These types are the 'normal' problem gambler, emotionally disturbed gamblers, and those defined by the presence of neurological or neurochemical dysfunction reflecting impulsivity. Blaszczynski[12] notes that while all three subgroups are affected by environmental variables, conditioning and cognitive processes, 'from a clinical perspective, each pathway contains different implications for managing treatment strategies and treatment interventions'.

From this recognition of the heterogeneity of the population for whom interventions are designed, it will be obvious that indicators of change will vary in relation to each of these subpopulations, as will indicators derived from prevention, early intervention and late intervention frameworks, and indicators derived from the explanatory model of the behaviour that is used. For example, whether abstinence or control is set as a goal of intervention, will vary according to the primary model used to explain the aetiology of problem gambling – an addictions approach associated with a 'medical model' or a contrasting biopsychosocial model.[13,14]

As well as there being debate about the nature of the populations and the goals of intervention, there is also debate, naturally, about how long these changes will take to achieve. If there is a paucity of comparative intervention data across similarly modeled treatment intervention programs, as there is,[11] there is even less relating to prevention programs where take up of gambling is the targeted behaviour, or to early intervention or problem recognition intervention programs, although a small amount of data on community education programs, where problem recognition and help-seeking is the focus, is now becoming available.[15]

Defining and measuring problem gambling

There has been considerable disagreement within the problem gambling research literature and among those involved in the regulation of gambling and provision of problem gambling interventions as to the selection and use of the most appropriate measurement tools.[16] This debate impacts upon the resolution of issues such as 'how serious and widespread is problem gambling within the community?' and 'what should we do about it?' The debate surrounding the measurement of problem gambling has been complicated by the varied, disparate and, perhaps mutually exclusive, objectives and purposes pursued by the developers of the respective measurement instruments purported to measure gambling and problem gambling. A detailed content analysis of these tools suggests that there is a concerning lack of clarity as to the actual stated objective described within existing tools.[4]

Problem gambling has been defined as 'any pattern of gambling behaviour that negatively affects other important areas of an individual's life, such as relationships, finances or vocation. The mental disorder of 'pathological' gambling lies at one end of a broad continuum of problem gambling behaviour'.[17] It has also been defined as 'a chronic failure to resist gambling impulses that results in disruption or damage to several areas of a person's social, vocational, familial or financial functioning. Excessive gambling is used to describe a level of gambling expenditure that is considered to be higher than can be reasonably afforded relative to the individual's available disposable income and as a result produces financial strain'.[18] This definition is one of the few to include explicit mention of both an underlying condition and its symptoms and consequences.

Although there is now a substantial international literature on the prevalence of problem and pathological gambling within the community, there remains considerable uncertainty as to the actual rates of problem gambling within different communities and jurisdictions, due in no small part to variations in definitions of problem gambling as well as methodological issues and problems in the conduct of the survey research. This situation arises out of the lack of conceptual clarity and agreement as to whether problem/pathological gambling is best construed as a dimensional behaviour (i.e. something that is a continuum along which people vary in extent) or a categorical disorder (i.e. something that you either have or do not have).

The core component defining a 'problem gambler' is impaired control although there is some level of circularity in argument inherent in these definitions. The problem gambler develops negative consequences because of an inability to control behaviour, and negative consequences arise because the gambler has no control over behaviour. There is a further group of gambling problems that has sometimes escaped attention. This is the situation where existing non-gambling related problems or conditions, such as relationship disharmony, are aggravated by gambling behaviours and their consequences, such as time and money lost.

A focus on harm as the foundation of a measure may be deemed appropriate for the purpose of determining the socioeconomic impact of gambling and excessive gambling within a community. It may also be useful in screening for individuals who have or may be at risk for developing into a problem gambler. The original purpose of the South Oaks Gambling Screen (SOGS),[19] for example, was to identify possible problem gamblers attending a drug and alcohol facility, and selecting these out for further diagnostic testing. In this regard, half of the SOGS items are directed to the presence of harm as manifested by the need to borrow money. However, its use as a diagnostic tool to identify a 'case' of a problem gambler is of questionable validity and its use as the screen of choice in multiple surveys has only served to overestimate prevalence rates. This point is well-exemplified in a comparative study of reliability, validity and classification accuracy of the SOGS, conducted by Stinchfield.[20]

The Productivity Commission[21] has estimated that 2.1% of Australians had 'significant problems with their gambling' and that 2.0% of Victorians fell into this category. The sixth and seventh Community Gambling Patterns and Perceptions Surveys conducted for the VCGA in 1998 and 1999 showed quite divergent rates of gamblers 'at risk' with rates of 1.5% and 0.8% respectively in the two studies. Comparable figures have been found in a wide range of jurisdictions, including Nebraska,[22] Minnesota,[23] and Quebec[24] and a range of United States communities.[25,26]

Whether we consider problem gambling to be a dichotomy or on a continuum is fundamental to the way we measure it. The Productivity Commission report[21] provides an especially clear discussion of this issue: 'The difficulty of identifying the "right" threshold for problem gambling stems from the fact that cases are only defined fuzzily when the severity of the problems varies along a continuum. In some areas of public health it is easy to define a case. For instance, someone either has HIV or they do not. But in problem gambling (and a range of other possible areas, such as obesity or diabetes) it is not clear where along the continuum people can be said categorically to have a problem. If the threshold is set low then obviously a lot of people are said to be "problem" gamblers . . .' (pp. 6.18–19).

Gambling participation and problem gambling prevalence in particular subpopulations

Adolescents

Studies have shown that despite their participation in many forms of gambling being illegal,[27] adolescents are as likely to participate in gambling as previous generations of youth experimented with tobacco and alcohol.[28–30] Research suggests that adolescent prevalence rates of pathological gambling generally range from 4–8%, which represents approximately two to four times prevalence rates in the adult population,[30–33] with up to 14% being described as 'at risk', 'problem' or 'potential problem' gamblers.[34] There has recently been some debate, however, as to the accuracy of some of these earlier estimates and the utility of the measures used.[35]

Despite higher prevalence rates, few adolescents who are regular gamblers consider their gambling to be problematic, although one quarter reported having had problems associated with their gambling in two studies[36,37] and clinicians note that adolescents rarely perceive themselves as problem or pathological gamblers.[38]

Studies have indicated that young males are more likely to exhibit problem gambling behaviour,[39] with some studies suggesting that pathological gambling is twice as prevalent among males as females.[40–43] In a recent review of gambling literature, Rossen[44] identified that adolescent pathological gamblers are more likely to exhibit risk-taking behaviour, demonstrate poor performance at school, suffer high rates of depression and low self-esteem, have poorer coping skills and be at a greater risk of suicidal ideation. Adolescent problem gamblers are more likely to participate in other risk-taking behaviour,[39] to participate in criminal activities and antisocial or delinquent behaviour and show high levels of disengagement from school.[45]

Ethnic communities

Thomas and Yamine[46] have suggested that community surveys of gambling patterns have seriously under-represented the numbers of people from different cultural backgrounds for whom it was expected that there might be higher rates of problem gambling than in the general community. These expectations were fulfilled when the Thomas and Yamine study analysed answers to the SOGS from respondents of Greek, Vietnamese, Chinese and Arabic cultural background and found rates of problem gambling broadly five times greater than in the general community. Consultations conducted as part of this study emphasized the importance of the immigration experience itself in contributing to a propensity to gamble, a point made strongly by Duong & Ohtsuka,[47] and Au & Yu[48] who have argued that gambling may be understood in the context of migration adjustment problems, such as unemployment, underemployment, and threats to the self-esteem of Asian men in particular.

Women

In a thorough review of research materials published over a ten-year period, Martins et al.[49] have argued that most problem gambler studies are conducted with male subjects, despite the fact that one-third of problem gamblers are women. They note that in Brazil, a clinical sample found a male–female ratio of 1:1 a finding similar to that of reviews of problem gamblers presenting to Gambler's Help in Victoria, Australia.[50–52] Some authors suggest that problem gambler progression is faster in women.[53] In female gamblers, this telescoping effect 'occurs in two periods: in the interval between gambling intensification and the first gambling-related problems and between these first problems and the time they sought treatment'.[49] Martins et al.[49] suggest that since the telescoping effect is a phenomenon common to alcohol and drug addiction as well as problem gambling, studies that explore the physiopathology of these conditions could clarify the biologic (genetic and/or hormonal) and sociocultural factors that contribute to this accelerated course in women.

Problem gambling intervention models

The approach taken to treating gambling-related problems, particularly at the level of the individual and group is determined by the view taken of the 'causes' of problem gambling. Broadly speaking, there are three main schools of thought that have dominated discussion about the causes and consequent required treatment of problem gambling: the 'medical' model, the 'behavioural' model and the 'cognitive' model.[7]

The medical model sees problem gambling as an addiction, akin to alcohol and substance dependence; as a compulsion; or as an impulse-control disorder, which must be treated by interventions appropriate for an illness, with the end goal being abstinence from all gambling.[13,54,55] The behavioural model interprets problem gambling as a learned behaviour, motivated and/or reinforced by the personal experiences and social context of the gambler. Like any other problem of behaviour, the treatment focus is on 'unlearning' bad habits and learning how to minimize the harm arising from gambling through 'controlled gambling'.[56] Abstinence, although theoretically consistent with this approach, is not usually specified as an endpoint. Cognitive theories of gambling suggest that problem gambling behaviours are maintained by irrational beliefs and attitudes about gambling.

To date, a great deal of the treatment literature has described clinical trials of various methods of intervention or efficacy studies, which in many cases have not yet been systematically translated into treatment programs.[57] Furthermore, of those established treatment programs that are described in the published literature, very few are accompanied by controlled effectiveness studies. The study undertaken by the US National Gambling Impact Study Commission[58] supports this. They concluded that few studies exist that measure the effectiveness of different treatment methods and those that do exist 'lack a clear conceptual model and specification of outcome criteria, fail to report compliance and attrition rates, offer little description of actual treatment involved or measures to maintain treatment fidelity by the counsellors, and provide inadequate length of follow-up'. The difficulty of evaluating the appropriateness of various treatment programs – for whom, at what level of problem intensity, for what type of problems, for what types of gamblers, in what mode of service delivery – is further complicated by the fact that there are 'no internationally established models of best practice in existence'.[11,59]

Community-based models

Community-based centres reported in the literature are somewhat similar in nature to the Gambler's Help system of service provision in Victoria, in that free specialist support is available through generalist community-based organizations, such as community health centres.[60] Community-based service models appear to provide accessible support for individuals with problems with their own gambling and support for family members experiencing gambling-related problems. In addition, the multi-modal approach to treatment adopted in this community model acknowledges the multi-faceted nature of problem-gambling behaviour in terms of impact. A review of community-based models of practice in Victoria has suggested that a majority of counsellors in Gambler's Help have adopted an eclectic approach to counselling, consistent with current trends in counselling and psychotherapy. Cognitive behavioural therapy (CBT) has been identified by the majority of Gambler's Help agencies as a major component of their theoretical and practice framework, along with broad psychosocial approaches. This orientation is reflective of best practice in community-based services reaching a client base heterogeneous in terms of gambling type and severity.[11,61,62]

The Gambler's Help Program is producing high levels of positive resolution in all defined problem areas[63] with these results being achieved with relatively small numbers of counselling sessions.[64]

Methods for measuring 'success', other than client and worker self-report, as in the Gambler's Help Study, are found in other community-based service models, but so are problems in follow-up. Walker et al.,[65] for example, report in their review of 130 counsellors in 75 agencies in New South Wales, that 42% of counsellors follow-up all clients, while an additional 27% follow-up those who gave permission to be followed up, those who completed treatment, or a random sample of clients.

Hospital inpatient and outpatient models

A range of hospital inpatient/outpatient models of treatment have also been reported. The Johns Hopkins Center for Pathological Gambling,[66] for example, became the first treatment centre for problem gamblers in the United States that was open to the general public, providing two types of treatment programs: an intensive residential treatment program and an outpatient program. The underlying therapeutic philosophy of the Center was that the most effective intervention for problem gamblers comprises an individual with a personal understanding of the problem, teamed with a suitably qualified counsellor. The primary objective of the program was to educate the client about the 'illness', initiate rehabilitation, and to eventually, refer the client for two years of outpatient work with a private practitioner and/or Gamblers Anonymous. Couple and family therapy as well as legal and financial counselling were available in the belief that both play an important role in the treatment of problem gamblers. One of the few Australian examples of a hospital model was the Behaviour Therapy Unit, Prince of Wales Hospital, later located at Liverpool Hospital, Sydney, Australia.[67] Treatment practice was informed by McConaghy's Behaviour Completion Mechanism Model,[68] and used imaginal desensitization. Details of treatment effectiveness from this program are detailed later in this chapter.

Self-help models

There are a small number of self-help models, which include Gamblers Anonymous, which uses a 12-step recovery process and abstinence treatment model based on the principles of Alcoholics Anonymous. Gamblers Anonymous accepts the disease model of problem-gambling behaviour, proposing that gambling is 'essentially incurable'.[69] Hence therapy is seen as an ongoing process. According to the Gamblers Anonymous model of treatment 'no member can afford to relax their guard against the urge to gamble', and therapy can only be successful if the gambler makes a sincere commitment to stop gambling.[69] The Free Yourself Program, Australia is a self-help model developed by a former problem gambler, which aims to free people of their 'addiction' to gambling, based on improving their physical, mental and spiritual wellbeing. The program was developed as an alternative to approaches used by Gamblers Anonymous and conventional problem gambling counselling and has been seen as particularly appealing to women problem gamblers.[11]

Methodological issues in determining problem gambling intervention outcomes

In examining intervention outcomes, it is apparent that there are numerous methodological issues in the definition and measurement of treatment outcomes of problem gambling programs making it difficult to generalize often about behavioural change in this context. A number of these are discussed here. The first issue is that of sample selection. Selection criteria and procedures for the inclusion of gamblers into treatment programs are often poorly delineated with samples characterized by heterogeneity of subjects. Many studies report the presence of co-existing primary Axis I psychiatric disorders, usually psychoactive substance abuse, and/or fail to ascertain whether therapy for gambling was the primary reason for referral.[70,71]

Another sampling issue is that few studies distinguish treatment effect related to different forms of gambling. Usually no attempt is made to distinguish those participating exclusively in one form as compared to multiple forms of gambling. There is no justified a priori reason to assume that factors influencing aetiology and persistence in gambling apply equally to all forms of gambling. In fact, empirical evidence points to the contrary view. For example, participation in low skill games such as EGMs is accompanied by a narrowing of attention acting as an emotional escape from daily stresses.[14,72] On the other hand, high skill games of cards and horse racing contribute to an elevation of mood in dysphoric/depressed gamblers.[73]

A second methodological problem relates to treatment outcome. Criteria of success based on the dichotomous global ratings of abstinence and non-abstinence typical of 'addictions'-oriented programs, fail to take into account significant improvement in other areas of functioning including reduced frequency, urge, ability to control gambling once initiated, and improved social, financial and interpersonal functioning. Taber et al.,[74] Blackman et al.,[75] and Blaszczynski,[76] for example, have found that gamblers showed clear signs of post-treatment improvement in many areas even though they continued gambling, albeit at reduced levels.

It is apparent that despite one or more lapses gamblers may continue to regard themselves as abstinent over the longer time frame. To suggest that a lapse constitutes treatment failure because it violates the criteria of abstinence is excessively rigid and has the potential to lead the gambler to regard such lapses as a total failure causing them to lose motivation to re-instate control.[76] The offer or option of controlled gambling as an alternative outcome may have an added advantage of enticing borderline motivated gamblers into treatment at a much earlier stage of their career. Lower treatment rejection and attrition rates may be achieved for gamblers who find complete cessation difficult or its notion unacceptable.[76–79]

A third methodological problem relates to treatment outcome criteria. Many studies do not present data on rejection (refusal to enter a program) or attrition (drop-out from programs), but where this information is available, high rates have been reported. Excluding non-starters or dropouts from statistical analyses results in an over-estimate of the likelihood of success. This tendency to ignore cases is equally pertinent when reporting on subjects lost to follow-up. Apart from Taber et al.[74] who achieved a rate of 86 percent from a sample of 66 gamblers at six months, follow-up data is generally obtained on approximately 50–60% of subjects initially treated and irrespective of the length of follow-up; 60% at two months to two years,[80] 48% at 12 months,[81] and 52% at five years follow-up.[73]

A fourth problem is the attribution of treatment effects. It is sometimes difficult to identify the impacts of primary interventions, in situations where a number of interventions are used simultaneously, for example, individual counselling and group therapy. Indeed, in some multi-modal programs there may not be a designated primary intervention, but a collection of interventions including individual counselling using a cognitive, behavioural or cognitive–behavioural approach for the person experiencing problems with their own gambling behaviour; couple or relationship counselling; financial counselling and legal advocacy to reduce the stress caused by excessive debt, etc. In this sort of program, it is often difficult to identify with certainty what intervention or combination of interventions, performed by whom, had what effect.

A fifth methodological concern is that it is not always clear in studies whether reliable and valid measures of change are being used, or how concepts such as 'improvement' are measured,[71,81,82] while a further methodological challenge relates to the definition of success on discharge. Few studies report on the status of the gambler at discharge preferring to provide assessments at six or 12 months follow-up. Much can happen in the intervening period between discharge and follow-up causing positive change independent of treatment received. In Blaszczynski's clinical experience,[11] gamblers at discharge have reported no perceived change in urge to gamble but at one month and after exposure to gambling cues have come to recognize significant positive changes in their behaviour and emotions.

A seventh methodological issue concerns the lack of clear-cut definitions of lapse and relapse and their relationship to treatment failure. While it is clear that some people fail to respond to treatment and continue to engage in unchanged levels of uncontrolled gambling, others exhibit periods of gambling against a background of abstinence, while others substitute more innocuous forms of gambling, Blaszczynski et al.[82] have shown that lapses do not invariably lead to a resumption of pathological gambling habits. A final methodological issue somewhat related to this, is the variation in post-treatment follow-up intervals, which often vary generally from six months to two years, although to adequately account for a full understanding of 'lapse' and 'relapse' behaviour, longer follow-up periods, say five years, may be more useful.

Treatment approaches and outcomes

A broad range of interventions has been employed in the treatment of problem gambling. Psychodynamic formulations appeared in the early turn of this century with behaviourally based interventions emerging in the 1960s. By the 1980s multi-modal programs came into vogue while in the 1990s the emphasis shifted toward cognitive–behavioural interventions, cognitive interventions and, increasingly in the 2000s, psychopharmacological regimes, alongside multi-modal and cognitive or cognitive/behavioural interventions.

Psychoanalytic formulations

Early psychoanalytic explanations of pathological gambling emphasized the sexual equivalence of the gambling situation and considered gambling an expression of an underlying psychoneurosis related to a regression to pre-genital psychosexual phases.[83–86] Although Freud did not intend his analysis to apply to all gamblers his writings lay the foundation for subsequent psychodynamic descriptions and treatment.[87–91]

Psychoanalytic explanations, however, have been considered as inherently weak and considered doubtful as a useful explanation of the pathogenesis of pathological gambling[92] and the effectiveness of psychodynamic treatments is difficult to evaluate. Little credibility can be apportioned to the myriad of single case reports on populations, heterogeneous in terms of psychological state. Generally, treatment goals have been unspecified and no measure of gambling severity or outcome described.[87,93–95] Only Bergler[88] reported on an appreciable sample of 80 patients selected from a larger pool of referrals. Taken as a proportion of those who commenced treatment, 75% achieved successful outcome, but this represents less than one fifth of the initial total pool of referrals.

Psychoanalytical formulations may in the future inform some work with couples, based on object relations theory and some individual work with women, where the association between excessive gambling and a history of childhood sexual abuse is being explored.

Self-help organizations

Despite the many barriers to examining its effectiveness a number of researchers have provided participant observational reports and carried out systematic observations of Gamblers Anonymous attendance rates. Scodel[96] and Cromer[97] provided participant observational reports outlining relevant processes emerging within the group structure but emphasized the inherent difficulties in identifying the crucial therapeutic ingredients underpinning positive outcome. Insight or personality changes did not emerge in the context of attendance.[96] Custer and Custer[70] surveyed 150 Gamblers Anonymous members and found that the mean period of attendance at GA meetings was seven years and three months. Forty-two percent reported no gambling since attending, 32% one lapse, 10% two lapses, and 16% more than two lapses.

Brown[77] carried out a systematic five-year retrospective and a three-month prospective study of GA attendance rates. In the retrospective phase of the study, only 7.3% of members met the required criteria of two-year abstinence. Results revealed that 22.4% of the initial total cohort of 232 gamblers dropped out after one meeting with 70% so doing by their tenth meeting. Reducing the period of abstinence to one year did not alter the success rate. In the prospective phase, Brown[77] observed a 50 percent attrition rate by the third week of attendance with a 12 months abstinence rate of 7.5%. Brown recognized that a stringent one to two-year abstinence rate potentially underestimated the full impact of GA, noting that those dropping out after even one meeting may well have benefited considerably from that experience. It has also been noted that the proportion of gamblers who participate in GA meetings during treatment in hospital settings and after discharge, appear to do significantly better in terms of continued abstinence.[74]

Behavioural treatments

Most behavioural treatments have used operant or classic conditioning aversive techniques to counter-condition the arousal/excitement associated with gambling. The most frequent early form of aversion was electric shocks in isolation[98,99] or in conjunction with supportive therapy[100] or covert sensitization.[101] Covert sensitization in which aversive imagery is substituted for electric shock stimuli was later combined with rational emotive therapy[102] and stimulus control and exposure.[103] Salzmann[104] reported the only use of a chemical substance, apomorphine, in an aversive therapy paradigm while Greenberg and Rankin[103] supplemented exposure to gambling cues with a rubber-band technique in which self-inflicted pain is produced by snapping a rubber band over the wrist. Most studies of behavioural interventions, however, have failed to operationally define outcome criteria, and that under these circumstances, consideration of treatment effectiveness and successful outcome is often governed by an arbitrary choice of liberal versus stringent criteria. Overall, as the NCETA[10] review argued, there is some evidence that imaginal desensitization is superior to aversion therapy and that cue-exposure/response prevention therapies are producing improvement rates in terms of control, comparable with alcohol treatment programs using the same methods.

Controlled gambling

The prospect of controlled gambling has been largely ignored despite Dickerson and Weeks'[78] report of successful application of behavioural counselling in a case of a 40-year-old male and a report by Rankin[79] using a similar approach in the treatment of a 44-year-old gambler with a 20-year history. Except for three lapses, control was reputedly maintained 'for almost all of the two-year follow-up period'.

Contrary to expectation, controlled gambling does not appear to increase the probability of relapse into uncontrolled gambling.[73,76,103,105] Russo et al.,[81] for example, found 21% of their sample who reported abstinence in the month preceding follow-up interview had earlier experienced gambling lapses without resurgence of pathological gambling behaviour patterns. Lapses may be beneficial in enhancing the learning process of identifying and subsequently coping with or avoiding situation and emotional determinants leading to gambling relapse.[82]

Cognitive therapy

Cognitive theories have been proposed to explain the apparent contradictions manifested in pathological gambling behaviour. These have variably emphasized notions of the illusion of control,[106] biased evaluation,[107,108] erroneous perceptions[109–111] and irrational thinking processes.[69]

Recently treatment studies have emerged explicitly based on a cognitive theory of problem gambling. Ladouceur et al.,[111] in a controlled clinical trail, evaluated the efficacy of a cognitive treatment package for pathological gambling. Sixty-six gamblers, meeting DSM-IV criteria for pathological gambling, were randomly assigned to treatment or waitlist control conditions. Thirty-five people completed treatment of up to 20 one-hour sessions (mean 11.03). Cognitive correction techniques were used first to target gamblers' erroneous perceptions about randomness and then to address issues of relapse prevention. The dependent measures used were the SOGS, the number of DSM-IV criteria for pathological gambling met by participants, as well as gamblers' perception of control, frequency of gambling, perceived self-efficacy, and desire to gamble. Post-test results indicated highly significant changes in the treatment group on all outcome measures, and analysis of data from six- and 12-month follow-ups revealed maintenance of therapeutic gains. The authors suggest that this treatment outcome study shows that a cognitive treatment can significantly improve pathological gambling, as demonstrated by the fact that 86% of the treated participants were no longer considered pathological gamblers, as measured by DSM-IV, at the end of treatment. In addition, those completing treatment had greater perception of control of their gambling problem as well as an increased self-efficacy in high-risk gambling situations. This study is important, in illustrating the effectiveness of theory-driven practice, and the effectiveness of a cognitive intervention targeting a specific cognitive error, namely the gambler's beliefs about randomness and their belief that they can control the outcome of random events.

Dickerson and Baron[112] have also argued for specific targeting of interventions, particularly a focus on the construct of choice or subjective control over gambling. Despite the conceptual difficulties that may be associated with the variable of self-control, they suggest that these may be overcome because contemporary research into the addictive behaviours has demonstrated considerable success in the definition and measurement of control and related themes such as craving, restraint and temptation.

Multi-modal therapies

A potential criticism of some behavioural and cognitive techniques is that they target only the specific reduction in the frequency of gambling without addressing significant ancillary issues. Although their aetiological significance is obscure, co-existing problems of depression, substance abuse, marital discord, legal action and employment problems are important but tend to be neglected on the presumption that they are secondary to the gambling.

These are expected to improve without direct intervention if gambling ceases. However, emotional stresses produced by the effects of gambling may themselves act as risk factors in persistence at gambling or in precipitating relapse episodes. This is pertinent where co-morbid substance abuse disorders exist and where disinhibition caused by alcohol may affect self-control resulting in impulsive or binge episodes. Financially, pressing debts may also prompt further gambling as the only perceived available alternative option to obtain funds to meet financial commitments. Clearly, multi-modal approaches with a focus on insight, group therapy and personal development seem an attractive proposition in the holistic management of pathological gambling.[74,75,81]

Lesieur and Blume[71] reported on the outcome of 72 patients at 6 to 14 months following completion of a combined alcohol, substance abuse and compulsive gambling treatment program. The multi-modal program consisted of individual and group psychotherapy, education on the impact of alcohol, drugs and gambling, family counselling, attendance at Alcoholics, Narcotics and Gamblers Anonymous meetings and psychodrama. Special groups for health professions, law enforcement agencies and employee assistance programs were offered with post-discharge continuity of care achieved through weekly group, individual or family sessions as required. Results were consistent with those of Taber and colleagues in that 64% of followed up subjects remained abstinent since treatment with the figure increasing to 94.4% if the more liberal criterion of overall improvement was used. Importantly, no substitution of one addiction for another was noted in the gambling group. Only 9.7% of the sample, however, indicated that the program as a whole was beneficial, with 51% singling out group therapy as the most useful contributor to outcome. Fifteen percent considered the disease concept itself, and the educational component, as the most helpful.

Comparable positive outcome rates are found in the European literature[113] on programs including such therapies as medical intervention, group therapy, individual treatment, occupational therapy, work therapy, hydrotherapy, autogenic training, sports and gymnastics, family group therapy, cognitive therapy, and health education. The multi-modal programs reported appear effective in 20–50% of cases over one to two years, but, methodologically, all were uncontrolled studies with no random allocation of patients or blind ratings of outcome. Analyses of these interventions suggested that less costly and briefer methods of behavioural intervention needed to be explored.

This has been done by Hodgins et al.[114] who compared two brief treatments for problem gambling with a waiting-list control in a randomized trial. Eighty-four percent of participants ($N = 102$) reported a significant reduction in gambling over a 12-month follow-up period. Participants who received a motivational enhancement telephone intervention and a self-help workbook in the mail, but not those who received the workbook only, had better outcomes than participants in a one-month waiting-list control. Participants who received the motivational interview and workbook showed better outcomes than those receiving the workbook only at three- and six-month follow-ups. At the 12-month follow-up, the advantage of the motivational interview and workbook condition was found only for participants with less severe gambling problems. Overall, these results were deemed to support the effectiveness of a brief telephone and mail-based treatment for problem gambling, and echo the Dickerson et al.[115] study on the use of a self-help manual with and without interview.

Early pharmacological interventions

From 1980 a number of case studies appeared in the literature describing the effective use of medication in the control of pathological gambling. The rationale for such use had not been theory-driven but, rather, based on attempts to simply block reinforcing affective 'thrill' components inherent in gambling[116] or on innovative clinical judgement in which analogies had been drawn between the manifestations of repetitive gambling behaviour and obsessive–compulsive disorders.[117]

Moskowitz[116] reported successful outcome in two of three pathological gamblers treated with 600 mg lithium carbonate t.d.s. The outcome of the third case report was not clearly elucidated, and it was not clear as to whether abstinence or reduced gambling was achieved by subjects over the unspecified follow-up periods. However, evidence that manifest pathological gambling behaviours coincided with cyclical episodes of affective excitability and impulsivity suggested the possibility that the pathological gambling was secondary to a primary diagnosis of manic-depressive illness. Therefore, the utility of lithium carbonate in pathological gamblers in general not displaying evidence of a cyclical affective disturbance remained uncertain.

Certain similarities in the nature of obsessive–compulsive disorders and repetitive impulse control disorders have led a number of authors to speculate on the possibility that impulse control disorders including gambling[117] are in some way related to a dimension of impulsivity/obsessive–compulsive disorders rather than a disorder of 'addiction'. This speculation has prompted the use of obsessive–compulsive medications such as the serotonin re-uptake blockers clomipramine and fluoexetine in the management of gambling problems[117] as well as, for example, body dysmorphic disorder,[118] and trichotillomania [119].

Later pharmacological interventions: Fluvoxamine and naltrexone

Figgitt and McClellan[120] note, of the more recently used selective serotonin re-uptake inhibitor (SSRI), fluvoxamine, that it is both potent and that it has little or no effect on other monoamine reuptake mechanisms. They report that in randomized, double-blind trials, fluvoxamine 100 to 300 mg/day for six to ten weeks significantly reduced symptoms of obsessive–compulsive disorder (OCD) compared with placebo. Response rates of 38 to 52% have been reported with fluvoxamine, compared with response rates of 0 to 18% with placebo. In patients with OCD, fluvoxamine had similar efficacy to that of clomipramine and, in smaller trials, the SSRIs paroxetine and citalopram, and was significantly more effective than desipramine.

Hollander et al.[121] assessed the effectiveness and tolerability of fluvoxamine in the treatment of pathological gambling in a 16-week randomized double-blind cross-over design that ensured that each participant received eight weeks of fluvoxamine and eight weeks of a placebo. Fifteen gamblers entered the treatment program, with ten completing. They found that fluvoxamine resulted in a significantly greater percent improvement in overall gambling severity on the PG Clinical Global Impression (PG-CGI) scale. There was a significant treatment effect on gambling urge and behaviour as measured by the PG modification of the Yale–Brown Obsessive Compulsive Scale and PG-CGI scale improvement scores. Interestingly, they also found a significant interaction of treatment effect with the order of administration of the drug and placebo. Post hoc analysis, treating each phase as a separate trial, demonstrated a significant difference between fluvoxamine and the placebo in the second phase of the trial, but not in the first, indicating a reduction of early placebo effect.

Bianco et al.,[122] in their pilot placebo-controlled study of fluvoxamine for pathological gambling did not find as positive a response as Hollander et al.[121] Thirty-two patients were treated for six months in a double-blind, placebo-controlled study of fluvoxamine 200 mg/day. Outcome measures included reduction in both money and time spent gambling per week. Longitudinal mixed effects models and treatment completers analyses were used for estimation and hypothesis testing. Fluvoxamine was not statistically significantly different from placebo in the overall sample. However, fluvoxamine was statistically significantly superior to placebo in males and in younger patients. Although the power of the study was limited by the high (59%) placebo-response rate, the authors note that fluvoxamine may be a useful treatment for certain subgroups of patients with pathological gambling. Again, further testing is warranted with a more diverse population of gamblers, with longer follow-up times, than end of treatment.

Zimmerman et al.[123] evaluated the effectiveness of citalopram in the treatment of pathological gambling through an open-label trial for 12 weeks of 15 adults who had met the DSM-IV criteria for pathological gambling. At treatment end, patients reported significant improvements on all gambling measures including the number of days gambled, the amount of money lost gambling, preoccupation with gambling, and urges to gamble. From this study, it appears that the SSRI citalopram is an effective treatment for pathological gambling, and that this benefit was independent of its antidepressant properties. As found in the Zimmerman et al. trial,[123] depressive symptoms are found in many, if not the majority of pathological gamblers. Given the fact that clomipramine and fluoexetine, for example, are robust antidepressants,[124] it has been necessary to exclude the possibility that the effectiveness of these medications may act through their mood-altering properties. Crockford and el Guebaly[125] report the effects of naltrexone on an alcohol-dependent EGM player also treated with fluoxetine for depression, who had been abstinent for one month (gambling) prior to being prescribed naltrexone. There was no relapse over the next month, and the authors suggest that the 'endogenous opioid system acts as a common pathway in regulating cravings'.

Further studies of naltrexone as a treatment for pathological gambling have confirmed the effects reported by Crockford and el-Guebaly.[125] Kim and Grant[126] report the results of a study designed to test the short-term efficacy and safety of naltrexone in the treatment of pathological gambling disorder in seventeen subjects (seven men, ten women) in a six-week open naltrexone flexible dose trial. Naltrexone reduced urges to gamble and gambling behaviour and men responded to naltrexone as well as women. These results have also been produced in a further double-blind naltrexone and placebo comparison study.[127] Using random regression analysis, Kim et al.[127] noted significant improvement in a number of gambling symptom measures, including patient-rated Clinical Global Impression; clinician-rated CGI; and Gambling Symptom Rating Scale.

What can we conclude about pharmacological interventions?

As we can see, several types of medication have been demonstrated to be effective in some cases of pathological gambling: seretonin re-uptake inhibitors; opoid antagonists; and mood stabilizers. The encouraging reports of the efficacy of clomipramine, fluoexetine and fluvoxamine in impulse control disorders suggests the possibility that repetitive, driven, or compulsive urges are characteristic features which may link pathological gambling, sexual paraphilias and obsessive–compulsive disorders. Such a proposition warrants further investigation for, if so, the reconceptualization of pathological gambling away from an addictive disorder to that of a variant of an 'obsessive–compulsive' illness may prove a more fruitful avenue of pursuit especially in respect of treatment.

Additional developments in pharmacological approaches to the management of problematic gambling behaviour, and developments in the way we understand the role of memory and decision-making, for example, may also stem in the future from ancillary areas of research in which brain function is implicated in gambling-related behaviours such as in the Stout et al.[128] study on decision making in Huntington's disease (HD) using a laboratory-based simulated gambling task which had been used to quantify decision-making deficits in ventromedial frontal lobe damaged participants.

Help–seeking and problem gambling interventions

In a previous study of problem gambler's progression, Tavares et al.[129] noted that on average five years elapsed between the experience of the first problem caused by gambling and the first attempt to have treatment, less than the nine years identified by the Productivity Commission,[21] in its study on Australia's Gambling Industries. In an adaptation of Sobell et al's[130] work on alcoholics, Hodgins and el-Guebaly[131] investigated a range of potential reasons for not seeking treatment among non-treated pathological gamblers. The gamblers' desire to handle the problem on their own was the main factor identified. The others were embarrassment, stigma, inability to share problems, and failing to regard gambling as a problem.

In attempting to answer the question of why problem gamblers delayed seeking treatment, Tavares et al.[132] aimed to gather objective evidence of the impact of delaying factors on treatment-seeking, while controlling for gambling severity, and cohort effects from changes over time in public awareness and treatment availability. The study found that the more recent the problem with gambling the less likely the subject was to delay treatment-seeking, due, the authors believe, to greater public awareness and treatment availability being available prior to the study taking place, thus concurring with earlier research on the effects of public education on problem gambling in terms of help seeking.[15] Two factors showed as the strongest predictors for treatment delay – shame and secrecy, and chasing losses/lonely efforts at self-control.

Data from this study also suggest that once problems begin, the process that will lead gamblers to treatment is independent from gender and type of game, although the influences of both of these factors have been shown elsewhere to be important in populations of help-seeking problem gamblers.[50,133] A recent modest report on barriers to help seeking for those with gambling-related problems, from a random community telephone survey[134] suggests that issues of access and perceived availability, perceived effectiveness and cost may all influence those with such problems from seeking help.

Some interesting findings complementing our understanding of help-seeking have been made concerning treatment completers and non-completers. Leblond et al.[135] have found that program participants who dropped out of an individual cognitive-oriented treatment had significantly higher scores on impulsivity than completers. They suggest that clinicians should consider problem gamblers exhibiting higher impulsivity to be at greater risk for prematurely dropping out and should therefore closely monitor the progress of these clients, and offer additional motivational enhancing interventions.

Group-level interventions

A small number of group and family interventions for problematic gambling have been reported. Haustein and Shurgers[136] describe a treatment program designed for problem gamblers that involved individual and group therapy as well as a voluntary group program. Throughout the sessions the therapist guided the discussion towards three basic issues: (1) what can the gambler do in their everyday life to make it as hard as possible for them to get to the slot machine; (2) what had happened just prior to relapse; and (3) parallel to these topics, the gamblers were asked exactly how they felt before, during and after gambling. Taber and Chaplin[137] reviewed some of the group psychotherapy techniques, ranging from rational–emotive psychotherapy to Zen philosophy based treatments, in their work with problem gamblers. They proposed that most pathological gamblers seem to have great potential to profit from short-term group psychotherapy, if the group is managed by a skilled professional, and if the group is homogenous with respect to the gambling problem.

The way forward: A model for the design of effective interventions

The model outlined below is presented as a way of conceptualizing the behaviours involved in problematic gambling and the range of intervention foci available in an integrated multi-level approach to dealing with problematic gambling behaviour.[138] It suggests that gambling uptake for individuals is influenced by varying intrinsic propensities to gamble and the availability of gambling products to that individual. It is further suggested that the outcomes and consequences of gambling are influenced by gambling uptake and that various protective, moderating and risk factors impact upon propensity to gamble, the availability of gambling products and also the outcomes and consequences of gambling uptake upon gamblers, their families and the community. This seems to be a useful way of tying together much that we know, some of which has been presented in this chapter, about where and how to intervene effectively in this complex behaviour.

Interventions may be targeted at influencing the propensity to gamble; restricting or modifying supply of gambling products; and/or ameliorating the negative outcomes and consequences of problematic gambling, at the level of the individual, family or community.

The inter-relationship of these intervention targets is illustrated in Fig. 11.1.

Propensity to gamble

In the model it is assumed that people vary in their propensity and desire to gamble and that this propensity to gamble may be influenced by a variety of factors such as impulsiveness and risk-taking. It may also be affected by other behavioural issues[139] such as psychiatric problems.[140] Evidence for intrinsic factors affecting gambling behaviour is provided by a study of 3359 twin

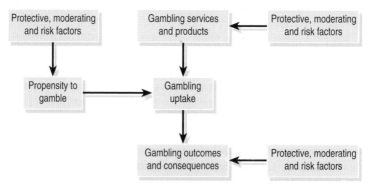

Fig. 11.1   A model of influences on gambling behaviours and outcomes.[138]

pairs[141] in which it was argued that familial factors, including both genetic inheritance and experiences shared by twin siblings, explained 62% of variation in the study sample in the diagnosis of pathological gambling disorder and lower amounts of variance in the elevated but 'normal' ranges of gambling behaviour. Although much of the research views the issues from a psychological and/or psychiatric framework, and thus focuses on the personal characteristics of the individual gambler, there is some research from a sociological perspective on the social and contextual factors associated with the propensity to gamble, such as family, as noted above[36,142]; living in isolated communities, particularly for women[143] and socioeconomic status.[144] All of these issues present challenges to the development of appropriate interventions at an individual and community level.

Gambling products

Gambling uptake and participation patterns are, of course, influenced by the availability of gambling products. The impact of geographical distribution of EGMs upon gambling uptake and rates of problem gambling has been reported, for example, by the Productivity Commission.[21] That study hypothesised a positive and statistically significant relationship between gambling-related problems and accessibility to gambling, particularly the number of gaming machines, and high average annual expenditure on gaming machines. Government can impact upon the rates and distribution of gambling product uptake through regulating the distribution of gaming products and the nature of such products within its jurisdiction. Product and placement issues so addressed may include high denomination note acceptors on electronic gaming machines (EGMs), clock displays, the removal of automatic teller machines (ATMs) from gaming areas, betting limits, the machine display of amounts wagered rather than units and enforced breaks in play.[145]

Self-exclusion as an intervention has also been given some attention.[146,147] A review of self-exclusion in Victoria, Australia[148] concluded that these programs are, overall, a useful adjunct to responsible gambling policies self-initiated by either the industry or mandated by government. O'Neil et al.'s[148] study, however, also suggests that the potential of self-exclusion programs is severely undermined by ineffective implementation and the problems associated with enforcing bans from multiple venues such as hotels and clubs, rather than from the single venue casinos reported in the literature.

Gambling uptake

The model suggests that gambling uptake is influenced by both the personal characteristics of the gambler, i.e. propensity to gamble, and contextual factors such as the availability of services and products for them to exercise these propensities. Uptake can be modelled demographically and also spatially to examine uptake of different products and services.

Protective and risk factors for gambling propensity, uptake and consequences

Each of the major model elements – gambling propensity, uptake, and outcomes and consequences – has associated with it a set of related protective, moderating and risk factors. It is important to understand these factors in order to be able to design appropriate interventions at each level and also to be able to target services and assistance to those who most need them. For example, we can target the propensity to gamble and the propensity to become a 'problem gambler' by targeting at-risk groups with appropriate communications in the mass media and in community settings. Although the effectiveness of this sort of intervention has been little studied in relation to gambling,[15] it has been widely demonstrated as effective in relation to a range of impulse control-related and health compromising behaviours.[149–153]

Social and family supports or the lack of them also appear to be important protective and risk factors for negative outcomes of gambling activity.[154] For example, people who are divorced or separated have been shown to appear at twice the expected rate in presentations to specialized problem gambling services.[52] While this may be either a cause or a consequence of the problem gambling, it is very well-known from other research literatures that familial and community social supports are a key protective factor for adversity.[155,156]

CONCLUSION

This multi-level intervention framework, it is suggested, could provide a useful device with which to design effective interventions for problem gambling, based on the best evidence available. We have seen that much more is known about interventions and associated behavioural changes which are aimed at individuals, less about small groups and very little about communities. Daughters et al.,[157] however, have also provided us with a timely reminder of how much we still need to know about what contributes to positive change in individuals but a program design framework such as this could provide a major step forward in meeting the challenges of the knowledge and practice gaps.

References

1. Mullen E. Research utilization in the social services – innovations for practice and administration. Social Work 1995; 40(2):282–283.
2. Davies H, Nutley S, Smith P. What works? The role of evidence in public sector policy and practice. Public Money and Management 1999; 19(1):3–5.
3. Walter I, Nutley S, Davies H. Research impact: A cross sector review. St Andrews: Research Unit on Research Utilisation; 2003.
4. Thomas SA, Jackson AC, Blaszczynski AP. Measuring problem gambling: Evaluation of the Victorian gambling screen. Melbourne: Gambling Research Panel; 2003.
5. Wiebe J, Single E, Falkowski-Ham A. Measuring gambling and problem gambling in Ontario. Ontario: Canadian Centre on Substance Abuse and Responsible Gambling Council; 2001.

6. Ferris J, Wynne H, Seigle E. Measuring problem gambling in Canada. Final Report Phase 1. Ottawa: Interprovincial Taskforce on Problem Gambling; 1999.

7. Petry NM, Armentano C. Prevalence, assessment, and treatment of pathological gambling: A review. Psychiatric Services 1999; 50(8):1021–1027.

8. Culleton RP. The prevalence of pathological gambling: A look at methods. Journal of Gambling Behaviour 1989; 5(1):22–41.

9. el-Guebaly N, Hodgins D. Pathological gambling: The biopsychological variables and their management – Interim Report. Alberta: Alberta Gaming Research Institute; 2000.

10. National Centre for Education and Training on Addiction. Current 'best practice' interventions for gambling problems: A theoretical and empirical review. Melbourne: Victorian Department of Human Services; 2000.

11. Jackson AC, Thomas SA, Blaszczynski AP. Best practice in problem gambling services. Melbourne: Gambling Research Panel; 2003.

12. Blaszczynski AP. Pathways to pathological gambling: Identifying typologies. Electronic Journal of Gambling Issues [serial online] 2002 [cited 2004 Jul]; Mar(1):14pp. Available from: URL: www.camh.net/egambling/issue1/feature/2002.

13. Bianco C, Moreyra P, Nunes EV, Saiz-Ruiz J, Ibanez A. Pathological gambling: addiction or compulsion? Seminars in Clinical Neuropsychiatry 2001; 6(3):167–176.

14. Blaszczynski AP, McConaghy N. The medical model of pathological gambling: current shortcomings. Journal of Gambling Behaviour 1988; 5(1):42–52.

15. Jackson AC, Thomas SA, Thomason N, Ho W. Longitudinal evaluation of the effectiveness of problem gambling counselling services, community education strategies and information products. Volume 3: Community education strategies and information products. Melbourne: Victorian Department of Human Services; 2000.

16. Dickerson M, McMillen J, Hallebone E, Volberg R, Woolley R. Definition and incidence of problem gambling, including the socio-economic distribution of gamblers. Melbourne: Victorian Casino and Gaming Authority; 1997.

17. Volberg RA, Moore WL, Christiansen EM, et al. Unaffordable losses: estimating the proportion of gambling revenues derived from problem gamblers. Gaming Law Review 1998; 2(4):349–360.

18. Blaszczynski AP, Walker M, Sagris A, Dickerson M. Psychological aspects of gambling behaviour: An APS Position Paper. Australian Psychological Society; September 1997.

19. Lesieur HR, Blume SB. The South Oaks Gambling Screen (SOGS): A new instrument for the identification of pathological gambling. American Journal of Psychiatry 1987; 144(9):1184–1188.

20. Stinchfield R. Reliability, validity, and classification accuracy of the South Oaks Gambling Screen (SOGS). Addictive Behaviors 2002; 271(1):1–19.

21. Productivity Commission. Australia's Gambling Industries. Canberra: AusInfo; 1999. Report No. 10.

22. Abbott DA, Cramer S. Gambling attitudes and participation: A Midwestern survey. Journal of Gambling Studies 1993; 9(3):247–265.

23. Emerson MO, Laundergan JC. Gambling and problem gambling among adult Minnesotans: Changes 1990 to 1994. Journal of Gambling Studies 1996; 12(3):291–304.

24. Ladouceur R. Prevalence estimates of pathological gambling in Quebec. Canadian Journal of Psychiatry – Revue Canadienne de Psychiatrie 1991; 36:732–734.

25. Volberg RA, Steadman HJ. Refining prevalence estimates of pathological gambling. American Journal of Psychiatry 1988; 145(4):502–505.

26. Volberg RA, Steadman HJ. Prevalence estimates of pathological gambling in New Jersey and Maryland. American Journal of Psychiatry 1989; 146:1618–1619.

27. Jacobs DF. Illegal and undocumented: A review of teenage gambling and the plight of children of problem gamblers in America. In: Shaffer HJ, Stein SA, Gambino B, Cummings TN, eds. Compulsive gambling: theory, research and practice. Massachusetts: Lexington Books; 1989.

28. Radecki TE. The sales of lottery tickets to minors in Illinois. Journal of Gambling Studies 1994; 10:213–218.

29. Rosenstein J, Reutter R. Gambling: An adolescent activity. Journal of Adolescent Health Care 1980; 1(2):180.

30. Shaffer HJ, Hall MN. Estimating prevalence of adolescent gambling disorders: A quantitative synthesis and guide toward standard gambling nomenclature. Journal of Gambling Studies 1996; 12:193–214.

31. Gupta R, Deverensky JL. Adolescent gambling behaviour: A prevalence study and examination of the correlates associated with excessive gambling. Journal of Gambling Studies 1998; 14:227–244.

32. Deverensky JL, Gupta R. Youth gambling: A clinician and research perspective. eGambling: The Electronic Journal of Gambling Issues 2000(2):6–19.

33. Fisher S. Gambling and pathological gambling in adolescents. Journal of Gambling Studies 1993; 9(3):277–287.

34. Jacobs DF. Juvenile gambling in North America: An analysis of long term trends and future prospects. Journal of Gambling Studies 2000; 16(2–3):119–152.

35. Derevensky JL, Gupta R, Winters K. prevalence rates of youth gambling problems: Are the current rates inflated? Journal of Gambling Studies 2003; 19(4):405–425.

36. Govoni R, Rupcich N, Frisch RG. Gambling behaviour of adolescent gamblers. Journal of Gambling Studies 1996; 12(3):305–317.

37. Kearney CA, Roblek T, Thurman J, Turnbough PD. Casino gambling in private school and adjudicated youngsters: A survey or practices and related variables. Journal of Gambling Studies 1996; 12(3):319–327.

38. Hardoon KK, Deverensky JL, Gupta R. An examination of the influence of familial, emotional, conduct, and cognitive problems, and hyperactivity, upon youth risk-taking and adolescent gambling problems. Montreal: R&J Child Development Consultants; 2002.

39. Gupta R, Deverensky JL. An examination of the differential coping styles of adolescents with gambling problems. Ontario: Ministry of Health and Long Term Care; 2001.

40. Lesieur HR, Cross J, Frank M, Welch M, White CM, Rubenstein G, et al. Gambling and pathological gambling among university students. Addictive Behaviors 1991; 16:517–527.

41. Moore SM, Ohtsuka K. Gambling activities of young Australians: Developing a model of behaviour. Journal of Gambling Studies 1997; 13(3):207–236.

42. Stinchfield R. Gambling and correlates of gambling among Minnesota public school students. Journal of Gambling Studies 2000; 162(2–3):153–173.

43. Stinchfield R, Winters KC. Gambling and problem gambling among youths. Annals of the American Academy of Political and Social Sciences 1998; 556:172–185.

44. Rossen F. Youth gambling: A critical review of the public health literature. Auckland: The University of Auckland, New Zealand; 2001.

45. Jackson AC, Patton G, Thomas SA, Wyn J, Wright J, Bond L, et al. The impacts of gambling on adolescents and children. Melbourne: Victorian Department of Human Services; 2000:92 pp.

46. Thomas S, Yamine R. The impact of gaming upon specific cultural groups. Melbourne: Victorian Casino and Gaming Authority; 2000.

47. Duong T, Ohtsuka K. Vietnamese Australian gamblers' view on luck and winning: A preliminary report. In: McMillen J, Laker L, eds. Developing Strategic alliances: Proceedings of the 9th National Association for Gambling Studies Conference. Gold Coast, Queensland: The National Association for Gambling Studies; 1999: 151–160.

48. Au P, Yu R. Working with Chinese problem gamblers: Integrating cultural diversities and treatment theories. In: Jacobs DF, ed. Problem gambling among Asians in Canada and the USA: A new challenge for intervention. Symposium conducted at the 10th International Conference on Gambling and Risk-Taking. Montreal, Canada; 1997.

49. Martins SS, Lobo DS, Tavares H, Gentil V. Pathological gambling in women: A review. Revista do Hospital das Clinicas; Faculdade de Medicina da Universidade de Sao Paulo 2002; 57(5):235–242.

50. Crisp BR, Thomas SA, Jackson AC, Thomason N, Smith S, Borrell J, et al. Sex differences in the treatment needs and outcomes of problem gamblers. Research on Social Work Practice 2000; 10(2):229–242.

51. Crisp BR, Thomas SA, Jackson AC, Thomason N. Not the same: A comparison of female and male clients seeking treatment from problem gambling counselling services. Journal of Gambling Studies 2004; 20(3):283–299.

52. Jackson AC, Thomas SA. Analysis of clients presenting to problem gambling counselling services, July 1, 1999 to June 30, 2000. Client and Services Analysis. Melbourne: Victorian Government Publishing Service; Report No. 6, 2001.

53. Grant J, Kim S. Gender differences in pathological gamblers seeking medication treatment. Comparative Psychiatry 2002; 43(1):56–62.

54. Hollander E, Buchalter AJ, DeCaria CM. Pathological gambling. Psychiatric Clinics of North America 2000; 23(3):629–642.

55. Wedgeworth R. The reification of the 'pathological' gambler: An analysis of gambling treatment and the application of the medical model to problem gambling. Perspectives in Psychiatric Care 1998; 34(2):5–13.

56. Petry N, Roll J. A behavioral approach to understanding and treating pathological gambling. Seminars in Clinical Neuropsychiatry 2001; 6(3):177–183.

57. Blaszczynski AP, Silove D. Cognitive and behavioural therapies for pathological gambling. Journal of Gambling Studies 1995; 11(2):195–220.

58. National Opinion Research Centre. Gambling impact and behavior study: Report to the National Gambling Impact Study Commission: National Gambling Impact Study Commission; April 1999.

59. Elliot Stanford and Associates. Evaluation of the Gamblers Rehabilitation Fund Final Report. Adelaide: Department of Human Services; 1998.

60. Horodecki I. The treatment model of the guidance center for gamblers and their relatives in Vienna/Austria. Journal of Gambling Studies 1992; 8(2):115–128.

61. Jackson AC, Thomas SA, Thomason N, Borrell J, Crisp BR, Enderby K, et al. Longitudinal evaluation of the effectiveness of problem gambling counselling services, community education strategies and information products. Volume 1: Service design and access. Melbourne: Victorian Department of Human Services; 2000.

62. Jackson AC, Thomas SA, Thomason N, Borrell J, Crisp BR, Ho W, et al. Longitudinal evaluation of the effectiveness of problem gambling counselling services, community education strategies and information products. Volume 2: Counselling interventions. Melbourne: Victorian Department of Human Services; 2000.

63. Smith S, Thomas SA, Jackson AC. An exploration of the therapeutic relationship and counselling outcomes in a problem gambling counselling service. Journal of Social Work Practice 2004; 18(1):99–112.

64. Crisp BR, Jackson AC, Thomas SA, Thomason N, Smith S, Borrell J, et al. Is more better? The relationship between outcomes achieved by problem gamblers and the number of counselling sessions attended. Australian Social Work 2001; 54(3):83–92.

65. Walker MB, Blaszczynski A, Sharpe L, Enersen K. A Report for the Casino Community Benefit Trustees. The National Association for Gambling Studies Journal 2002; 14(1):23–40.

66. Politzer R, Morrow J, Leavey S. Report on the cost–benefit/effectiveness of treatment at the Johns Hopkins Center for Pathological Gambling. Journal of Gambling Behaviour 1985; 1(2):131–142.

67. Blaszczynski AP. Juego patologico: Una revision de los tratamientos. Psicologia Conductual 1993; 1:409–440.

68. McConaghy N. Behavioural completion mechanisms rather than primary drive maintain behavioural patterns. Activas Nervosa Superior (Prague) 1980; 22:138–151.

69. Walker MB. The psychology of gambling. Oxford: Pergamon Press; 1992.

70. Custer R, Custer L. Characteristics of the recovering compulsive gambler: A survey of 150 members of Gamblers Anonymous. In: Paper presented at the Fourth National Conference on Gambling and Risk Taking; 1978; Nevada: Reno; 1978.

71. Lesieur HR, Blume SB. Evaluation of patients treated for pathological gambling in a combined alcohol, substance abuse and pathological gambling treatment unit using the Addiction Severity Index. British Journal of Addiction 1991; 86(8):1017–1028.

72. Anderson G, Brown IF. Real and laboratory gambling, sensation seeking and arousal: Towards a Pavlovian component in general theories of gambling and gambling addictions. British Journal of Psychology 1984; 75(Pt 3):401–411.

73. Blaszczynski AP, McConaghy N, Frankova A. Control versus abstinence in the treatment of pathological gambling: A two to nine year follow-up. British Journal of Addiction 1991; 86(3):299–306.

74. Taber JI, McCormick RA, Russo AM, Adkins BJ, Ramirez LF. Follow-up of pathological gamblers after treatment. American Journal of Psychiatry 1987; 144(6):757–761.

75. Blackman S, Simone R, Thoms D. Letter to the editor: Treatment of gamblers. Hospital and Community Psychiatry 1986; 37(4):404.

76. Blaszczynski AP. Clinical studies in pathological gambling: Is controlled gambling an acceptable treatment outcome? [Doctoral dissertation]. Sydney: University of New South Wales; 1988.

77. Brown RIF. The effectiveness of Gamblers Anonymous. In: The Gambling Studies: Proceedings of the Sixth National Conference on Gambling and Risk Taking. Reno: Bureau of Business and Economic Administration, University of Nevada; 1985.

78. Dickerson MG, Weeks D. Controlled gambling as a therapeutic technique for compulsive gamblers. Journal of Behavior Therapy and Experimental Psychiatry 1979; 10:139–141.

79. Rankin H. Control rather than abstinence as a goal in the treatment of excessive gambling. Behaviour Research and Therapy 1982; 20(2):185–187.

80. Koller K. Treatment of poker machine addicts by aversion therapy. Medical Journal of Australia 1972; 1(15):742–745.

81. Russo AM, Taber JI, McCormick RA, Ramirez LF. An outcome study of an inpatient treatment program for pathological gamblers. Hospital and Community Psychiatry 1984; 35(8):823–827.

82. Blaszczynski AP, McConaghy N, Frankova A. A comparison of relapsed and non-relapsed abstinent pathological gamblers following behavioural treatment. British Journal of Addiction 1991; 86(11):1485–1489.

83. Kris E. Ego development of the comic. International Journal of Psychoanalysis 1938; 19:77–90.

84. LaForgue R. On the eroticization of anxiety. International Journal of Psychoanalysis 1930; 11:312–321.

85. Simmel E. On the psychoanalysis of the gambler. Internationale Zeitschrift fur Psychanalyse 1920; 6.

86. von Hattinger H. Analerotik, Angslust und Eigensinn. Internationale Zeitschrift fur Psychoanalyse 1914; 2:244–258.

87. Bergler E. The gambler: a misunderstood neurotic. Journal of Criminal Psychopathology 1943; 4:379–393.

88. Bergler E. The psychology of gambling. New York: Hill and Wang; 1957.

89. Greenberg HR. Psychology of gambling. In: Kaplan H, Freedman A, Saddock B, eds. Comprehensive textbook of psychiatry, 3rd edn. Baltimore: Williams and Wilkins; 1980:347–357.

90. Herman RD. Gamblers and gambling. New York: Harper Row; 1976.

91. Israeli N. Outlook of a depressed patient interested in planned gambling. American Journal of Orthopsychiatry 1935; 5(1):1–23.

92. Rosecrance J. Controlled gambling: A promising future. In: Shaffer HJ, Stein SA, Gambino B, Cummings T, eds. Compulsive gambling: theory, research and practice. Lexington, MA: Lexington Books; 1989:147–160.

93. Greenson R. On gambling. American Imago 1947; 4:61–77.

94. Matussek P. On the psychodynamics of the gambler. Journal of Psychology and Psychotherapy 1955; 1:232–252.

95. Harris H. Gambling and addiction in an adolescent male. Psychoanalytic Quarterly 1964; 33:513–525.

96. Scodel A. Inspirational group therapy: A study of gamblers anonymous. American Journal of Psychotherapy 1964; 18:115–125.

97. Cromer G. Gamblers Anonymous in Israel: A participant observation study of a self-help group. International Journal of the Addictions 1978; 13(7): 1069–1077.

98. Barker JC, Miller M. Aversion therapy for compulsive gamblers. Journal of Nervous Mental Disorders 1968; 146(4):285–302.

99. Goorney AB. Treatment of compulsive horse race gambler by aversion therapy. British Journal of Psychiatry 1968; 114(508):329–383.

100. Seager C. Treatment of compulsive gamblers using electrical aversion. British Journal of Psychiatry 1970; 117(540):545–553.

101. Cotler SB. The use of different behavioural techniques in treating a case of compulsive gambling. Behaviour Therapy 1971; 2:579–584.

102. Bannister G. Cognitive behaviour therapy in a case of compulsive gambler. Cognitive Therapy and Research 1977; 1(3):223–227.

103. Greenberg D, Rankin H. Compulsive gamblers in treatment. British Journal of Psychiatry 1982; 140(4):364–366.

104. Salzmann MM. Treatment of compulsive gambling. British Journal of Psychiatry 1982; 141:318–319.

105. Baucum D. Arguments for self-controlled gambling as an alternative to abstention. In: Proceedings of the Sixth National Conference on Gambling and Risk Taking. University of Nevada: Reno; 1985.

106. Langer EJ. The illusion of control. Journal of Personality and Social Psychology 1975; 32:311–321.

107. Gilovich T. Biased evaluation and persistence in gambling. Journal of Personality and Social Psychology 1983; 44(6):1110–1126.

108. Gilovich T, Douglas C. Biased evaluations of randomly determined gambling outcomes. Journal of Experimental Social Psychology 1986; 22:228–241.

109. Coulombe A, Ladouceur R, Desharnais R, Jobin J. Erroneous perceptions and arousal among regular and occasional video poker players. Journal of Gambling Studies 1992; 8(3):235–244.

110. Griffiths MD. Teenage gambling: A pilot study. Psychological Reports 1990; 68(3 Pt 1): 946.

111. Ladouceur R, Sylvain C, Boutin C, Lachance S, Doucet C, Leblond J, et al. Cognitive treatment of pathological gambling. Journal of Nervous Mental Disease 2001; 189(11):774–780.

112. Dickerson M, Baron E. Contemporary issues and future directions for research into pathological gambling. Addiction 2000; 95(8):1145–1159.

113. Schwartz J, Lindner A. Inpatient treatment of male pathological gamblers in Germany. Journal of Gambling Studies 1992; 8(1):93–109.

114. Hodgins DC, Currie SR, el-Guebaly N. Motivational enhancement and self-help treatments for problem gambling. Journal of Consulting and Clinical Psychology 2001; 691(1):50–57.

115. Dickerson M, Hinchy J, Legg England S. Minimal treatments and problem gamblers: A preliminary investigation. Journal of Gambling Studies 1990; 61(1):87–103.

116. Moskowitz JA. Lithium and Lady Luck; use of lithium carbonate in compulsive gambling. New York State Journal of Medicine 1980; 80(5):785–788.

117. Hollander E, Frenkel M, DeCaria C, Trungold S, Stein DJ. Treatment of pathological gambling with clomipramine. American Journal of Psychiatry 1992; 149(5):710–711.

118. Hollander E, Wong C. Body dysmorphic disorder, pathological gambling, and sexual compulsions. Journal of Clinical Psychiatry 1995; 56(Suppl 4):7–12.

119. Winchel RM, Jones JS, Stanley B, Molcho A, Stanley M. Clinical characteristics of trichotillomania and its response to fluoxetine. Journal of Clinical Psychiatry 1992; 53(9):304–308.

120. Figgitt DP, McClellan KJ. Fluvoxamine: An updated review of its use in the management of adults with anxiety disorders. Drugs 2000; 60(4):925–954.

121. Hollander E, DeCaria C, Finkell J, Begaz T, Wong C, Cartwright C. A randomised double-blind fluvoxamine/placebo crossover trial in pathologic gambling. Biological Psychiatry 2000; 47(9):813–817.

122. Bianco C, Petkova E, Ibanez A, Saiz-Ruiz J. A pilot placebo-controlled study of fluvoxamine for pathological gambling. Annals of Clinical Psychiatry 2002; 14(1):9–15.

123. Zimmerman M, Breen R, Posternak M. An open-label study of citalopram in the treatment of pathological gambling. Journal of Clinical Psychiatry 2002; 63(1):44–48.

124. Stahl SM. The current impact of neuroscience on psychotropic drug discovery and development. Psychopharmacology Bulletin 1992; 28(1):3–9.

125. Crockford DN, el-Guebaly N. Naltrexone in the treatment of pathological gambling and alcohol dependence. Canadian Journal of Psychiatry 1998; 43(1):86.

126. Kim S, Grant J. An open naltrexone treatment study in pathological gambling disorder. International Clinical Psychopharmacology 2001; 16(5):285–289.

127. Kim S, Grant J, Adson D, Shin Y. Double-blind naltrexone and placebo comparison study in the treatment of pathological gambling. Biological Psychiatry 2001; 49(11):914–921.

128. Stout J, Rodawalt W, Siemers E. Risky decision making in Huntington's disease. Journal of the International Neuropsychological Society 2001; 7(1):92–101.

129. Tavares H, Zilberman M, Beites FJ, Gentil V. Gender differences in gambling progression. Journal of Gambling Studies 2001; 17(2):151–159.

130. Sobell LC, Sobell MB, Leo GI, Cancilla A. Reliability of a timeline method: assessing normal drinkers' reports of recent drinking and a comparative evaluation across several populations. British Journal of Addictions 1988; 83(4):393–402.

131. Hodgins DC, el-Guebaly N. Natural and treatment-assisted recovery from gambling problems: A comparison of resolved and active gamblers. Addiction 2000; 95(5):777–789.

132. Tavares H, Martins SS, Zilberman ML, el-Guebaly N. Gamblers and treatment-seeking: Why haven't they come earlier? Addictive Disorders and Their Treatment 2002; 1(2):65–70.

133. Petry NM. A comparison of treatment-seeking pathological gamblers based on preferred gambling activity. Addiction 2003; 98(5):645–655.

134. Rockloff MJ, Schofield G. Factor analysis of barriers to treatment for problem gambling. Journal of Gambling Studies 2004; 20(2):121–126.

135. Leblond J, Ladouceur R, Blaszczynski A. Which pathological gamblers will complete treatment? British Journal of Clinical Psychology 2003; 42(Pt 2):205–209.

136. Haustein J, Shurgers G. Therapy with male pathological gamblers: Between self-help group and group therapy – Report of a developmental process. Journal of Gambling Studies 1992; 62:131–142.

137. Taber J, Chaplin M. Group psychotherapy with pathological gamblers. Journal of Gambling Behaviour 1988; 4(3):183–196.

138. Thomas SA, Jackson AC. Influences on gambling behaviours and outcomes: A model for the design of effective interventions. Gambling Research 16, 2, Nov. 41–53.

139. Spunt B, Dupont I, Lesieur H, Liberty HJ, Hunt D. Pathological gambling and substance misuse: A review of the literature. Substance Use and Misuse 1998; 33(13):2535–2560.

140. Black DW, Moyer T. Clinical features and psychiatric co-morbidity of subjects with pathological gambling behavior. Psychiatric Services 1998; 4911:1434–1439.

141. Eisen SA, Lin N, Lyons MJ, Scherrer JF, Griffith K, True WR, et al. Familial influences on gambling behaviour: An analysis of 3359 twin pairs. Addiction 1998; 93(9):1375–1384.

142. Winters KC, Stinchfield RD, Fulkerson J. Patterns and characteristics of adolescent gambling. Journal of Gambling Studies 1993; 9:371–386.

143. Brown S, Johnson K, Jackson AC, Fook J, Wynn J, Rooke C. Healthy, wealthy and wise women: The health impacts of gambling on women in Melbourne's Western Metropolitan Region. Melbourne: Women's Health West; 2000.

144. Welte JW, Barnes GM, Wieczorek WF, Tidwell MO, Parker JC. Risk factors for pathological gambling. Addictive Behaviours 2004; 29(2):323–335.

145. Blaszczynski AP, Sharpe L, Walker M. The assessment of the impact of the reconfiguration on electronic gaming machines as harm minimisation strategies for problem gambling. Sydney: University of Sydney Gambling Research Unit; 2001.

146. Nowatzki N, Williams. Casino self-exclusion programmes: A review of issues. International Gambling Studies 2002; 2(Jul):3–25.

147. Ladouceur R, Jacques C, Giroux I, Ferland F, Leblond J. Analysis of a casino's self-exclusion program. Journal of Gambling Studies 2000; 16(4):453–460.

148. O'Neil N, Whetton S, Dolman B, Herbert M, Giannopoulos V, O'Neil D, et al. Evaluation of self-exclusion programs. Melbourne: Gambling Research Panel; 2003.

149. Bracht N, Kingsbury I. Community organisation principles in health promotion: A five stage model. In: Bracht N, ed. Health Promotion at the Community Level. Newbury Park: Sage Publications; 1990.

150. Budd J, Gray R, McCron R. The Tyne Tees Alcohol Education Campaign: An Evaluation. Newcastle England: Centre for Mass Communication Research; 1982.

151. Carleton R, Lasater T, Assat A, Feldman H, McKinley S. The Pawtucket Heart Health Program: community changes in cardiovascular risk factors and projected disease risk. American Journal of Public Health 1995; 85:777–785.

152. Puska P, Nissinen A, Tuomilehto J. The community-based strategy to prevent coronary heart disease: Conclusions drawn from the ten years of the North Karelia Project. Annual Review of Public Health 1985; 6:147–153.

153. Wallack LM. Drinking and driving: toward a broader understanding of the role of mass media. Journal of Public Health Policy 1984; 5(4):471–496.

154. Ciarrocchi J, Reinert D. Family environment and length of recovery for married male members of Gamblers Anonymous and female members of GamAnon. Journal of Gambling Studies 1993; 9(4):341–351.

155. Fobair PA, Zabora JR. Family functioning as a resource variable in psychosocial cancer research: Issues and measures. Journal of Psychosocial Oncology 1995; 131(2):97–113.

156. McCubbin MA, McCubbin HI. Resiliency in families: A conceptual model of family adjustment and adaptation in response to stress and crises. In: McCubbin HI, Thomson AI, McCubbin AL, eds. Family assessment: resiliency, coping and adaptation – inventories for research and practice. Madison: University of Wisconsin System; 1996.

157. Daughters SB, Lejuz CW, Lesieur H, Strong DR, Zvolensky MJ. Towards a better understanding of gambling treatment failure: Implications for translational research. Clinical Psychology Review 2003; 23(4):573–586.

CHAPTER **12**

Crash and injury prevention

Brian Fildes
Nicola Pronk

INTRODUCTION

Health issues and programs to address road crashes and injuries will be reviewed and discussed in this chapter. It sets out to address the scope of the problem, the evidence-based approach, interventions typically used to prevent or treat road crash injuries with strong reliance on evidence of the most effective prevention strategies and treatments in the short and longer term and the philosophies associated with injury prevention. This chapter aims to provide a background for those interested in an evidence-based approach to behavioural change in road safety.

EPIDEMIOLOGY OF ROAD CRASHES

In 1996, the Global Burden of Disease[1] noted that road traffic crashes were the 9th leading cause of disability-adjusted life years (DALYs) lost among adults aged 15–44 across all countries in 1990 and the fourth for developed countries. Moreover, they predict that by 2020, road traffic crashes will become the third leading cause of disease or injury DALYs across the world (see Table 12.1) essentially from an increasing burden of road traffic problems in developing countries.

Table 12.1   Rank ordering of the 15 leading causes of DALYs lost for 1990 and 2020 prediction[1]

1990	Percentage total	2020	Percentage total
Lower respiratory infection	1	Ischaemic heart disease	1
Diarrhoeal diseases	2	Unipolar major depression	2
Conditions arising during the perinatal period	3	Road traffic accidents*	3
Unipolar major depression	4	Cerebrovascular disease	4
Ischaemic heart disease	5	Chronic obstructive pulmonary disease	5
Cerebrovascular disease	6	Lower respiratory infection	6
Tuberculosis	7	Tuberculosis	7
Measles	8	War	8
Road traffic accidents*	9	Diarrhoeal diseases	9
Congenital abnormalities	10	HIV	10
Malaria	11	Conditions arising during the perinatal period	11
Chronic obstructive pulmonary disease	12	Violence	12
Falls	13	Congenital abnormalities	13
Iron-deficiency anaemia	14	Self-inflicted injuries	14
Anaemia	15	Trachea, bronchus and lung cancers	15

*The term crash is generally preferred today as 'accident' implies an event that is beyond the scope of human intervention.

In the Western world,[2] road safety has been something of a success story over the last 30 or 40 years as shown in Fig. 12.1. The fatality rate fell from around 9 to 1.5 deaths per 10 000 vehicles from 1960 to 1995 in spite of a substantial increase in the numbers of vehicles on the road and an increase in the average distance travelled. Similar improvements are also apparent in the rate of fatalities per 100 000 of population in Fig. 12.2.

THE EVIDENCE–BASED APPROACH

This impressive improvement in safety on the road occurred primarily because of the adoption of an evidence-based approach to injury prevention. In the 1960s, the physician and epidemiologist, Dr William Haddon, introduced a new approach to improving road safety when he first published the 'Haddon Matrix', an evidence-based systematic account of categorizing problems and identifying effective solutions to address these problems.[3] Haddon's Matrix (see Table 12.2) breaks the injury prevention task into pre-crash (preventing the crash), crash (preventing the injuries) or post-crash (minimizing the trauma) and separates the driver from the road and the vehicle. Adopting

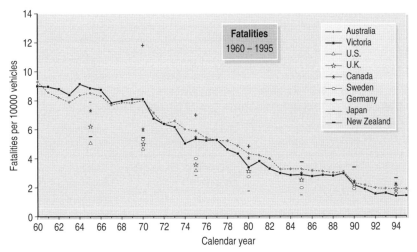

Fig. 12.1 Rate of fatalities per 10 000 vehicles in Victoria and Australia compared to other Western Countries (1960 to 1995).

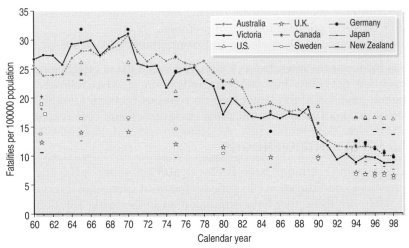

Fig. 12.2 Rate of fatalities per 100 000 population in Victoria and Australia compared to other Western Countries (1960 to 1998).

this approach enabled the practitioner to focus attention on major problem areas and effective solutions, using evidence-based best practice. A more detailed and comprehensive account of the history of road safety can be found in Trinca et al.[4]

The use of the evidence-based approach led to the identification of a number of innovative and effective solutions to a range of major road safety problems, including:

Table 12.2 Haddon's Matrix[3]

	Human	Vehicle	Roads
Pre-crash	Drink-drive programs Speed reduction Aggressive behaviour	Better handling Improved braking Increased visibility	Road engineering Black-spot treatments Better delineation
Crash	Wearing seat-belts Cycle helmets Protective clothing	Crashworthiness Airbags, seat-belts Other safety features	Frangible poles Roadside barriers Black-spot treatments
Post-crash	First-aid knowledge Medical details	Easy access for recovery Hospital alarms	Rapid triage systems Rapid alert mechanisms Helicopter access

- Seat-belts to restrain occupants inside the vehicle in a crash.
- Improved roadways (and dual carriageways) to minimize the likelihood of vehicles colliding.
- Improved crashworthiness of passenger cars and an increase in vehicle safety technology.
- Substantial reductions in drink-driving behaviour and attitudes.
- More effective police enforcement methods.
- Greater community knowledge and commitment to road safety.

This is by no means intended as a comprehensive list of effective road safety intervention programs but rather an indication of what followed a major change in road safety thinking based on rigorous problem identification and solutions using a sound scientific research approach and best evidence.

ROAD SAFETY INTERVENTIONS

Road safety interventions have been categorized as the 3-Es: Engineering, Enforcement and Education.[5] In general, the most successful interventions in road safety are those that have stipulated an Engineering solution or those involving heavy Enforcement. Attempts to modify behaviour through Education have been less successful in general, although in fairness, it is often more difficult to evaluate the effects of education in the short term, compared to the others.

Road safety interventions can be loosely categorized as those applying to an individual, a group of individuals or the community at large. The selection of a particular intervention or intervention category depends very much on the problem at hand and what is most likely to yield optimal benefits. A review of some of these follows.

Individual interventions

It is a truism to say that all road safety countermeasures must have some effect on individual road users if they are to be successful. However, there are a number of road safety intervention programs that are more directly delivered at the individual level, and these commonly involve either enforcement or education campaigns.

There are a number of examples of individual interventions aimed at modifying errant behaviour including licence suspensions and demerit point penalties for persistent offenders, vehicle interlocks to prevent unfit drivers from starting their vehicle, and defensive driving courses to teach motorists safe driving practices. Two individual interventions, namely motor vehicle sanctions and rehabilitation programs for recidivist drivers will be discussed in more detail.

Motor vehicle sanctions

Penalties for persistent lawbreakers on the road range from fines, demerit point penalties, and suspension of one's license to drive, up to periods of imprisonment in jail. Evaluations of these interventions have shown mixed success. A recent intervention against those who continue to drive while unlicensed involves preventing access to one's vehicle through either confiscating their vehicle in a police or council compound or 'wheel-locking' the vehicle at the individual's home. Several of these vehicle sanction programs have been evaluated recently.

Compounding a person's vehicle when they continue to flaunt the law has been tried in some states in the USA and in New Zealand. It is defined as the temporary removal of property or withholding access to property. In the USA,[6] seven states allow for the immobilization of a vehicle when the driver has driven while intoxicated or while suspended following a drink-drive offence. Immobilization can take several forms including wheel locking the vehicle in the offender's own driveway or garage. Ten US states also allow for physical impoundment of vehicles, again after driving while intoxicated or suspended, while 25 states allow for the forfeiture and sale of vehicles primarily for multiple offences of drink-driving.[6] Vehicle sanctions are also widely used throughout Canada.[7]

Land Transport in New Zealand introduced impoundment of vehicles for disqualified or unlicensed drivers in May 1999.[8] When a car is impounded at the roadside, the police officer calls for a tow truck to take the vehicle away to a storage yard. The owner of the vehicle has to pay the tow and storage fees at the end of 28 days before they can get the vehicle back. The owner has little recourse to the sentence as he or she is obligated to ensure that anyone who drives his or her vehicle is licensed.

In the two years following its introduction, more than 25 000 vehicles were impounded in New Zealand and the number of unlicensed driver fatalities fell from 10% to 6.9% (a 45% improvement). There was also a one-third reduction in the number of driving-while-disqualified offences.[9] The results have also shown that between 40% and 50% of the vehicles are unclaimed at the end of the impoundment period (often unroadworthy vehicles) so a beneficial side effect has been the removal of a large number of unroadworthy vehicles from the road.

The New Zealanders also permanently confiscate vehicles for serious drink- or drug-driving offences, driving while disqualified or suspension, dangerous or reckless driving causing injury or death and involvement in a criminal offence (e.g. aggravated robbery, burglary or drug trafficking). These vehicles are subsequently sold at auction and all associated costs are deducted from the proceeds before returning the remaining funds to the vehicle owner. In the years since 1996 when vehicle confiscation was introduced, there have been over 4500 cases of vehicle confiscation (the confiscation rate is about 1 in 10 of all eligible cases). For the most part, confiscation was equally divided between driving with excessive alcohol or while disqualified.[9]

Land Transport New Zealand note that their vehicle sanction program is not the total answer to safety enforcement, but is part of a comprehensive deterrence package, including random breath testing, speed enforcement and appropriate public education.

Rehabilitation programs

Rehabilitation has also been tried as a road safety initiative for recidivist drivers, especially in the area of drink-driving. Two landmark meta-analyses were published in 1995 that examined the efficacy of remediation programs for drink-driving offenders.[10,11] Most of the 215 studies in the meta-analysis were from the USA, although 20% came from elsewhere, including Australia and New Zealand. To be included in the analysis, studies had to include drink-drive samples and had to compare either remediation with no remediation groups or two or more different remediation treatments.

Notwithstanding the difficulties of comparing results across different studies, the authors reported a robust reduction in recidivist and alcohol-involved crashes of at least 7–9% for those who undertook remediation treatments over those who did not. The found that the combination of rehabilitation with licensing sanctions to be the most optimal combination for reducing crashes and infringements. Multiple treatment modalities[12] combining counselling, education and probation was also shown to be more effective than single modality approaches in other studies.

A recent Californian study[13] looked at the effectiveness of rehabilitation, licence sanctions and imprisonment in reducing drink-drive recidivism. The study examined the effectiveness of three levels of outpatient alcohol education and treatment programs, targeted at first, second and third or more offenders, with other sanctions. The results suggest that the combinations of treatment with licence suspension was associated with the lowest recidivist rate for first time and multiple drink-drive offenders, consistent with the findings reported above.

It appears then that rehabilitation programs can have a significant road safety benefit for a small proportion of recidivist drink drivers. It has been suggested[14] that effective rehabilitation programs for drink-driving and other traffic offenders needs to include the following criteria:

- A thorough and valid assessment of all program referrals.
- Their assessment results should help guide the level of care and type of program developed.
- Each client needs to have an individualized treatment plan.
- Programs should be multi-modal.
- Each specific group needs an individually trained counsellor.
- Treatment and program goals should be clear and evaluated.
- Programs should include after-care and long-term follow-up.

The degree of the program success will depend heavily on the extent to which these factors are taken into account in its development.

Group interventions

The next category of safety intervention is that where group dynamics are used as part of the delivery method. These include such things as road safety educational programs, young driver licensing regimes and programs for teaching children 'safe routes to school'. Two additional Australian group interventions, 'Walk-With-Care' for seniors, and Fleet Safety programs for companies, are reviewed here as examples of evidence-based interventions to bring about behavioural change.

The Walk-With-Care pedestrian program

This program was introduced in Melbourne during the early 1990s to address the growing number of seniors who are involved in pedestrian crashes in this country. It is a three-staged process aimed at educating older people in the dangers of pedestrian behaviour and outlining suggestions for them in safe walking practices.[15] It comprises a planning phase, an educational phase (combining publicity and discussion components) and an advocacy phase.

Recruits to the program are elicited from surveys conducted in targeted high-crash municipalities to identify specific problems in these regions. Workshops are then arranged for between 10 and 20 participants who agree to attend them. A number of activities are focused on during these workshops[15] including:

- The facts, simple up-to-date crash statistics presented in a non-threatening way.
- How to make crossing the road easier.
- Reducing (exposure) time on the road.
- Pedestrian visibility (day and night).
- Anticipating unexpected events.
- Understanding right-of-way at confusing traffic situations.

Program materials comprise posters, various teaching aides, an educational video, and giveaways. The results from the information provided on local pedestrian 'black-spots' is subsequently used as part of the advocacy activity to initiate improved on-road treatments.

Walk-With-Care is aimed at improving the safety of older pedestrians. It focuses on high crash locations and relies on an integrated approach to tackling well-defined local problems.[16] There does not appear to be an evaluation of its crash benefits, presumably because of insufficient crash data being available.[17] A review of the efficacy of the program[15,18] highlighted a number of problems with the way the program was staffed, implemented and the use of outdated materials. While it is understood that many of these have since been addressed, its benefits in terms of crash savings and acceptability still need to be assessed.

Vehicle safety policies

A number of companies are beginning to realize the burden, or potential burden, that road trauma can have on their industry. Estimates of the cost of work-related road trauma across countries are significant; in Australia, estimates vary between 0.5 and 1 billion dollars annually and more than $17 billion in the USA.[19] Crash statistics are even more alarming for work-related trauma as shown in Table 12.3.

It can be said that employers who ensure that their employees drive the safest vehicles are not only protecting their most valuable resources but also providing the safest workplace environment for their workers. They are also reducing the likelihood of a major Occupational Health and Safety (OHS) claim for failure to provide adequate protection for their on-road workers.[20]

Murray[21] listed ten barriers to successful fleet safety based on evidence from UK and Australia. These included:

- Limited extent and purpose of the journey data.
- Operational procedures and structures.
- Senior management commitment.
- Integration between fleet safety and OHS.
- Companies following 'claims-led' procedures.
- Lack of crash investigations.
- Inappropriate standard definitions and conventions.
- Reactive focus on injury prevention.
- Inflexible attitudes to change.
- Poor management practices.

Table 12.3 Fleet safety statistics from various studies[19]

Statistic	Australia	UK	France	USA
Increased risk of fleet crash	3×	2×		
Percentage work deaths while driving	58%	55%		
Percentage work road deaths c.f. all road deaths	14%		10%	
Percentage work fleet crashes annually	10–50%	19%		20%
Journeys for business	33%			
Crash costs c.f. total fleet costs				13–15%

Fleet budget and management incentives are also issues that work to prevent fleet managers from buying the safest vehicles for their employees. Mechanisms to ensure that transport and OHS policy makers work together would also help instill greater fleet safety in the community.[21]

There have been a number of interventions introduced in an attempt to improve fleet safety. The most common approach is for organizations to adopt corporate behaviour strategies that include safety as a major criterion when purchasing fleet vehicles. In Sweden, for instance, Folksam Insurance who rent a sizeable fleet of vehicles have a policy only to rent cars that feature highly in crash tests or safety ratings based on their claims as well as those that exceed national targets for fuel consumption.[22]

One of the most stringent fleet buying policies is that specified by the Monash University Accident Research Centre in Melbourne, Australia[23] where suppliers are required to meet ten safety criteria to sell cars to this organization (see Box 12.1).

These criteria are based on the best evidence available of likely safety benefits for their inclusion. Similar policies are beginning to appear in a number of other Australian organizations. Interestingly, though, one Australian vehicle manufacturer[19] claimed that only 'Blue Chip' corporations or the government sector generally specified their 'safety vehicle' as a matter of purchase policy currently.

Community interventions

Community-wide measures are the final category of evidence-based behavioural interventions reviewed here. Examples include enforcement and mass-media campaigns programs aimed at speeding, drink-driving, seat-belt wearing, fatigue and so on, as well as widespread engineering road treatments (e.g. black-spot programs) and mandatory vehicle regulations. It is only possible to review two such programs here, namely speed enforcement and advertising, both of which tend to be based on the latest research evidence of effectiveness in bringing about a change in community behaviour. It should be pointed out that community-based interventions are the most

---

Box 12.1   Fleet safety–buying criteria used by MUARC[23]

High scores in consumer tests (or statistical ratings)
Dual front supplementary restraint system (SRS) airbags
Side airbags in the front seating area
Three-point seat-belts in all positions (pre-tensioners on front belts)
Head restraints in all positions (four position adjustment on front seats)
Curb weight over 1300 kg
Cargo barriers fitted for station wagons (estates)
Manufactured in Australia (Monash University requirement)

difficult to gain substantial behavioural change because of the large numbers of people associated. Nevertheless, there is good evidence of change as a result of some of these programs.

Speed enforcement

Speed cameras have become a major weapon in the fight against excessive speeding on roads in the United Kingdom, New Zealand and Australia (other countries also use speed cameras to stop speeding but evidence of their effectiveness was either missing or more difficult to obtain). In the UK, speed cameras tend to be used at fixed locations, essentially to induce a local or regional speed reduction. In Australia (and New Zealand), though, they are more likely to be used randomly from mobile vehicles using both overt and covert operations.

Speed cameras have been used in the UK since the early 1990s and several independent studies have demonstrated their effectiveness. To improve their effectiveness, a recent pilot study was conducted in eight regions in England, Wales and Scotland to improve their cost-benefits.[24] In the first two years since their introduction, average speed reduced by approximately 10%, the numbers exceeding the speed limit fell by two-thirds, and excessive speeding at these sites was virtually eliminated. There was a significant 35% crash reduction at the six fixed-camera sites (two cameras were used randomly) over that two-year period and a 56% reduction in pedestrian casualties.[24] They note the need to use cameras at locations with the worst casualty history to gain maximum benefits.

The Victorian government in Australia introduced mobile cameras fitted to cars as a general speed reduction program in 1989, which led to an immediate reduction in casualty crashes of between 28% and 40% in the following 18 months.[25] More recent estimates suggest that casualty crash reductions could be even greater in later years[26,27] (see Fig. 12.3). Current plans are to increase the number of cameras, adoption of 'point-to-point camera technology, shift to covert operations and the use of new speed and encroachment cameras at intersections.

The effectiveness of mobile cameras used overtly (visible to passing motorists) and covert (hidden inside an unmarked vehicle) was examined by the Land Transport Safety Authority in New Zealand.[28,29] They reported a significant overall reduction in speeds of around 2%, an 11% reduction in the number of crashes and an 8% reduction in casualties due to the introduction of their hidden speed camera program. These reductions were in addition to those accruing from their overt camera program.[28] Moreover, they found that these reductions were sustained over a two-year period.[29]

In justifying the use of such an aggressive enforcement approach to elicit a behavioural change, government agencies must rely on evidence-based research findings to convince the public of the worthiness of these measures. Speed cameras do produce considerable revenue for governments. Media and the public are quick to criticize governments, claiming that cameras are

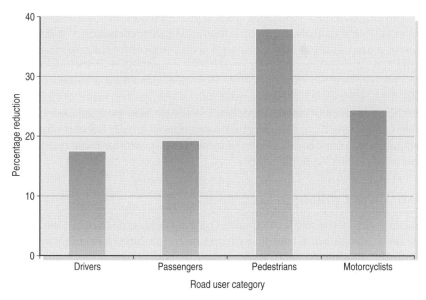

Fig. 12.3   Crash reductions in Victoria, Australia, 2001 and 2002.[27]

nothing more than a means of collecting additional revenue without clear and positive evidence of the societal benefits. Even so, there is clearly a case for ensuring that a sizeable proportion of the revenue is returned to the community through new and proven road safety interventions to maintain public support for these programs.

Mass media campaigns

Mass media campaigns serve several purposes. First, they help support safety campaigns such as speed cameras by elucidating the considerable road safety benefits. They also serve to inform the public of these programs and to outline the conditions, constraints, penalties, etc. Moreover, they can be an effective road safety intervention program themselves, aimed at changing behaviour.

The Institut National de Recherche sur Transports et Leur Sécurité (INRETS) conducted a meta-analysis of some 265-road safety media campaigns in 17 European, North American and Asian countries.[30] They found a significant reduction overall of up to 15% in crashes for the after-period of the campaigns they reviewed. They argued that the more effective campaigns are those carried out at a local or regional level. Similar benefits have been found in other meta-analyses.[31] A general conclusion from both these studies is that the most effective campaigns were those based on an explicit theoretical framework.[27,30,31]

One point stressed in these meta-analyses reports has been the quality of many of these studies and the range of outcome measures employed. Many of the evaluations fail to enable costs and benefits to be calculated, thereby not permitting a comparison with other road safety measures.[27] A theoretical basis for a road safety media campaign is also important for ensuring that the results can be meaningfully interpreted.[30] Campaigns that include publicity with enforcement are more effective than just mass media campaigns[32] and those that use persuasive or emotional language are more effective than rational or informational approaches.[31,32] Elliott also pointed out that Australian campaigns have been slightly more effective than US and other world campaigns,[31] a point he attributes to more directly aiming these campaigns at influencing safe road behaviours.

ROAD SAFETY PHILOSOPHIES

In recent years, there are signs that the past successes in reducing the road toll may have plateaued. Current measures seem to have less effect now than they did originally and there seems to be no magical new interventions on the horizon to ensure continuing road safety improvements. A growing movement believes that it is time to re-examine the way we approach road safety today and whether past theories and philosophies are still suitable, given that we are in a period of diminishing returns and that future savings will be even more difficult to justify using conventional approaches.

Traditional safety models

Safety philosophy has for many years adopted what can be termed a 'transportation model'.[34] Under this model, safety is seen as a tradeable commodity against mobility. We accept that mobility is important and desirable within our society and that safety must be traded-off against allowing people access to an unlimited range of mobility options. Indeed, there is clear evidence that the community desires the right to move around in our environment unimpeded.

The transportation model stresses the need to find the right balance between safety and mobility. 'Safety at Reasonable Cost' is a statement that reflects this philosophy.[34] Benefit–cost analysis is the means by which we achieve this balance. We cost safety benefits and mobility losses in terms of dollars and cents and discount potential savings in human trauma against losses in mobility. If a potential safety countermeasure does not produce a sufficiently high benefit–cost ratio, discounted of course for traffic delays, the safety initiative is generally overlooked.[34]

Underlying this model, whether we believe it or not, is the implicit assumption that a degree of road trauma is acceptable. The transportation model inevitably specifies that there will be people killed and seriously injured on our roads in the interest of maintaining existing or even higher levels of mobility in our society. The transportation model has gained widespread acceptance in this country by politicians, industry, government agencies, researchers and indeed the community itself.

Safety as a health problem

A new approach to road safety philosophy has emerged from Europe. It is essentially a health model, placing absolute emphasis on the value of human life and suffering. Philosophies such as 'Vision Zero' in Sweden and 'Sustainable Safety' from the Netherlands state that no crash should be more severe than what the human can tolerate.

Vision Zero

The Vision Zero model, developed in Sweden by Claes Tingvall and his colleagues at the Swedish Road Administration, argued the need to radically change the current traffic system to achieve future road safety improvements.[36,37] They claim that the present road transport system is a global public health problem, and compared to other man/machine systems, traffic safety systems around the world are underdeveloped. Vision Zero adopts a strong ethical stance on the issue of serious injury. It argues that it is totally unethical to consider that human life is tradeable. The system must place priority on preventing death and serious injury ahead of all other considerations.

Another point of departure from the transportation model is the issue of blame or fault. Tingvall and his colleagues claim that it is too easy to simply attribute fault to the driver when in fact the system may well have contributed to the crash.[36] Blaming the driver often glosses over the real fault, which is more likely to be the system or environment in which the human operates. It is true that humans are fallible and often make errors of judgment while driving. However, they argue that it is more appropriate to consider how the environment can adversely influence human decisions rather than attribute blame solely to the vehicle operator. Tingvall notes that, 'we must build a system that is forgiving to human mistakes and misjudgments'.[37]

Vision Zero is very much a systems-wide approach to road safety; the system as a whole must be more forgiving to the likely mistakes of drivers. This raises the notion of a 'crashworthy system' where improving road safety means examining the complete driving environment (vehicles, roads, the surrounding environment, traffic mix, and so on) and ensuring that crash energy is optimally managed within the system.[36,37] Vision Zero accepts that there will always be crashes as a consequence of mobility. However, it stresses that crashes should only be allowed if they do not lead to severe trauma. Managing crash energy must consider the biomechanical tolerance of humans. This introduces the notion of a dose/response approach to safety (see Fig. 12.4).

It is usual for the number of crashes on our roads to be higher at low crash severity and lower at high severity. Tingvall calls this the exposure to violence or the dose curve. Fortunately, the biomechanical tolerance of humans to violence is greater at low crash forces (lower crash severity)

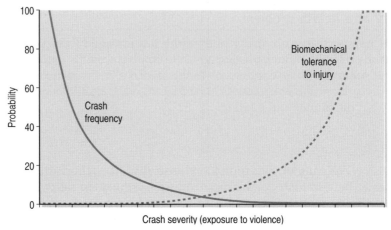

Fig. 12.4 Dose–response curve for injury outcome.

than at higher ones. This is reassuring as it means that the higher exposure events occur at levels where the human is best able to tolerate them. However, a proportion of crashes do occur at levels beyond human tolerance, and these are the ones that generally produce severe injury and fatal outcomes. To achieve Vision Zero objectives, then, it is critical that there are no crashes at unsustainable high levels of crash violence. That is, the dose must be kept below the energy levels leading to a severe injury response.

Sustainable safety

The Netherlands has developed the notion of 'sustainable' safety as a road safety philosophy.[38,39] Sustainable safety explicitly presents itself as an initiative that sets out to re-design the transport system. As with Vision Zero, it adopts a strong ethical basis as its starting point noting that 'The adverse consequence of today's mobility demands should not present a burden for future generations'.[40] The Dutch society does not want to hand over a road traffic system to the next generation in which there is an acceptance that road transport causes thousands of deaths and tens of thousands of injuries.[41] Sustainable safety has two main axioms:[41]

1. That man is the reference standard. A sustainable safety system must be able to adapt to the limitations of the human through proper design of the road system.
2. That the means are available to substantially reduce the costly and largely avoidable casualty problem.[39]

Wegman[40] noted that the key to a sustainably safe system lies in the systematic and consistent application of three principles of safety:

- The functional use of the road network (preventing unintentional use of roads).
- The homogenous use of the roads (minimizing large differences in vehicle speed, direction and mass at moderate to high speeds).
- The predictable use of the road system (enhancing predictability of the road and thus preventing uncertainty among road users).

Potential contributions of the new approach

These new philosophies do offer scope for considerable further improvements in road safety over traditional methods in this area. First, they both call for a system-wide approach where the need for intervention is a holistic process involving specialists in the road, vehicle and driver behavior working together to develop innovative new approaches involving all aspects of a safe road system. They claim that no longer is it acceptable for agents to provide unimodal solutions to problems that might not be optimal for the system as a whole. Reduced speed limits without consideration of engineering and perceptual support to enhance driver acceptance is one example of the misuse of such an approach[37] (see Figs 12.5 and 12.6).

Second, they place much greater emphasis on road safety as a health problem where safety is paramount and not to be traded against mobility. The consequences for a new safety solution might mean reduced mobility but this should

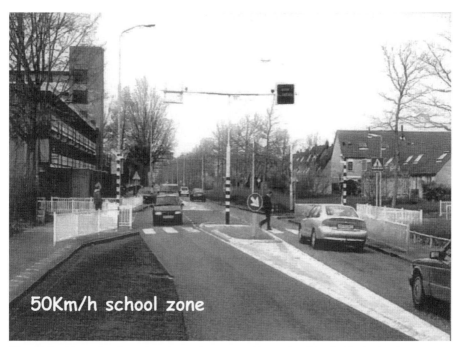

Fig. 12.5   Example of a reduced speed zone outside a school in the Netherlands.

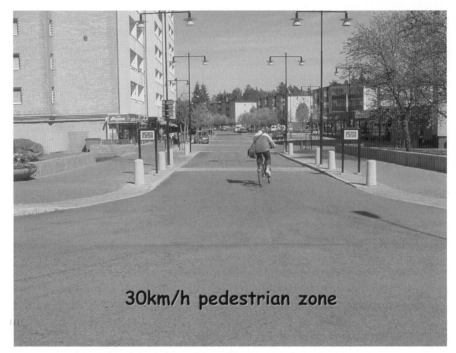

30km/h pedestrian zone

Fig. 12.6   A reduced speed zone in a busy shopping precinct in Sweden.

not detract from implementing this solution. For instance, research evidence (and basic physics) clearly show that high impact speed is injurious and that safety benefits could be achieved for the whole community by either improving the infrastructure to prevent the most serious crashes or reducing travel speed. The latter would inevitably mean increased travel time to some degree. To achieve the desired health outcome, supporters argue that we must accept these (relatively minor) mobility penalties; it is no longer acceptable to trade-off safety benefits for slight increases in mobility costs.[36] (There is also a growing concern that mobility costs used in benefit–cost analyses are artificially high, as the supposed savings do not reflect real benefits to the community.)

Finally, the thrust of these new philosophies is against the common practice today of simply blaming the driver for road crashes: in many cases, it is the system that has failed the road user, not the reverse. A more productive approach is to examine all of the associated factors involved in the crash and address all of these. Of course, there will always be a need for drivers, riders and pedestrians to act safely on the road but opportunities for safety improvement must look beyond blame and address ways in which the road environment can be more forgiving.

The future role of the evidence–based approach

These new approaches to road safety do not negate the need for the evidence-based approach; rather, they call for more reliance on sound scientific evidence in making decisions. It is clear that adopting a more rigorous scientific basis to road safety strategies and countermeasures has been an enormous advantage for road safety over the years as was argued earlier. Hence, we need to be careful not to throw out the evidence-based approach in any new initiative but rather extend the use of rigorous scientific evidence in developing new safety programs.[3]

Safety research and policy has relied heavily on the availability of extensive crash data and scientific analysis for highlighting road safety problems and aiding decision-making. In most countries, this commonly involves using data from the police and insurance companies as a basis for intervention. The wealth of data usually available and the ability to examine the extent of crashes and injury accurately advantage these databases. However, they are usually limited in their amount of detail, can only provide scant details on causal factors and are usually of variable quality given the range of people and systems involved.

For new innovative solutions, there is clearly a need for more informative crash data than that currently available to the road safety practitioner. Data must provide more detailed information on the multiple factors involved in the crash and the level of injuries sustained by the people involved than what is generally available. Important factors such as crash and injury severity are paramount to enable analysts to conduct rigorous analyses to tease out causation factors and identify effective and realistic scientifically valid solutions to today's safety problems.

SUMMARY AND CONCLUSIONS

This chapter has reviewed how the evidence-based approach to developing health interventions has contributed to improved road safety through positive behavioural change. Various examples of successful interventions, aimed at the individual, to groups of individuals, as well as to the community at large were discussed in terms of their evidence of how a change in behaviour led to fewer crashes, injuries or aberrant behaviour. Finally, the theoretical basis for adopting road safety programs and initiatives was considered and why there is a need for adopting more of a health than a transportation model in future to ensure continuing success in reducing fatalities and serious injuries on our roads.

There is overwhelming evidence that adopting an evidence-based approach has been successful in addressing what is and continues to be a major safety and health problem, worldwide. The need to take a systematic approach when confronting a serious community epidemic (as road safety is) has been well-substantiated in other health circles. The epidemiologist, William Haddon, had the vision back in the 1960s to adopt such an approach for solving road safety's problems and consequently, many lives and serious injuries have been saved, courtesy of his vision. It has been argued that the time is right now for a re-think of the emphasis we still place on mobility and safety if we hope to continue to see the number of people killed and seriously injured on our roads decline.

While it is comforting to look back on the successes of the past, it should be noted that road safety still continues to be one of the major health epidemics today and will only get worse in the years ahead without new innovations and initiatives. While crash rates have fallen to around five or six deaths per 100 000 people in the better Western societies, it is not so impressive generally, especially in developing regions. We must be on our guard not to rest on our pass successes and continue to search for new evidence showing ways in which errant behaviour can be modified to improve road safety.

Adopting a European model such as Vision Zero or Sustainable Safety would seem to have considerable merit. We can no longer continue to trade human lives and suffering for the privilege of unrestricted freedom in the way we drive our automobiles. While preventing crashes is still important, they will unfortunately continue to occur; our challenge is to ensure that when they inevitably happen, no one experiences life-threatening impact forces. This will require radical thinking in future and a consorted effort by all of us to behave more safely. There is no doubt that this will present enormous challenges if we are serious about achieving Vision Zero outcomes. Our success in even getting close to this desirable outcome is likely to mean substantial investments in infrastructure, a new collaborative or systems-wide approach to addressing road safety issues and problems and a massive change in community attitude. Continuing to adopt an evidence-based approach will be essential, both in terms of countermeasure development and community acceptance. We hope for the sake of our children and future generations that we are able to achieve such an admirable objective.

References

1. Murray CJL, Lopez AD. The Global Burden of Disease: Harvard University Press; 1996.
2. Australian Transport Safety Bureau. Road crash data and rates, Australian States and Territories 1925 to 2001. Canberra: Department of Transport and Regional Services; 2002.
3. Haddon W. A logical framework for categorizing highway safety phenomena and activity. Journal of Trauma 1972(12):193–207.
4. Trinca G, Johnston I, Campbell B, Haight F, Knight P, Mackay M, et al. Reducing traffic injury – a global challenge. Melbourne: Massina & Co; 1988.
5. Evans L. Traffic safety and the driver. New York: Van Nostrand Reinhold; 1991.
6. Levy M, et al. A review of research on vehicle sanctions in the USA. In: International conference on alcohol, drugs, and traffic safety. Sweden; 2000.
7. Beirness D, et al. Evaluation of administrative licence suspension and vehicle impoundment programs in Manitoba. Ottawa, Ontario: Traffic Injury Research Foundation of Canada; 1997.
8. Langford J, Pronk N. Benefits of vehicle sanction programs. Canberra: National Library of Australia; 2003.
9. Frith W. Motor vehicle sanctions in New Zealand. Tasmania: Tasmanian Road Safety Council; 2002.

10. Wells-Parker E, Bangert-Drowns R, McMillen R, Williams M. Final results from a meta-analysis of remedial interventions with drink/drive offenders. Addiction 1985; 90:907–926.
11. McNight J. Meta-analysis of remedial interventions with drink-drive offenders: a useful clarification of what is and is not known. Addiction 1985; 90:1591–1592.
12. Ferguson M, Sheehan M, Davey J, Watson B. Drink-driving rehabilitation: The present context, Report CR 184. In. Canberra: Australian Transport Safety Bureau [online] [access 2004 August]. Available from URL: http://www.atsb.gov.au/road/pdf/cr184.pdf; 1999.
13. DeYoung D. An evaluation of the effectiveness of alcohol treatment, driver license actions and jail terms in reducing drunk driving recidivism in California. Addiction 1997; 90:907–926.
14. Pronk N, Langford J. Road safety impact of various rehabilitation programs for traffic offenders. In: Langford J, Fildes B, eds. Road safety handbook. Canberra: Austroads; 2003.
15. Kent S, Fildes B. A review of Walk-With-Care: An education and advocacy program for older pedestrians, Report 109. Melbourne: Monash University Accident Research Centre; 1997.
16. Cairney P. Pedestrian safety in Australia Report FHWA-RD-99-093. McLean, VA: Federal Highway Administration; 1999.
17. Tziotis M. Pedestrian crashes in Melbourne's central activity district. Melbourne: Victorian State Institute; 1995.
18. Couch M, McCutcheon A, Cirocco B. Older pedestrians: Moving from a high recognition of problems to an effective local response. In: Road Safety Research, Policing and Education Conference; 2000; Brisbane; 2000.
19. Haworth N, Tingvall C, Kowadlo N. Review of best practice road safety initiatives in the corporate and/or business environment, Report 166. Melbourne: Monash University Accident Research Centre; 2000.
20. Seljak R, Maddock S. Workplace health and safety in the road transport industry: a sleeping giant. In: Symposium on work-related road trauma and fleet risk management in Australia. Canberra: Australian Transport Safety Bureau.
21. Murray W. Overcoming the barriers to fleet safety in Australia. In: Symposium on work-related road trauma and fleet risk management in Australia. Canberra: Australian Transport Safety Bureau; 2001.
22. Folksam Research. How safe is your car? Sweden: Folksam Insurance; 1999.
23. Monash University Accident Research. Policy for purchase and use of vehicles at MUARC. In: Victoria: Monash University Accident Research Centre [online] [access 2004 August] Available from URL www.general.monash.edu.au/muarc/carpolcy.htm; 2000.
24. Gains A, Humble R, Heydecker B, Robertson S. Cost recovery system for speed and red-light cameras – two year pilot evaluation. London: Department For Transport, Road Safety Division; 2003.
25. Cameron M, A. C, Gilbert A. Crash-based evaluation of the speed camera program in Victoria 1990–1991. Report 42. Clayton: Monash University Accident Research Centre; 1992.
26. Cameron M, Delaney A, Diamantopoulou K, Lough B. Scientific basis for the strategic directions of the safety camera program in Victoria, Preliminary Draft Report. Victoria: Monash University Accident Research Centre; 2003.
27. Howard E. Improving road safety outcomes: 'Arrive-alive' Victoria's road safety strategy 2002–2007. In: TRAFINZ Street Safe Conference, New Zealand; 2003.

28. Keall M, Povey L, Frith W. The relative effectiveness of a hidden versus a visible speed camera programme. Accident Analysis and Prevention 2001; 33:277–284.

29. Keall M, Povey L, Frith W. Further results from a trial comparing a hidden speed camera with visible camera operations. Accident Analysis and Prevention 2002; 34:773–777.

30. National Institute of Research on Transport and their Safety (INRETS). Evaluated road safety media campaigns: An overview of 265 evaluated campaigns and some meta-analysis on accidents. Gadget Project RO-97-SC.2235. Brussels: European Commission, 4th Framework Programme; 1999.

31. Elliott B. Road safety mass media campaigns: A meta analysis. Report CR118. Canberra: Department of Transport and Regional Services; 1993.

32. Haworth N. Maximising the road safety impact of advertising, in Fildes B and Langford J (eds). Road Safety Handbook, Austroads, Canberra, Australia; 2003.

33. Delaney A, Lough B, Whelan M, Cameron M. A review of mass media campaigns in road safety. Report for the Swedish National Road Administration. Borlänge, Sweden; 2003.

34. Fildes B. Vision Zero – a dream or reality? In: Zero-Toll symposium. Hobart: Australasian Transport Research Forum; 2001.

35. National Road Safety Committee. Road Safety Strategy 2010: A Consultation Document. Wellington, New Zealand: Land Transport Safety Authority; 2000.

36. Elvik R. Can injury prevention efforts go too far? Reflections on some possible implications of Vision Zero for road accident fatalities. Accident Analysis and Prevention, 1999; 31:265–286.

37. Johansson R, Lie A, Tingvall C. The Vision Zero; what is it and what has it done in Sweden. In: Traffic Safety Summit, Kananaskis, Canada; 1998.

38. Vaa T. Vision Zero and Sustainable Safety: A comparative discussion of premises and consequences: Swedish National Road Administration; 1999.

39. Van Vliet P, Schermers G. Sustainable safety a new approach for road safety in the Netherlands. The Netherlands: Traffic Research Centre, Rotterdam; 2000.

40. Wegman F. The concept of a sustainable safe road traffic system, Report D-27-2. Lidschendam, The Netherlands: Institute for Road Safety Research; 1997.

41. Institute of Transport Economics. Vision Zero and Sustainable Safety: A comparative discussion of premises and consequences. Working Paper O-2506. Swedish: National Road Administration.

CHAPTER **13**

Self-management and chronic illness

Amanda Weeks
Hal Swerissen

CHAPTER CONTENTS

INTRODUCTION

Chronic illness is a significant issue for industrialized countries and a rapidly emerging one for developing countries. The management of chronic illness introduces a number of challenges for people with these conditions, their carers and the health-care professionals with whom they interact. It is arguable that current treatment, care and support for this group is inadequate and could be significantly improved.

Most recently there has been considerable interest in the development of more participatory approaches to the management of chronic illness which involves the development of partnerships between professionals, carers and those who have a chronic illness. The development of programs to teach self-management skills has been an important initiative in this emerging picture.

EPIDEMIOLOGY

According to the World Health Organization[1] chronic illnesses will be the leading cause of disability by 2020. This has not always been the case; until the nineteenth century, infectious diseases and injury dominated the health of world populations. In the 1900s, six out of 10 leading causes of death were infectious diseases or diseases related to infectious processes, e.g. tuberculosis, influenza, pneumonia, and diphtheria.[2] In industrialized countries, infectious disease mortality has decreased from about 36 per 100 deaths by approximately six per 100 deaths in the past 100 years.[3] There has been a corresponding increase in the prevalence of chronic disease and, for these countries, they are now the main cause of mortality and morbidity.

DEFINITION AND CHARACTERISTICS OF CHRONIC ILLNESS

Much of the literature uses the terms 'chronic illness', 'chronic disease' and 'chronic condition' interchangeably with no distinction made in the use of them.[4] In general most common definitions are both medically and disease-oriented, with little consideration of the role or experience of the person with the chronic illness. Definitions often imply incurability, dependency, non-compliance and expense to the health-care system.[5,6] This can be problematic insofar as definitions influence the way in which people with a chronic illness are treated.[7]

This is a common problem with most earlier definitions of chronic illness.[8–10] More recent definitions are less prescriptive, medically focused and pessimistic about the course of chronic illness. Table 13.1 illustrates how definitions have changed over the past 50 years.

Current definitions of chronic illnesses cover an enormously broad range of health concerns. According to the World Health Organization[1] chronic illnesses include: non-communicable diseases, persistent communicable diseases, long term mental disorders and ongoing physical/structural impairments.

The illnesses within these categories vary from country to county. For example, cardiovascular disease, mental disorders, injury and cancer disease have the greatest impact on the health and quality of life of Australians and place the largest financial burden on the health system.[11] In Africa HIV/AIDS has the greatest impact, followed by lower respiratory infections, malaria and tuberculosis.[1]

While each of these categories and the illnesses within them are seemingly very different they all share the same fundamental characteristics:

- Most chronic illnesses are long-term (in that they last for a period of six months or more) and persistent, leading to a gradual deterioration in health. Their onset is usually gradual.
- Most chronic illnesses are not immediately life-threatening, yet they are the most common and leading cause of premature mortality.

Table 13.1   Definitions of chronic illness: Advantages and disadvantages

Date	Author	Definition	Advantages	Disadvantages
1949	Commission of Chronic Diseases[85]	'All impairments or deviations from normal which have one or more of the following characteristics: are permanent, leave residual disability, are caused by non-reversible pathological alteration, require special training of the patient for rehabilitation, and/or may be expected to require; long period of supervision, observation or care' (p. 1)	Concise Generally applicable	Medically based Not flexible
1972	Abram[10]	Any impairment of bodily function over a period of time requiring general adaptation (summarized).	Behaviourally oriented Concise Flexible	Brief Medically based
1974	Feldman[19]	Ongoing medical condition with spectrum of social, economic and behavioural complications that require meaningful and continuous personal and professional involvement (summarized).	Allows for multi-disciplinary action Holistic Recognizes role of patient Flexible	
1979	Buergin et al.[86]	Symptoms and signs caused by a disease within a variable period of time that runs a long course and from which recovery is only partial (summarized).	Concise Traditional	Medically oriented
1981	Cluff[8]	A condition not cured by medical intervention requiring periodic monitoring and supportive care to reduce the degree	Recognizes role of patient in self-care	

Continued

Table 13.1 Definitions of chronic illness: Advantages and disadvantages—*cont'd*

Date	Author	Definition	Advantages	Disadvantages
		of illness, maximize the person's functioning and responsibility for self-care (summarized).		
1982	Mazzuca[87]	A condition requiring a high level of self-responsibility for successful day-to-day management (summarized).	Recognizes role of patient in self-care	Too brief
1986	Curtin & Lubkin[4]	'Chronic illness is the irreversible presence, accumulation, or latency of disease states or impairments that involve the total human environment for supportive care and self-care, maintenance of function, and prevention of further disability' (p. 6)	Recognizes role of patient in self-care Allows for multi-disciplinary action	
1988	Corbin & Strauss[33]	'They are long-term; they follow an uncertain course, often requiring large efforts at palliation; they are disproportionately intrusive upon the lives of the ill and their families; and they are expensive to treat and manage' (p. 11)		Implies patient to be dependent, passive recipients of treatment, who are expensive to treat and who contribute little to society
2001	Common-wealth Department of Health and Ageing, Australia[88]	Chronic illnesses are those which are long-term (lasting more than 6 months) and can have a significant impact on a person's life	Not prescriptive (room for change)	Too brief
2002	World Health Organization[1]	'Are health problems that require ongoing management over a period of years or decades' (p. 11)	Enable wide range of conditions Not prescriptive (room for change)	Too brief

- Most chronic illnesses significantly compromise quality of life through activity limitations and may require assistance from others over an extended period of time. Furthermore most chronic illnesses are not necessarily illnesses of ageing but can occur across all stages of the life cycle.[12]

In industrialized countries chronic illness is the most significant contribution to the overall burden of illness for the population. In Australia, for example, it is estimated that chronic illnesses are responsible for approximately 80% of the total burden of disease with an estimated three million Australians suffering from one or more chronic illnesses.[12] According to the Australian Institute of Health[12] and the National Health Survey[13] this means that at least 10% of the population suffer from a chronic illness. In dollar terms, chronic diseases account for 40% or $12.6 billion of total health expenditure, with $5.9 billion (46%) being spent on chronic illnesses in the hospital sector alone.[11]

THE CHRONIC ILLNESS EXPERIENCE

People suffering from chronic illness are affected in different ways. Some are severely restricted in performing basic activities of daily living, for example those affected by Parkinson's disease, while others experience intermittent episodes of ill health of varying intensity and duration. Pain, discomfort, functional limitations and the need for ongoing treatment have social, psychological, behavioural and economic effects. In many respects it is these consequences that define the nature of chronic illness.

Social impacts

Families often influence how a family member defines illness and when and how to seek medical care.[14] The emotional reactions, beliefs and behaviours of families also influence the response a family member has to being diagnosed with a chronic illness. Often they provide the majority of treatment and care informally. This is particularly true for women.[15] Often having a family member take on the role of carer means a change in the family structure as the ill family member's capacity to perform his or her usual role in the family changes. This may in turn lead to role tensions, emotional, physical and financial strain; inconvenience, anxiety and depression for both the carer and the family member for whom care is provided.[15,16] Responses to chronic illness can be thought of as a continuum or illness trajectory that changes over time. Figure 13.1 illustrates this process.

Over time, people with a chronic illness adapt to their social circumstances. The outcomes of this process of adaptation may be thought of as taking on a role. For people who are acutely ill, this has been conceptualized by Parsons[17] as the 'sick role'. According to the Parsonian model, an individual who is sick is: (1) not responsible for their condition; (2) exempt from normal social role responsibilities and has the right to be cared for; (3) obligated to get well or to do what can be done to obtain maximum functional ability; and (4) obligated

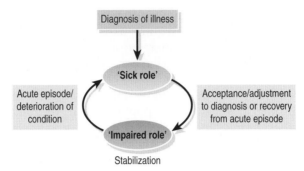

Fig. 13.1   Illness behaviour continuum. Adapted from Corbin & Strauss[33] and Lubkin.[15]

to seek and accept professional care. These conditions are clearly violated by chronic illness, often with problematic social consequences.

On the one hand, Falvo[18] suggests chronic illness can often result in 'discrimination, social isolation, disregard, depreciation, devaluation, and, in some instances, even threats to safety and wellbeing'. Such factors can have a profound impact on an individual's ability to maintain functional capacity when suffering from a chronic illness.

On the other hand, it is clear that there may also be gains for individuals who remain in the sick role.[19-21] These so-called 'secondary gains' may include avoidance of normal responsibilities, increased attention, and increased personal and psychological support. Maintenance of sick role behaviours often prevents the chronically ill individual from taking over the management of their own care which for the carer can lead to emotional strain. This can manifest in many ways, including feelings of isolation, anxiety, guilt, resentment and frustration.[22] Over time commitment to caring responsibilities may be undermined.

It is important to recognize that the Parsonian 'sick role' is a normative statement of expectations about sickness behaviour and attitudes. It is what the 'good patient' should do. Alternative statements of our normative expectations for those with a chronic illness have been proposed. Gordon[23] for example suggests the 'impaired role for people with more ongoing problems'. In the impaired role an individual is not expected to 'want to get well' but rather encouraged to function within their limitations. The impaired role assumes individuals will engage in rehabilitation and maximization of wellness, which requires them to focus on the maintenance of their condition, prevent of complications, and resume 'normal' role responsibilities.[21] More recently, there has been a significant development of the concept of social rights for people who have chronic illness and disability.

Psychological impacts

The psychological effects of chronic illness are usually associated with an individual's ability to adapt to their condition and their attempts to cope with the illness.[24] Leventhal et al.[25] have suggested that there are two coping processes attributable to chronic illnesses: (1) is coping with the illness and (2) coping with the emotional reactions of the illness (see Fig. 13.2).

An individual's fears and attempts to cope with the illness are usually determined by their own perception of the illness and their own perception of their capacity to deal with it. Falvo[18] has identified a variety of cognitive coping mechanisms employed by chronic illness sufferers, including denial, regression, compensation and diversion of feelings.

Emotional reactions to illness may include depressive or phobic reactions. According to Johnson,[24] depressive reactions are more likely at the acute stages of the illness such as at onset of illness, a time of relapse or deterioration, or an acute episode requiring hospitalization or extra care and are not necessarily related to severity of condition. Such reactions are considered in terms of 'learned helplessness'. Clinical manifestations of a depressive reaction may include moods of sadness, hopelessness, self-deprecation, reduced activity and social interaction, insomnia, changes in appetite and weight, lack of libido and so forth. Phobic reactions occur when the person suffering from the chronic illness becomes fearful of symptoms or situations associated with symptoms and may learn to avoid any situation that may elicit symptoms.

Economic impact

Chronic illness has significant economic effects. Income for the majority of people suffering from chronic illnesses is derived from Government benefits, partly because of social attitudes towards employment of the chronically ill and partly because of the fact that many chronic illness sufferers are of or beyond retirement age.[1] In Australia, for example, the Disability Support Pension is the main Government benefit provided to people with chronic illness. There were over 600 000 recipients in 2000 and expenditure on the payment totalled $5.2 billion.[11]

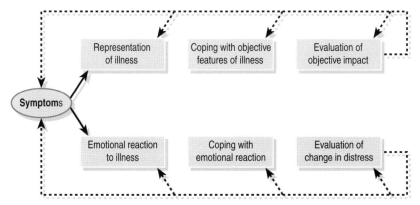

Fig. 13.2   Coping processes for chronic illness. Adapted from Leventhal et al.[25]

For those people with a chronic illness who are able to maintain employment it has been noted that their earnings are often considerably lower than those who do not suffer from a chronic illness.[26] In general the more severe the illness, the lower the earnings from work. In addition to having to contend with lower earnings, they are also often liable for the higher cost of medical care and prescriptions, as a result of not having a health-care card which would entitle them to subsidised prescriptions, ambulance coverage and a wide range of other government benefits. Such costs can have a major impact. In Australia individuals spend on average $360 million dollars on hospital related care, $636 million on generalist medical services and approximately $1.5 million dollars on pharmaceuticals.[27]

HEALTH-CARE SYSTEM TREATMENT OF CHRONIC ILLNESS

Meeting the complex needs of patients with chronic illness or impairment is one of the greatest challenges facing the health-care system. Glazier,[28] Lubkin[15] and Cluff[8] have noted that there are a variety of reasons why the current health-care system has problems in managing chronic conditions. The basis for these reasons lie in the intrinsic differences between acute and chronic conditions (see Table 13.2).

The acute care system often does not encourage physicians to attempt to foster health maintenance behaviours among their patients which is an essential requirement for conditions that are permanent or long term, where the patient needs to learn to live with their condition. Additionally, the nature of acute care makes it difficult to address ongoing psychological coping and family support issues.

A large proportion of people suffering from chronic illnesses do not receive effective therapy, have poor disease control and are unhappy with the care they are receiving. This has led to calls for a new approach to the provision of

Table 13.2   Differences between acute illness and chronic illness

Acute illness	Chronic illness
Patient is passive, dependent, regressive Illness temporary and results of treatment seen relatively rapidly	Positive dependency Illness permanent or long-term
Patient has limited experience with this role	Patient knowledgeable about role since illness is full time
Decision making by staff	Patient retains much decision making power; wants familiar patterns followed
Doctor responsible for patient health management	Doctor directs care plan but not responsible for it
Doctor held accountable for care by patient	Doctor holds patient accountable for managing own care

Adapted from Glazier[28], Lubkin[15] and Cluf.[8]

treatment and support for people with chronic illness. New means of delivering care which emphasize the person with a chronic illness as co-partner in the delivery process have been advocated to replace approaches which view these individuals as inexperienced and passive recipients of medical care.[29] Schofield et al.[30] suggest that health-care providers should, in their treatment of chronic illnesses aim for the prevention of complications of the disease rather than its cure; aim to encourage patients to take responsibility for their own illnesses; aim to minimize the degree of handicap the patients' disabilities cause them; and aim to help families adjust and adapt to one of their members having a chronic illness (p. 65). The implications of this for health service delivery, care of patients and health resources would be vast.

One method for enhancing chronic illness management is through self-management. Results of many randomized control trials show that effective self-management programs can achieve better outcomes than the usual care currently being offered by our health-care system.

SELF-MANAGEMENT OF CHRONIC ILLNESS

The term self-management emerged as a result of the self-care movement of the 1960s and 1970s. One of the first to use the term was Thomas Creer in an article on asthma self-care in the mid 1970s.[31] Creer[31] felt that self-management guaranteed that the patient was an active participant in their treatment. Since the 1970s, the term self-management has been used widely and has mainly referred to patient education programs. Unfortunately, while the term is used widely, it has not been well conceptualized or defined.

In an effort to rectify this Gruman and Von Korff[32] conducted a comprehensive literature review of over 400 articles on self-management. They propose that self-management 'involves [the person with the chronic illness] engaging in activities that protect and promote health, monitoring and management of symptoms and signs of illness, managing the impacts of illness and functioning, emotions and interpersonal relationships and adhering to treatment regimes' (p. 1).

Corbin and Strauss[33] identified three sets of tasks commonly dealt with by people with chronic illnesses. The first, involves the medical management of the illness such as the patient taking medications, doing prescribed exercises, following a prescribed diet etc. The second set of tasks involves maintaining, changing and/or creating new meaningful life roles. The final set of tasks requires individuals to deal with the emotional effects of having a chronic illness. Corbin and Strauss conclude that self-management programs must include content that addresses all three tasks.

However, most self-management programs do not address these three tasks. In the main most self-management programs address the medical management of the illness but ignore the emotional effects and the need to change or create new life roles. For instance, a literature search using Medline on chronic illnesses such as diabetes and asthma showed that self-management was largely concerned with the development of action plans, self-monitoring, access to health professionals and information.

In addition to the tasks outlined by Corbin and Strauss,[33,34] Lorig[34] notes that effective self-management is characterized by the ability to adapt to the condition stating that that self-management is about enabling:

> *Participants to make informed choices, to adapt new perspectives and generic skills that can be applied to new problems as they arise, to practise new health behaviours, and to maintain or regain emotional stability. The result of these activities is improved health status or the slowing of deterioration. A secondary outcome of self-management is the reduced utilization of health-care services (p. 11).*

Moreover, Lorig emphasizes that self-management should not be viewed as an alternative to medical care but that the two should be seen as complementary strategies. Wagner et al.[35] suggest that this could be achieved by integrating self-management activities into the medical care system through the use of explicit plans and protocols, practice redesign to meet follow-up needs of patients, ready access to expert systems and the development of supportive information systems. Von Korff et al.[36] and Clark et al.[37] suggest that an essential component of the two complementing one another is the need for collaboration among chronically ill patients, their families and health-care providers and that for successful collaborative management patients and care providers must have 'shared goals, a sustained working relationship, mutual understanding of roles and responsibilities, and requisite skills for carrying out their roles' (p. 1097). This relies on the shared goals being based on what the patient perceives as the problem rather than what the health professionals think patients should know and do.[29,33]

Self-management is therefore a complementary strategy to usual medical care that involves the individual, family and health professional working in partnership to maximize the potential health benefit of any medical intervention by teaching individuals the skills they need to:

- Participate effectively in treatment regimes.
- Engage in activities that protect and promote health.
- Monitor and manage symptoms and signs of illness.
- Manage the impact of illness on day-to-day functioning, emotions and personal relationships.
- Create new and meaningful life roles.

Theoretical basis for self-management programs

A number of programs to facilitate self-management skills for people with chronic illness have been developed. The theoretical underpinnings for these programs include the Theory of Reasoned Action,[38] the Health Belief Model[39] and Social Learning Theory[40,41] and more recently the Stages of Change Model[42] (see also Ch. 2).

The Health Belief Model and self-management

The Health Belief Model (HBM) was one of the first models that adapted theory from the behavioural sciences to health problems. It was originally introduced in the 1950s by psychologists working in the US Public Health Service to explain the way a person's beliefs about health and illness can predict health service use and personal health decisions. According to this model, decisions are based on the clients perception of their level of susceptibility to the illness, the severity of the consequences of the illness (physical or social), the potential benefits derived by a given health action and the balancing of physical, psychological, financial, or other barriers related to the health action against the benefit (see Fig. 13.3).

Social Learning Theory and self-management

There is increasing recognition that social learning theory, in particular perceived self-efficacy, is critically important to promoting effective self-management of chronic illness.[34,43,44] According to Tobin et al.[45] there are three principle therapeutic goals in social learning theory through which self-management of chronic illness can be achieved: '(1) self-control skills are learned; (2) beliefs likely to promote changes in health behaviour are enhanced (e.g. efficacy expectations); and (3) environmental conditions (including

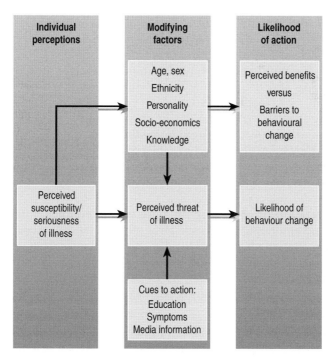

Fig. 13.3   The Health Belief Model. Adapted from Egger et al.[84]

family and social networks) that promote the self-control of chronic illness are created' (p. 32). Another important treatment goal of self-management is to enhance the beliefs, or levels of personal efficacy, that promote the effective performance of self-management skills.[45]

Self-efficacy is defined as a person's confidence or belief that they can change and regulate a specific behaviour or cognitive state in order to produce given attainments.[46] According to Bandura[46,47] personal efficacy will affect life choices, level of motivation, quality of functioning, resilience to adversity and vulnerability to stress and depression. Thus, when applying social learning theory to self-management programs the program itself should not only be concerned with teaching the skills needed to successfully self-manage, but should also incorporate mechanisms in which a participant's beliefs that he can successfully perform those skills are increased.

One of the strengths of the self-efficacy framework is its direct applicability to the practice of modifying health behaviours by specifying mechanisms that enhance learning and also increase motivation. As individuals successfully adapt strategies for their own circumstances their perceptions of self-efficacy, control and empowerment increase and they are more likely to apply and generalize the skills and techniques they have learnt in their everyday lives. Bandura[47] states that a person's beliefs in their efficacy are developed and enhanced through the following four efficacy enhancing mechanisms:

- **Skills mastery.** Skills mastery is generally achieved through the experience of attempting behaviour. The success of attempting a behaviour will raise efficacy judgments and failure will normally lower them, especially if the failure occurs early and is associated with substantial effort. Self-management programs can assist in providing people with the skills to ensure success by having the person attempt a behaviour by breaking it into small manageable tasks and then making sure that each small task is successfully completed.
- **Modelling.** Seeing people similar to oneself manage task demands successfully and having them provide feedback on the effectiveness of the strategies they have developed to achieve this can increase self-efficacy.
- **Persuasion.** Persuasion can take many forms and can be achieved through many mechanisms such as presentation of knowledge, information and argument.
- **Reinterpretation of physiological signs and symptoms.** Inferences from somatic and emotional states indicative of personal strengths and vulnerabilities are often made by people with chronic illnesses. Often these inferences are irrational and prevent people from reaching their full potential. Self-management programs can assist in changing these behaviours by providing people with the skills needed to identify the irrational belief and to subsequently reinterpret it.

Self-efficacy is not a static concept but rather is influenced by changes in situation, task, social context and individual development.[48] Bandura[47] notes that perceived efficacy can improve from the point when people begin to contemplate changes and continues to improve as they undertake strategies to change. The theory underlying the various stages at which a person's perceived efficacy can improve is best explained by the 'Stages of Change' or, as it is also referred to, the Trans-Theoretical Model of Change.

Stages of Change Theory and self-management

The Stages of Change Model outlines how people change behaviour, either on their own or within an intervention program and is based on the premise that behaviour change is a process and not an event, and that individuals are at varying levels of motivation or readiness to change. Prochaska et al.[42] have identified five basic stages of change (see Fig. 13.4). At any stage within this model relapse may occur. This is not necessarily seen as a negative event, for each time a stage is repeated the person learns from the experience and gains new skills to help them move on to the next.

The content of self-management programs

Following an extensive review, Wagner et al.[35] outlined a general program model for successful self-management interventions. This model outlined four essential elements needed to facilitate a successful self-management program:

- **Collaborative problem definition:** Programs that enable the patient to define their problems in conjunction with their health professional.
- **Targeting, goal setting and planning:** Programs should target the issues that are of greatest importance to the patient and health-care provider, set realistic goals, and develop a personalized care plan or action plan. Programs are successful if the process is guided by a consideration of the consumer's readiness to change and self-efficacy.
- **Self-management training and support services:** Programs that include instruction on disease management, behavioural support programs,

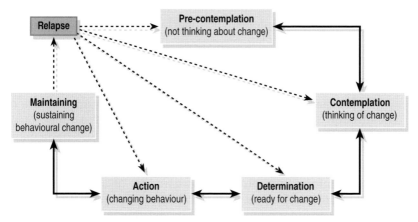

Fig. 13.4   Stages of Change Model. Adapted from Prochaska et al.[42]

physical activity and interventions that address the emotional demands of having a chronic condition.

- **Active and sustained follow-up:** Evidence shows that reliable follow-up at regular intervals, initiated by the provider, leads to better health outcomes.

A number of strategies and techniques for teaching self-management skills have been developed. These include action, or as they are sometimes referred to, care plans; monitoring diaries; and information provision.

Action/care plans

The literature demonstrates that a central and effective feature of many self-management programs is the patient-generated short-term action plan.[32,49-51] Action plans have been used in the management of many chronic illnesses, particularly in the management of asthma. Action plans are developed by patients as something they want to do. They are not provided by health-care professionals or chosen from a list of options. The purpose of action plans is to give patients confidence in managing their illness, confidence that fuels internal motivation. Self-efficacy theory holds that the successful achievement of the action plan is more important than the plan itself.

Monitoring diaries

Monitoring diaries are widely recommended in the literature and are completed using either a device (e.g. peak expiratory flow [PEF], blood sugar level [BSL]) or through subjective interpretation of symptoms (e.g. pain, amount of exercise). According to the Flinders University Health Behaviour and Health Research Unit (2001) monitoring diaries are essential for three reasons: (1) 'triggers for symptom or physiological worsening are ascertained; (2) symptom action plans are devised based on information contained in the diary; and (3) ongoing use of a diary motivates the use of action plans'.

Research using monitoring diaries has shown that this method is rarely effective for managing symptoms when used in isolation and is best used in conjunction with an action plan.[52,53]

Information provision

Information provision to support self-management programs is more often than not through verbal instruction. However, there are a range of other mediums in which additional information is made available to participants of self-management programs. These include books, videos, CD-ROMs, and the Internet. Very few evaluations have been conducted that demonstrate the effectiveness of information provision as a means of assisting in the self-management of chronic illnesses. Of the evaluations that have been conducted the information was reported to be useful in assisting with self-management and was also found to increase knowledge levels.[89,90]

Participant characteristics

According to Tobin et al.,[45] patients who one would expect to be most responsive to self-management exhibit the following characteristics: (1) a supportive environment; (2) a belief that the use of self-management skills can prevent or delay the onset of illness or effect symptomatic control to a significant degree; (3) the ability to accept a collaborative relationship with health professionals in which the responsibility for health change is shared; (4) no indications that easily administered and effective surgical or pharmaceutical interventions are preferred; (5) chronic illness with behavioural components that impact on the course of the disorder; (6) an absence of prior failure with self-management; and (7) the absence of significant physical dysfunction.

There are many barriers that may prevent an individual successfully managing their condition.[54] These include:

- Poor literacy skills.
- Disability.
- Lack of finance.
- Health-care provision.
- Level of self-efficacy.
- Motivation.
- Myths about self-management, e.g. self-management equates to self-treatment.
- Non-supportive family and friends.

Delivery of self–management programs: Professionally led or peer–led?

Two unique approaches to the implementation of self-management programs are emerging in Australia, Britain, China and the United States of America. They concern whether health-care professionals or peers deliver self-management programs.

The use of laypersons as providers of health care has been documented since the late 1960s. One of the earliest and most noteworthy examples is the Reach to Recovery Program developed by the American Cancer Society.[55] The program uses trained volunteers, all of whom are former mastectomy patients, to provide support and up-to-date information to patients who have been newly diagnosed with breast cancer. Information is also provided to spouses, children, friends, etc.

An evaluation of the Reach to Recovery Program was completed in 1995 to determine if cancer patients who received the program were satisfied with the program and to determine if participation in Reach to Recovery affected the quality of life of program participants compared to patients who did not receive the program. Ashbury et al.[56] found that participants were generally satisfied with the program they received and that the program has incremental benefits to the quality of life of patients with breast cancer. They conclude that peer-led support programs can be effective in enhancing quality of life.

More recently, the Stanford Arthritis Centre developed a self-management course that is taught by trained laypersons, of whom about 50% themselves have arthritis.[57] The program has consistently demonstrated improvements in knowledge, self-efficacy and the use of self-management behaviours.[34,58] Lorig et al.[57] has also conducted a comparative study of the arthritis program when taught by laypersons and professionals. They found that based on the results of this study, which demonstrated professional-taught programs achieved greater knowledge gain while lay-taught programs have greater changes in relaxation and a tendency toward less disability. They concluded that laypersons could teach self-management courses with results similar to those achieved by professionals.

Outside of the United States, both Britain and Australia have embraced the use of laypersons to deliver self-management programs. In Britain, the National Health Service (NHS) recently established an Expert Patients Task Force to design a new program that would bring together the work of patient and clinical organizations in developing self-management initiatives. Peer-leaders, in Britain, are more often than not referred to as 'expert patients.' What emerged from this task force was a plan, over a six-year period to intro-duce and integrate lay-led self-management training programs for patients with chronic diseases within the existing NHS provision of health care in England.[59] Prior to the formation of the task force there were a number of sim-ilar programs to that of Lorig et al.[57] developed by patient groups and repre-sentative organizations. These included the:

- **Challenging Arthritis Program (CAP)** that was developed by Arthritis Care. This is a user-led arthritis self-management program in which all senior staff, self-management trainers and volunteer course leaders are people with arthritis. In randomized controlled trials the CAP, and modi-fied versions of it, showed consistent improvements in knowledge, self-efficacy and the use of self-management behaviours, notably exercise.
- **Self-Management Training Programme (SMTP) for Manic Depression** was begun by the Manic Depression Fellowship in 1998. It is entirely user-devel-oped and user-led. The program has been designed to enable individuals with a diagnosis of manic depression to gain confidence in their own capaci-ties and to take control of their lives. This program was developed from a course that originated in Ohio. It is currently the subject of a randomized con-trolled trial (RCT) with good outcomes to date, including improvements in mood sustained three to six months after completion of the course.
- **Self-Management in Multiple Sclerosis Program** developed by The Mul-tiple Sclerosis (MS) Society. This program is based on the Lorig model, where trained laypersons with MS deliver a structured self-management course. The course content includes choosing treatment, managing fatigue, problem solving, accessing health services and communicating with health-care professionals.[59]

According to Lorig et al.,[57] there are several reasons for having laypersons or peers, as they are otherwise known, deliver self-management programs. The first is that they serve as successful role models. The importance of modelling and its relationship to improved health outcomes has been suggested by the theoretical work of Bandura on self-efficacy and has been demonstrated in several self-management programs. Secondly, laypersons provide a large pool of potential volunteers that may allow for mass delivery of self-management programs. Thirdly, there are significant savings to be made by using laypersons to deliver self-management programs.[59]

In summary, peer-led self-management programs share many characteristics with professionally led programs: (1) they are both evidence-based; (2) they have both demonstrated measurable effects in terms of outcomes; and (3) they both include medical management of conditions. How peer-led self-management programs differ, however, is that they (1) are driven by the patient rather than the health professional; (2) facilitate and promote patient efforts to manage chronic illness using the theory of self-efficacy; and (3) they are more cost-effective.

EVIDENCE OF EFFECTIVENESS

A number of studies have now investigated the impact of programs to teach self-management to people with a chronic illness on social, psychological, clinical and functional outcomes. Research in both the United States and Britain has shown that self-management programs can achieve positive outcomes across a range of indicators, such as health status, health behaviour and decreased health-care utilization. There is now a significant body of evidence suggesting these interventions may be a cost-effective complement to existing health-care provision.[60–62]

Lorig and her colleagues have conducted a number or randomized controlled trials which demonstrate outcomes of their self-management programs. Their studies have investigated the impact of the Arthritis Self-Management Program, the Spanish Arthritis Self-Management Program and the Back Pain Self-Management Program, which are condition-specific, and the Chronic Disease Self-Management Program, which is a program designed for people with a range of chronic illnesses. All of these programs have been evaluated in trials lasting from four to twelve months. Self-management on its own was able to give long-term benefits to participants; the benefits were more closely linked to improvements in self-efficacy rather than changing people's behaviours; and interventions were cost effective and demonstrated significant reductions in health-care utilization.[34,63–65]

Improvements in self-efficacy and self-management of chronic illness are a key outcome for many studies. Program impact on these indicators has been studied across a range of conditions. For example, Bartholomew et al.[66] studied the impact of self-management training for cystic fibrosis patients and their families. They found improved self-efficacy for patients' aged five to eleven years and for caregivers following intervention.

Similarly, Lenker et al.[67] attempted to address the question of which strategies were most effective by undertaking a content evaluation of an arthritis self-management course. Using a questionnaire containing both open-ended and structured questions about participants' perceptions of the course, the effect the course had on their lives and benefits experienced, Lenker et al.[67] confirmed that self-management courses do effect individual self-efficacy but do not elaborate on the strategies that achieve this.

Gibson et al.[68] have studied the impact of self-management education for people with asthma. They concluded that 'self-management education about asthma which involves self-monitoring by either PEF or symptoms, regular medical review and a written action plan, improves health outcomes for adults with asthma. There are major reductions in resource use and improvements in morbidity' (p. 2) and that 'less intensive interventions, particularly those without a written action plan, are less efficacious' (p. 12). The authors also state 'self-management education that involves a written action plan, self-monitoring and regular medical review should be offered to adults with asthma' (p. 12) and that 'either symptom diaries or peak expiratory flow measurement can be used for self monitoring' (p. 12). Similar studies have also demonstrated that the use of the action plans improves perceived control of asthma symptoms and levels of self-confidence to self-manage.[69–76]

A number of studies have investigated the impact of self-management training on functional outcomes and, in particular, increased physical activity. Increased physical activity is seen as an important indicator of improved outcomes because it is associated with both improved physical and psychological well-being. In general self-management education has been found to improve physical activity levels.[63,77,78]

There is an emerging body of evidence that self-management programs can reduce health service utilization.[79–82] Thoonen et al.[79] found that effective self-management can improve work productivity. Fries et al.[82] reviewed a number of randomized controlled trials which demonstrate that self-management has the potential to significantly lower service use. Gallefoss and Bakke[70] found improved coordination of services and greater adherence to treatment regimens.

Despite these positive findings, the research has a number of limitations. Methodologically, a number of studies are difficult to interpret because of their design limitations. Issues include recruitment procedures, randomization, self-selection, the measurement of outcomes, the lack of adequate controls and sustainability over time and across settings.[83] Even when designs are relatively rigorous, programs are often compared to waiting list controls which receive usual care. Comparisons between different approaches or with general consumer support groups are generally not made. Consequently, the effectiveness of specific components of self-management training is not known.

Similarly, although evidence for the effectiveness of self-management education across different groups of people with chronic illness is growing, further research is required to assess the impact of different conditions, health systems and cultural and social factors. In particular, further work needs to investigate the relationship between general self-management training and specific coaching and education in skills for particular treatment regimes.

More broadly, research on self-management is in the innovation and development stage. There are few well-funded, large-scale demonstration trials across substantial health-care systems. The majority of research is with small-scale, one-off samples which require special recruitment strategies and program delivery which is outside the mainstream health-care setting. It is difficult to evaluate the efficacy of self-management when its impact has not been tested in mainstream health-care settings as part of the overall delivery of treatment, care and support.

SUMMARY AND CONCLUSIONS

Chronic illness is a significant issue for industrialized countries and a rapidly growing issue for developing countries. Increased life expectancy and population ageing, growing health-care costs and increasingly more educated and assertive health-care consumers will place pressure on health systems to find more innovative approaches to the management of chronic illness.

Chronic illness, by its very nature, lends itself to the development of partnerships between the individuals who are ill, their carers and clinicians. This will require a shift in orientation and approach from one which sees people with chronic illness as patients who are the passive recipients of treatment, to one which views them as active partners in their own care and management. Self-management programs and techniques have been developed in response to this emerging trend.

The current indications are that self-management programs are a useful complement to usual care. They have been found to increase self-efficacy and self-management skills. They can improve physical activity and consumer involvement in the management of specific treatment modalities. They can lead to reductions in unnecessary health-care utilization and improvements in productivity. Moreover, those who participate in self-management programs report improved perceptions of health and wellbeing.

However, self-management programs have not yet been widely institutionalized as a systematic component of the overall management of chronic illness. To date the research has largely investigated the use of self-management with relatively small-scale, one-off samples over limited time periods. Inevitably this leaves questions about recruitment, applicability across different conditions, populations and settings and sustainability of programs and effects. Although self-management programs show promise, large-scale, systemic interventions are now needed to test the efficacy of self-management programs and techniques across a range of health-care settings.

References

1. World Health Organization. Innovative care for chronic conditions: building blocks for action (Global Report). Geneva: Non-Communicable Diseases and Mental Health, World Health Organization; 2002.

2. Matarazzo J. Behavioural health's challenge to academic, scientific, and professional psychology. American Psychologist 1982; 37(1):1–14.

3. Burish T, Bradley L. Coping with chronic disease. Research and Applications. New York: Academic Press; 1983.

4. Curtin M, Lubkin I. Chronic illness. Impact and interventions. Boston: Jones and Bartlett; 1986.

5. Walker C. Meanings of chronic illness. Usage of the term 'chronic illness' by clinicians, policy makers and consumers in current literature. Melbourne: Chronic Illness Alliance and Health Issues Centre; 1999.

6. Martin C, Peterson C. Transdisciplinary challenges for health services research and evaluation in general practice: The case of chronic disease management. Australian Journal of Primary Health Interchange 1997; 3(2&3):32–43.

7. Walker C. Recognising the changing boundaries of illness in defining terms of chronic illness: A prelude to understanding the changing needs of people with chronic illness. Australian Health Review 2001; 24(2):207–214.

8. Cluff L. Chronic disease, function and the quality of care. Journal of Chronic Diseases 1981; 34(7):299–304.

9. Commission on Chronic Illness. Guides to action on chronic illness. New York: National Health Council; 1956.

10. Abram HS. The psychology of chronic illness. J Chronic Dis 1972; 25(12):659–664.

11. Australian Institute of Health and Welfare. Health Expenditure Australia 2000–2001. Canberra: Australian Institute of Health and Welfare; 2002.

12. Australian Institute of Health and Welfare. Chronic diseases and associated risk factors in Australia, 2001. Canberra: Australian Institute of Health and Welfare; 2002.

13. Australian Bureau of Statistics. National Health Survey: First Results. Canberra: Australian Bureau of Statistics; 1997.

14. Dimond M, Jones S. Chronic illness across the life span. Connecticut: Appleton-Century-Crofts; 1983.

15. Lubkin I. Chronic illness: Impact and interventions. Boston: Jones and Bartlett; 1986.

16. Thomas E. Problems of disability from the perspective of role theory. Journal of Health and Social Behaviour 1966; 6(1):2–16.

17. Parsons T. The social system. London: Routledge; 1951.

18. Falvo D. Medical and psychosocial aspects of chronic illness and disability. Maryland: Aspen; 1991.

19. Feldman D. Chronic disabling illness: A holistic view. Journal of Chronic Diseases 1974; 27(6):287–291.

20. Mann SB. Being ill: Personal and social meanings. New York: Irvington; 1982.

21. Wu R. Behaviour and illness. Englewood Cliffs, NJ: Prentice Hall; 1973.

22. Crossman L, Kaljian D. The family: Cornerstone of care. Generations VIII 1984; 4:297–300.

23. Gordon G. Role theory and illness: A sociological perspective. Connecticut: College and University Press; 1966.

24. Johnston M. Psychological aspects of chronic disease. In: Hasler J, Schofield T, eds. Continuing care: The management of chronic disease. New York: Oxford University Press; 1990.

25. Leventhal H, Nerenz DR, Steele DJ. Illness representations and coping with health threats. In: Baum A, Singer J, eds. Handbook of psychology and health. Hillsdale, NJ: Erlbaum; 1984:219–252.

26. Townsend P. Disability and income. In: Walker A, Townsend P, eds. Disability in Britain. Oxford: Martin Robinson; 1981.

27. Australian Institute of Health and Welfare. Health resources and use of services. In: Australian Institute of Health and Welfare, ed. Australia's Health 2002. Canberra: Australian Institute of Health and Welfare; 2002:238–337.

28. Glazier W. The task of medicine. Scientific American 1973; 228(4):13–18.

29. Lorig K, Holman H. Self-management education: context, definition, and outcomes and mechanisms. In: Department of Health and Aged Care, ed. The National Chronic Disease Self-Management Conference: Sharing Health Care. Sydney, Australia; 2000.

30. Schofield T, Hasler J, Barnes G. Implications for practice. In: Hasler J, Schofield T, eds. Continuing care: The management of chronic disease, 2nd edn. Oxford: Oxford Medical Publications; 1990:64–83.

31. Creer T, Renne C, Christian W. Behavioural contributions to rehabilitation and childhood asthma. Rehabilitation Literature 1976; 37(8):226–232, 247.

32. Gruman J, Von Korff M. Indexed bibliography on self-management for people with chronic disease. Washington DC: Centre for Advancement in Health; 1996.

33. Corbin J, Strauss A. Unending work and care: Managing chronic illness at home. San Francisco: Jossey-Bass; 1988.

34. Lorig K, Holman H. Arthritis self-management studies: A twelve-year review. Health Education Quarterly 1993; 20(1):17–28.

35. Wagner E, Austin B, Von Korff M. Organizing care for patients with chronic illness. The Milbank Quarterly 1996; 74(4):511–544.

36. Von Korff M, Gruman J, Schaefer J, Curry S, Wagner E. Collaborative management of chronic illness. Annals of Internal Medicine 1997; 127(12):1097–1192.

37. Clark NM, Becker MH, Janz NK, Lorig K, Rakowski W, Anderson L. Self-management of chronic disease by older adults: A review and questions for research. Journal of Aging and Health 1991; 3(1):3–27.

38. Ajzen I, Fishbein M. The prediction of behavioural intentions in a choice situation. Journal of Experimental Social Psychology 1969; 5(5):400–416.

39. Maiman L, Becker M. The health belief model: Origins and correlates in psychological theory. Health Education Monographs 1974; 2(4):336–353.

40. Bandura A. Social foundations of thought and action: A social cognitive view. USA: Englewood Cluffs, Prentice Hall; 1986.

41. Rotter J. Social learning and clinical psychology. New York: Prentice Hill; 1954.

42. Prochaska JO, DiClemente CC, Norcross JC. In search of how people change: applications to addictive behaviors. American Psychologist 1992; 47(9):1102–1114.

43. Clark N, Zimmerman B. A social cognitive view of self-regulated learning about health. Health Education Research 1990; 5(3):371–379.

44. Taal E, Riemsma R, Brus H, Seydel E, Rasker J, Wiegman O. Group education for patients with arthritis. Patient Education and Counseling 1993; 20(2–3):177–187.

45. Tobin DL, Reynolds RVC, Holroyd KA, Creer TL. Self-management and social learning theory. In: Holroyd KA, Creer TL, eds. Self-management of chronic disease: Handbook of clinical interventions and research. Orlando: Academic Press; 1986.

46. Bandura A. Self-efficacy: The exercise of control. New York: WH Freeman; 1997.

47. Bandura A. Self-efficacy. In: Ramachaudran V, ed. Encyclopedia of human behavior. New York: Academic Press; 1994:71–81.

48. Berry J, West R. Cognitive self-efficacy in relation to personal mastery and goal setting across the life span. International Journal of Behavioural Development 1993; 16(2):351–379.

49. Watson P, Town G, Holbrook N, Dwan C, Toop L, Drennan CJ. Evaluation of a self-management plan for chronic obstructive pulmonary disease. European Respiratory Journal. 1997; 10(6):1267–1271.

50. Lorig K, Sobel D, Ritter P, Laurent D, Hobbs M. Effect of a self-management program on patients with chronic disease. Effective Clinical Practice 2001; 4(6):256–262.
51. Wilson S, Scamagasa P, German D, Hughes G, Lulla S, Coss S, et al. Controlled trial of two forms of self-management education for adults with asthma. American Journal of Medicine 1993; 94:564–576.
52. Blanchard E, Appelbaum K, Radnitz C, Morrill B, Michultka D, Kirsch C, et al. A controlled evaluation of thermal biofeedback and thermal biofeedback combined with cognitive therapy in the treatment of vascular headache. Journal Consulting Clinical Psychology 1990; 58(2):216–224.
53. Greene B, Blanchard E. Cognitive therapy for irritable bowel syndrome. Journal Consulting Clinical Psychology 1994; 62(3):576–582.
54. Flinders University Human Behaviour and Health Research Unit. What is Self-management? [online]. 2001 [cited 6 January 2003]. Available from: URL: http://som.flinders.edu.au/FUSA/CCTU/Self-management.htm.
55. Timothy FE. The reach to recovery program in America and Europe. Cancer 1980; 46(4 Suppl):1059–1060.
56. Ashbury FD, Cameron C, Mercer SL, Fitch M, Nielsen E. One-on-one peer support and quality of life for breast cancer patients. Patient Education and Counseling 1998; 35(2):89–100.
57. Lorig K, Feigenbaum P, Regan C, Ung E, Chastain R, Holman H. A comparison of lay-taught and professional-taught arthritis self-management courses. Journal of Rheumatology 1986; 13(4):763–767.
58. Lorig K, Chastain R, Ung E, Shoor S, Holman H. Development and evaluation of a scale to measure perceived self-efficacy in people with arthritis. Arthritis and Rheumatism 1989; 32(1):37–44.
59. Cooper J. Living with long-term illness (Lill) project. Four six-monthly reports (Report 4). London: Long-term Medical Illness Alliance; 2001.
60. Barlow J, Turner A, Wright C. Long-term outcomes of an arthritis self-management programme. Rheumatology 1998; 37(12):1315–1319.
61. Lorig K, Sobel D, Stewart A, Brown B, Bandura A, Ritter P, et al. Evidence suggesting that a chronic disease self-management program can improve health status while reducing hospitalization: a randomized trial. Medical Care 1999; 37(1):5–14.
62. Kruger JM, Helmick CG, Callahan LF, Haddix AC. Cost-effectiveness of the arthritis self-help course. Arch Intern Med 1998; 158(11):1245–1249.
63. Lorig K, Gonzalez V, Ritter P. Community-based Spanish language arthritis education program. A randomized trial. Medical Care 1999; 37(9):957–963.
64. Dongbo F, Hua F, McGowan P, Yi-e S, Lizhen Z, Huiqin Y, et al. Implementation and quantitative evaluation of a chronic disease self-management program in Shanghai. Unpublished manuscript. Shanghai; 2002.
65. Lorig K, Ritter P, Stewart A, Sobel D, Brown B, Bandura A, et al. Chronic disease self-management program: 2-year status and health care utilization outcomes. Medical Care 2001; 39(11):1217–1223.
66. Bartholomew L, Czyzewski D, Parcel G, Swank P, Sockrider M, Mariotto M, et al. Self-management of cystic fibrosis: Short-term outcomes of the Cystic Fibrosis Family Education Program. Health Education and Behaviour 1997; 24(5):652–666.
67. Lenker S, Lorig K, Gallagher D. Reasons for the lack of association between changes in health behaviour and improved health status: An exploratory study. Patient Education and Counseling 1984; 6(2):69–72.
68. Gibson P, Coughlan J, Wilson A, Hensley M, Abramson M, Bauman A, et al. The effects of limited (information only) patient education programs on the health

outcomes of adults with asthma (Cochrane Review): The Cochrane Library, Issue 4, 1997. Oxford: Update Software.

69. Abdulwadud O, Abramson M, Forbes A, James A, Walters EH. Evaluation of a randomised controlled trial of adult asthma education in a hospital setting. Thorax 1999; 54(6):493–500.

70. Gallefoss F, Bakke PS, Rsgaard PK. Quality of life assessment after patient education in a randomized controlled study on asthma and chronic obstructive pulmonary disease. Am J Resp Crit Care Med 1999; 159(3):812–817.

71. Klein JJ, van der Palen J, van den Hof S, Rovers MM. Self-treatment by adults during slow-onset exacerbations of asthma. Patient Education and Counseling 1997; 32(1 Suppl):S61–66.

72. Lucas DO, Zimmer LO, Paul JE, Jones D, Slatko G, Liao W, et al. Two-year results from the asthma self-management program: Long-term impact on health care services, costs, functional status, and productivity.[comment]. Journal of Asthma 2001; 38(4):321–330.

73. Martin Olmedo P, Leon Jimenez A, Benitez Rodrigueza E, Gomez Gutierrez JM, Mangas Rojas A. Comparison of two models of education for asthmatic patients [in Spanish]. Medicina Clinica 2001; 116(11):408–412.

74. Ratima MM, Fox C, Fox B, Te Karu H, Gemmell T, Slater T, et al. Long-term benefits for Maori of an asthma self-management program in a Maori community which takes a partnership approach. Australian and New Zealand Journal of Public Health 1999; 23(6):601–605.

75. Stevens CA, Wesseldine LJ, Couriel JM, Dyer AJ, Osman LM, Silverman M. Parental education and guided self-management of asthma and wheezing in the pre-school child: a randomised controlled trial.[comment]. Thorax 2002; 57(1):39–44.

76. van der Palen J, Klein JJ, Zielhuis GA, van Herwaarden CL, Seydel ER. Behavioural effect of self-treatment guidelines in a self-management program for adults with asthma. Patient Education and Counseling 2001; 43(2):161–169.

77. Harland J, White M, Drinkwater C, Chinn D, Farr L, Howel D. The Newcastle exercise project: A randomised controlled trial of methods to promote physical activity in primary care. British Medical Journal 1999; 319(7213):828–832.

78. Robertson M, Devlin N, Gardner M, Campbell A. Effectiveness and economic evaluation of a nurse delivered exercise programme to prevent falls. 1: Randomised controlled trial. British Medical Journal 2001; 322:697–701.

79. Thoonen B, Jones K, van Rooij H, van den Hout A, Smeele I, Grol R, et al. Self-treatment of asthma: possibilities and perspectives from the practitioner's point of view. Family Practitioner 1999; 16(2):117–122.

80. Gonon M, Soler M, Langewitz W, Perrochoud A. Is self-management practical in bronchial asthma? [in German]. Schweizerische Medizinische Wochenschreift 1999; 129(13):519–525.

81. Lahdensuo A. Guided self-management of asthma – how to do it. British Medical Journal 1999; 319(7212):759–760.

82. Fries J, Koop C, Sokolov J, Beadle C, Wright C. Beyond health promotion: Reducing need and demand for medical care. Health Reforms 1998; 127(2):70–84.

83. Lawlor D, Hopker S. The effectiveness of exercise as an intervention in the management of depression: systematic review and meta-regression analysis of randomised controlled trials. British Medical Journal 2001; 322(7289):763–767.

84. Egger G, Spark R, Lawson J. Health promotion strategies and methods. Sydney: McGraw-Hill; 1990.

85. Commission on Chronic Illness. Guides to action on chronic illness. New York: National Health Council; 1956.

86. Buergin P. In: Phipps W, Long B, Woods N, eds. Medical-surgical nursing, Chapter 29. St Louis, USA: C.V. Mosby; 1979.

87. Mazzuca S. Does patient education in chronic disease have therapeutic value? Journal of Chronic Diseases 1982; 35:521–529.

88. Commonwealth Department of Health and Ageing (2000, January 2005). Health Insite: Chronic conditions and injury [Website]. Population Health Division, Commonwealth Department of Health and Ageing. Available: http://www.healthinsite.gov.au/content/internal/page.cfm?ObjID=000DABEC-0520-1D2D-81CF83032BFA006D [2001, November].

89. Anderson R, Fitzgerald T, Funnel M, Barr P, Stepen C, Hiss R, Ambruster B. Evaluation of an active diabetes education newsletter. Diabetes Educator 1994; 20(1):29–34.

90. Jenkinson D, Davidson J, Jones S, Hawkin P. Comparison of effects of a self management booklet and audio cassette for patients with asthma. British Medical Journal 1988; 297:267–270.

CHAPTER **14**

Pushing the boundaries of evidence-based research: Enhancing the application and sustainability of health promotion programs in diverse populations*

Marcia G. Ory
Connie J. Evashwick
Russell B. Glasgow
Joseph R. Sharkey

* This chapter was conceived and written with the sponsorship of the Institute for Advanced Study, La Trobe University, Australia.

INTRODUCTION

A new science of translational research is emerging, which includes concentrated attention to concepts such as program reach, adaptation (re-invention), diffusion, and sustainability. This paper will build on the growing knowledge-base about effective public health programs for older adults by emphasizing the importance of these less commonly applied concepts for understanding true program impact. Health behaviour research can be conceptualized as involving different types of studies at each critical stage of discovery – starting with epidemiological studies, moving to process studies examining factors influencing health and illness behaviours, and culminating with the development and testing of theory-based interventions. Newer research traditions focus on evaluating public health impacts in real world settings and identifying strategies for enhancing actual adaptation and dissemination. Evidence-based intervention research is often built upon a common set of behavioural principles and understanding of the potential of older adults to engage in recommended lifestyle behaviours. This review will highlight those principles that help facilitate the translational research process for older adults. In addition to summarization of existing literature, a case study approach will be utilized to reflect on factors that affect research translation and strategies for improving the public health impact of evidence-based programs. While concepts are generalizable to many health promotion interventions, reported literature and case studies will primarily focus on physical activity and chronic disease management programs.

EVOLUTION OF HEALTH BEHAVIOUR RESEARCH IN PHYSICAL ACTIVITY

The epidemiological evidence supporting the linkage between physical activity and a myriad of health outcomes is indisputable, with physical inactivity currently identified as a major cause of premature death.[1-3] While research is documenting the physical activity–health relationship for different health and functional outcomes, more information is needed to specify precisely how much physical activity is necessary for which types of desired outcomes in different populations.[4-7] Whereas the original focus was on vigorous activity, the value of moderate activity has been increasingly recognized.[8] Similarly, there is a new emphasis on active living in addition to more traditional forms of 'exercise', or other structured activity as through sports.[9-11]

In addition to epidemiological and clinical studies, there have now been numerous studies examining the determinants or correlates of physical activity – or its converse, physical inactivity and sedentary lifestyles.[12-14] While barriers and facilitators at the individual psychosocial level have received the most study, contemporary research reports are taking a multi-level approach in examining influences using a social ecological framework.[15-17] Intrapersonal, interpersonal, organizational, community, and policy factors are all seen as potential influences and targets of intervention.

This growing body of evidence has led to a greater specification of a public health message calling for increased physical activity around the world.[18] For example, Americans are called upon to engage in thirty or more minutes of moderate physical activity on most (preferably all) days of the week.[19,20] Despite more inclusive definitions of leisure time activity, national studies still indicate that the majority of adults, and especially older adults, fail to meet these recommendations. For example, one quarter to one half of Americans over 50 years of age get no leisure time physical activity at all, and rates are highest among the oldest populations.[21] Instead of improvements in physical activity levels, trend data show that activity rates have not improved over the past decade, and, alarmingly, associated conditions such as obesity levels are actually rising.[22,23]

CHANGING VIEWS OF HEALTH PROMOTION AND AGING

Whereas older adults were once viewed as unlikely candidates for health promotion programs, these stereotypes of aging are giving way to an understanding of the importance of encouraging older adults to engage in recommended lifestyle behaviours and designing supportive environments to do so.[11,24-30] Despite persistent aging stereotypes, we now know that it is never too late to increase physical activity – and always too soon to quit.[30,31] Thus it is important to design and evaluate health promotion interventions appropriate for persons of all ages.

PRINCIPLES OF BEHAVIOUR CHANGE

Given the well-documented costs of sedentary lifestyles, there is renewed emphasis on testing the efficacy of theory-based interventions to encourage adults fifty and older to initiate and maintain more active lifestyles. Several principles of behaviour change research are emerging from this perspective.[32] These principles help inform choices related to theoretical application, study design, recruitment and retention activities, treatment implementation or fidelity activities, assessment issues, and targeted outcomes.

Behaviour change occurs within broader sociocultural contexts, whereby initiating and maintaining healthy behaviours are best accomplished through identifying multiple opportunities for intervention in people's physical and social environments. Interventionists need to better understand mechanisms and moderators of change, and target these variables.

The goals of healthy behaviour change are more successful when they are concrete and arrived at through collaboration between the interventionist and the relevant stakeholders (e.g. the individual participant, worksite population, or community). The goals of behaviour change should be conceptualized as moving targets based on initial performance levels, to be adjusted rather than absolutes. The adoption and maintenance of healthy behaviours require basic skills that can be taught, practised, and used effectively in 'real world' contexts. Adherence to and maintenance of healthy behaviours are influenced by different factors than those associated with initial establishment or initiation and typically benefit from planned 'boosters' (i.e. repeating or enhancing key parts of the initial intervention). Sustained change in target populations requires the development of a variety of interventions aimed, either singularly or in combination, at multiple levels of influence.

In sum, knowledge of these principles can help inform what variables should be measured and the optimal research designs to be applied (e.g. the importance of longitudinal designs to assess change over time with attention to maintenance or relapse issues). While there is a relatively strong measurement history for psychosocial mediators and behavioural physical activity outcomes, for other critical issues there is a dearth of rigorous investigation. For example, what are the best measures for contextual factors, such as neighborhood environmental factors or social cohesion, how does one measure capacity for sustainability, and indicate extent of program adaptability? Additionally, there is special difficulty of assessing trans-behavioural change – e.g. attempting multiple behaviour changes at one time.

BETTER SPECIFICATION OF PROGRAM DEVELOPMENT MODELS

Traditionally, program development models were viewed as stage-based describing a logical flow from program planning, program implementation, and program evaluation. We realize now that these processes are really more iterative and dynamic, with each program element involving complex processes. Yet, even a more dynamic view of this model is incomplete, as long as there is a lack of attention to the generalizability, adaptation and long-term maintenance of program results.

Fortunately a new public health model, the RE-AIM framework,[33] has been developed to address critical translational research topics such as program reach, adoption and sustainability. Figure 14.1 describes questions associated with each program element.

This model provides practitioners a systematic way to approach health behaviour promotion planning and design.[34] It can also assist researchers, practitioners, and policy decision makers in the evaluation of health behaviour interventions at both the individual and the setting level.[35] As a concrete example of the importance of these concepts,[36] most evidence-based studies evaluate programs in highly controlled settings with participants who are usually more advantaged than the general population. The goal of most translational research studies is to examine if programs can attract and thus benefit a more representative population. Public health impact will be increased when interventions reach broader populations, many of whom are at increased risk for sedentary lifestyles and can potentially achieve great benefits from health promotion interventions.

Table 14.1, prepared by RE-AIM investigators, describes common challenges encountered in evaluating health behaviour interventions and suggests some potential remedies.

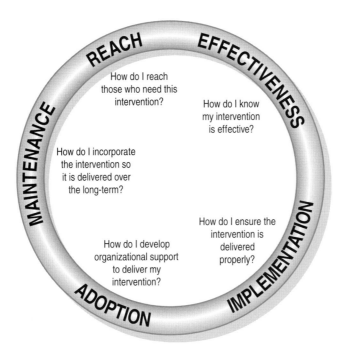

How do I reach those who need this intervention?

How do I know my intervention is effective?

How do I incorporate the intervention so it is delivered over the long-term?

How do I ensure the intervention is delivered properly?

How do I develop organizational support to deliver my intervention?

REACH

EFFECTIVENESS

MAINTENANCE

ADOPTION

IMPLEMENTATION

Fig. 14.1   RE-AIM framework. Cited with permission of authors. Retrieved from www. RE-Aim.org

Managed by the Kansas State University Research and Extension Community Health Institute, the RE-AIM website is an excellent source for interactive materials.[37] For example, there are tools for program planners and evaluators to calculate and report Program Reach and Adoption. In response to systematic literature reviews which indicate that few published studies of lifestyle interventions report program representation, adoption, or maintenance, the RE-AIM team is committed to encouraging researchers to include these elements in their program reports and have developed supplemental reporting items to be considered in CONSORT reporting[38] (see also related materials posted on the Health Maintenance Consortium Web-site available at: http://hmcrc.srph.tamhsc.edu/measures/ConsortPlus.pdf). Additionally, the RE-AIM team provides advice on strategies for designing practical clinical trails that can actually make a difference and be sustained in community or clinical settings.[39]

BALANCING PROGRAM FIDELITY WITH PROGRAM ADAPTATION

Most evidence-based research studies emphasize internal validity – stressing the importance that potentially confounding and alternative explanations for program outcomes be controlled through rigorous experimental designs and that interventions are delivered and implemented as designed.[36] This later

Table 14.1   Common challenges encountered in evaluating health behaviour interventions and remedies

RE-AIM dimension	Challenge	Remedy
Reach	Not studying a relevant, high-risk, or representative sample	Use population-based recruitment or over-recruit high risk subgroups Do not include too many exclusion criteria
Efficacy or effectiveness	Not thoroughly understanding outcomes or how they come about, e.g. no knowledge of mediators, conflicting or ambiguous results, or inadequate control conditions to rule out alternative hypotheses	Assess broad set of outcomes including possible negative ones Include measures of hypothesized mediators Conduct subgroup analyses or include different assessment points Select stringency of control condition to fit your question
Adoption	Program not ever adopted or endorsed – or only used in academic settings	Involve potential adoptees (real world) settings beginning with initial design phase Approach a representative or broad group of settings early on when you can still revise
Implementation	Protocols not delivered as intended (type III error)	Assess if Tx is too complicated, too intensive, or not compatible with other duties Involve potential (non-research) intervention agents in program design
Maintenance	Program or effects not maintained over time	Include maintenance phase in both protocol and in evaluation plan Leave Tx behind after study and plan for institutionalization

Table from www.re-aim.org[37]. Cited with permission from authors.

concept of treatment fidelity is important, with lack of treatment fidelity associated with Type 3 errors in research studies, or the assumption that interventions are not effective, when the problem is not the actual intervention itself but delivery failures.[40] Recent research has delineated different aspects of treatment fidelity and offered strategies for measuring and enhancing treatment fidelity in randomized clinical trials.[41]

Yet, there is often a tension between treatment fidelity and program adaptation when attempting to reach broader populations who do not resonate to programs as originally developed. The classic quote 'What good is science if it doesn't help us?'[42] reflects the frustrations some community members feel when presented with 'one size fits all' intervention strategies. It is important to understand as will be described in some of the case studies to be presented, that this is not an either/or situation. The identification and adherence to the core elements of what makes an intervention evidence-based, allowing for modifications in format and delivery, may be essential for getting individual or community buy-in. Community participatory-research methods[43,44] are seen as critical for implementing essential elements that are culturally acceptable and adoptable and can evoke the following sentiment: 'Science can help, but only when we work together'.[42]

CASE STUDIES DEMONSTRATING RESEARCH TRANSLATION, SUSTAINABILITY AND DISSEMINATION EFFORTS

To bring these research concepts alive, the authors will highlight how these issues are addressed in several ongoing or recently completed research projects familiar to the authors. In many cases, there are limited road maps for understanding how these concepts play out in practice. So these illustrious examples represent the authors' experiences and reflections in driving down some of these uncharted roads. Active for Life® provides an example of how evidence-based programs may need to be adapted to be widely adoptable in community settings. The discussion on sustainability will be informed by our Archstone Award study where we tried to ascertain factors related to program success and sustainability in twenty award-winning innovative programs. The widespread failures in dissemination of clinical guidelines into practice settings represents our third major area of exploration, one that we are just beginning to study in a new CDC-funded study. In addition to these examples, we bring the reader's attention to some related successes in research translation related to the emergent Active Living movement.

Understanding research translation: Active for Life®

Research-based interventions are often successful in research-based settings, but typically are never tested in real-world settings or may fail to translate effectively. By the same token, and due in large part to limited resources and lack of research trained staff, community-developed interventions are often not evaluated and thus their effectiveness is never demonstrated.

Active for Life research questions

Building on two decades of behaviour intervention research for adults in the middle and later years, Active for Life was designed to take research-based programs into community settings, provide structured social marketing support, and conduct independent evaluation to measure effectiveness. Initiated in 2000 with support from the Robert Wood Johnson Foundation®, Active for Life is a four-year initiative designed to increase the number of American adults age 50 and older who engage in regular physical activity (at least 30 minutes a day on most days). This initiative tests the added utility of a multi-pronged strategy that connects people to the places where they live, with an appreciation of the need for tailored interventions based on the diverse social, behavioural, environmental and functional circumstances of mid-life and older adults. The Active for Life National Program Office, housed at the School of Rural Public Health at The Texas A&M University System Health Science Center, is one of several programs in the RWJF Active Living Consortium.

In addition to National Program Office oversight, The University of South Carolina Prevention Research Center is evaluating the program. Information from a two-phase evaluation that integrates quantitative and qualitative approaches will help the physical activity and aging fields understand how the intervention models work in real-world settings, and the effectiveness of the models in encouraging people age 50 and older to initiate and maintain physical activity. The field of public health and successful aging can benefit from knowing how these research-based models may need to be adapted when implemented in the community, and for which subgroups of the age 50 plus population they are most effective.

In the process evaluation, we hope to learn the ways in which the two selected program models must be adapted to be acceptable to community organizations and intended constituents, and then determine whether the adaptation is consistent with the core elements of the original program. If the adaptation is an acceptable variation on the original, it should be added to the knowledge base about the model and shared with others who are struggling to translate the research into practice. If the adaptation is not an acceptable variation on the original, that needs to be shared as well, for quality control. The primary reason to conduct outcome evaluation at the new sites, once the pilot phase is over, is to understand the extent to which outcomes are similar in the new adaptations, and for whom?

The heart of the initiative is an $8.7 million dollar grant program that supports nine community-based organizations (with multiple sites) for a four-year period to test the effectiveness of two promising interventions to promote physical activity in the general population of mid-life and older persons at health risk because of their sedentary lifestyles. Several criteria were utilized to select two interventions for further testing: (1) prior success in increasing physical activity in the 50 plus population; (2) a behaviourally-based intervention that explicitly incorporated the principles of behavioural change research (i.e. more than an exercise training program alone); (3) a manualized program in terms of having program materials and facilitator's guide developed; and (4) tested previously in multiple settings with a variety of participants. Additional information about the two selected programs, Active Choices and Active Living Every Day, can be found on the Active for Life website www.activeforlife.info.

Reflections on translating research

While it is too soon to know the results of this program initiative, the initial pilot study demonstrates that community-based organizations are interested in improving the physical activity levels of their clients and can implement evidence-based protocols. National program and evaluation staff are currently debriefing grantees about their experiences in enrolling nearly 850 adults 50 and older from diverse ethnic backgrounds into one of the two Active for Life programs.

Communities want – and deserve – a say in research designs and evaluation methodologies. Randomized controlled designs may be the gold standard for academic researchers, but they are not often acceptable in community projects where emphasis is on serving all constituents. It is often hard to establish traditional control groups in field settings – since communities feel that everyone deserves something for being in the study. Similarly, individuals may be less motivated to come back for follow-up assessments if they don't see the immediate benefit for them. Moreover, the typical university-based Institutional Review Board paperwork requirements, new HIPAA regulations in the US, and increasingly legalistic stance often seem onerous to community-based organizations devoted to service delivery issues. That having been said, communities are very concerned about screening and safety protocols in terms of providing safe services for their clients and avoiding liability issues, as well as sensitivities in approaching their clientele.

Measurement batteries need to be substantially truncated – and culturally acceptable. This may be seen as problematic by researchers who think in terms of comprehensive multi-dimensional assessments that have superior psychometric properties. In a collaborative vein, we made some fundamental alterations based on feedback from community groups (e.g. simplification of screening assessment forms, etc). The key is to try to reach a compromise that is seen as acceptable for the researcher ('good enough') and yet 'do-able' and useful for the community organizations. There has been some related work[45] that summarizes criteria for the selection of practical lifestyle measures and actually identifies measures that can be used in primary care settings for baseline assessment and intervention tracking.

Communities know their current service constituents well and have an easier time accessing them than external researchers would. Researchers can help communities with strategies for reaching out to new populations and going beyond current comfort levels in assessments. However, an essential ingredient is community trust. After this is established, measurements that initially seem threatening may be able to be assessed with little reluctance (e.g. getting basic demographic information about ethnic characteristics that may initially be interpreted as sensitive data).

Due to logistical and cost issues, we had to drop the idea that everyone would get a physical functional assessment. However, several groups took this upon themselves to assess, since a functional assessment was seen as valuable feedback information for making the case for sustainability in their own settings. Our lesson learned is that community partners may be willing to 'buy in' to more extensive assessments if they see the value of such measurements for their constituency as well as their organization.

Researchers need to think in terms of creating tool kits and templates that can be widely used in community settings and are adjuncts to recruitment and program implementation. Especially needed are tools that help communities assess who they are actually reaching, and which help community organizations extend beyond the community segments that they typically reach to those who may be underserved though who may significantly benefit. Also critical is attention to cultural sensitivities, linguistic competencies, and opportunities for feedback to both providers and consumers. Some approaches may result in productive yields, but may not push programs beyond 'business as usual' with their current clientele. For optimum use and effectiveness, these toolkits should emphasize principles and guidelines, not mandated lock step protocols. The RE-AIM website[37] provides tools that enable clinicians and practitioners to identify and assess success in obtaining projected reach and other critical components of program implementation and evaluation.

Behavioural scientists/program developers need to realize that in the field, programs are often implemented in ways that depart significantly from the theory-based interventions as originally designed. The question is how much and what type of adaptation can be made and still have the program adhere to essential components. There is always a delicate balance between fidelity- and adaptation-reinvention to fit particular settings.[46] Communities can tell researchers what works and doesn't work in their settings. Testing an unacceptable intervention is not really a good test of program reach and effectiveness. It is critical to assess what adaptations are being made, and the rationale for such adaptations, and if essential program elements are actually implementable in field settings. This can help guide the next generation of applied intervention strategies. A comprehensive process evaluation can be quite useful in documenting these adaptations, reasons for the adaptations, and impact on outcomes.

Although not initially envisioned as community participatory research, from the beginning, grantee sites wanted to make changes to the programs. Some of those changes, such as adapting the layout and font size of program materials to improve readability were obviously helpful. Others, such as changing some of the physical activity tracking forms made sense, but determining how to change the forms proved to be complex. The forms needed to be adapted in a way that (1) made them easier to use for the participants; (2) captured the information that was important to the evaluation team; and (3) provided the educational and behavioural benefits to the participant that the program developers intended. Discussions between the grantee sites, program developers, evaluation team and grant coordinators have helped us understand the perspectives of each group. Through these discussions we recognized the need for an ongoing review process. This enables grantee sites to adapt programs relatively quickly, while assessing the potential effects of the proposed adaptations. All parties have a voice in the process. This should help insure that future adaptations will be collaborations between the grantee sites and program developers, with input from the grant coordinators and evaluation team when necessary.

Understanding factors associated with program sustainability: The Archstone Foundation Award Program

While there is a growing recognition of the importance of program sustainability among community practitioners, researchers, and funding agencies, research in this area is still in a nascent stage. Both conceptual and methodological challenges have been noted. There is a lack of definitional clarity with one recent review[47] identifying 11 related concepts related to the maintenance or continuation of an innovation, including terms such as confirmation, continuation, durability, incorporation, institutionalization, level of use, maintenance, routinization, sustainability, and sustained use. Sustainability is one of the most frequently used terms and is sometimes viewed as the generic concept. It is important to recognize that sustainability is a multi-faceted concept with several basic types being recognized, e.g. sustainability can refer to projects or programs, ideas, community capacity designed to promote the interventions, or the intended benefits.[48] There is no overarching conceptual model, although many studies cite the framework established by Shediec-Rizkallah and Bone[49] that helps organize potential factors related to sustainability in terms of (1) project design and implementation features; (2) factors within the organizational setting; and (3) factors within the broader community environment. The interaction or fit of these three factors are critical determinants of sustainability. Recent reviews[47,48,50–52] have highlighted several key points about sustainability: (1) sustainability is a dynamic process which should be attended to at the beginning of a project and not left to the end; (2) sustainability potential is based on the match between organizational setting and program characteristics; (3) both organizational routines and institutional standards are important aspects of sustainability; and (4) while there is a desire for programs to sustain, funding agencies have not always designed their grant-making to maximize sustainability. Additionally, although there are some scales to assess institutionalization, for the most part research has been limited by lack of strong measures or rigorous analytical techniques.[53]

Archstone Foundation Awards sustainability study

Understanding factors associated with promoting program sustainability is important for designing and evaluating program effects, as well as determining which types of innovations might be the best future investments in times of scarce resources. Toward this end, Evashwick and Ory[54] designed a study to address the following questions: What factors influence whether a community-based program for older adults can be sustained over time? Which innovative programs emanating from community-based organizations will become institutionalized into the core operations of their organizations? What types of organizational structures are most effective in fostering longevity of successful programs?

In Fall 2002, representatives from 20 projects awarded by the Archstone Foundation as an innovative program providing health and related social support services to older adults were interviewed using a structured questionnaire designed by the authors reflecting components in the Shediac-Rizkallah and Bone[49] framework.

The findings of the conceptual analysis of the interviews are quite consistent with existing organizational literature and support many of our initial hypotheses regarding factors associated with sustainability. The 'lessons learned' from the twenty Archstone Award winners relate to what professionals need to know to develop or fund health programs for seniors that they would like to have continue over time. They also offer insights about how to succeed in the complex health and social services environment of the United States in the twenty-first century. Specific lessons learned:

1. **Seek strong leadership.** Innovations come from visionary people and are implemented by charismatic leaders. All of these projects began small and with very limited resources. The charisma, skill, and dedication of the leader was often what kept them going until they reached maturity and were inculcated into the ongoing operations of a larger organization. This is consistent with our hypothesis that organizations that sustain will 'have a driving force or leader who remains present'. It modifies the prediction in that the leader did change in some circumstances, but the successor was an equal champion of the program.

2. **Involve communities and key stakeholders.** We also predicted that sustained organizations would engage in grassroots community involvement. The importance of community and stakeholder involvement, well-documented as cornerstones of successful community-based programs, were validated by the twenty Archstone Award winners. The principles of community organization seem well-known and automatically implemented by those starting new initiatives: almost all had a community advisory board of some type. Going beyond the typical lip-service nod to constituency interests, the projects were all based on needs of seniors clearly identified in the community or corporate hierarchy. The sense of commitment felt by the professional staff, the seniors participating in the program, and the community and corporate stakeholder organizations carried the projects forward even when the funding was questionable or the organization in flux. None of these twenty projects could be characterized as imposed on the community by external forces or initiated by a university strictly to investigate a research question.

3. **Build on a supporting organizational infrastructure.** Our predictions that sustainability would be related to large size, long organizational history, and dominant service were supported. The majority of the Archstone Award winners were community-based projects serving seniors. This often has the connotation of a grassroots, informal organization. However, we found that the size, scope, and longevity of a parent organization contribute greatly to the ultimate success of new community initiatives. All twenty of these innovative projects were housed in an established organization with

resources and expertise that no doubt contributed to the successful launch of the new service. We hope this finding does not discourage the entrepreneurial spirit in smaller, newer organizations.

4. **Engage in active outreach and informal marketing.** Only two of the twenty projects had formal marketing approaches, and these were lodged in corporate marketing departments that had broader responsibilities than just the innovative project. However, all twenty engaged in active outreach efforts. The techniques varied, but most were inexpensive, to keep the costs of the project low. Marketing included collaboration with other organizations to exchange referrals, ads at senior centres, flyers, and personal contacts of board members. Seeking external validation, such as applying for an award, was a valuable way of gaining recognition for the program and its value.

5. **Gather outcome data.** In contrast to the time when community-based organizations were not expected to document outcomes, the twenty winning Archstone Award projects all kept data and conducted some type of evaluation, process, outcome, or both. They used the information for several purposes: to refine the service, to market, to secure additional funding, to contribute to the relevant body of research. Several of those being interviewed mentioned, unsolicited, that gathering process and outcomes measurements and other evaluations had been seminal to attaining stability. These results supported our hypothesis that sustainability is related to documenting concrete outcomes measures. Several mentioned the importance of a university connection, particularly at the outset of the project, to tap into research and evaluation expertise and resources.

6. **Achieve financial self-sufficiency.** The concept of community-based programs serving seniors as a gesture of good will has evolved into a business model. These twenty innovative projects have endured because they met a need and achieved financial stability in meeting it. In several instances, organizational arrangements have changed in order to achieve the financial support needed to maintain the service. Some have achieved financial stability by becoming a core service of the parent organization, and thus are funded internally, but nonetheless have achieved predictable funding. For those projects funded initially by grants, interviewees discussed the importance of converting from soft money to permanent funding, without relying on continued grant support that might be difficult to continue to secure over time. The study confirmed our prediction that financial self-sufficiency was essential to stability.

7. **Maintain a shared organizational vision.** Relationships among organizations were important for many of the projects and the services they provided. Having a shared vision enables organizations to work together without formal agreements. Moreover, these informal relationships can be sustained over many years – especially where there are charismatic leaders involved. A forum for discussion was mentioned as important in order to

work out operational problems and allow the service to continue. This feature was not predicted per se by the model, but is consistent with having a strong leader and a well-established organization that knows its mission and goals.

8. **Recognize and employ principles of behavioural and organizational change.** To support start-up, an organization must recognize that time and patience are essential. For programs targeted at seniors, the community, as well as the professionals, must understand that seniors can and do indeed change. Thus, a program that promotes healthy lifestyles for seniors can have an impact. Similarly, the organization must believe that theory can work when applied, but the organization must be receptive and able to translate academic-generated concepts into applied principles and operations. Several of those interviewed mentioned the importance of their commitment to the idea they were trying to implement and the need for time and patience before judging outcomes too quickly.

Redefining the Model of Sustainability

The survey of the Archstone Foundation Innovative Projects Award winners demonstrates that the Model of Sustainability proposed by Shediac-Rizkallah and Bone[49] can be operationalized. The results of the study, in turn, have contributed to a critique of the model, particularly in offering suggestions of how the model can be enhanced when applied.

Organizational evolution and expansion The programs had evolved and expanded in a variety of ways. More people were being served, more services were offered, and/or more geographical and organizational settings were reached. For example, a program starting out in a hospital was diffused into public health settings; a program delivered in one part of a city was expanded to other surrounding communities. Programs that focused initially only on older adults added caregivers or younger disabled to their target audiences. Although most programs grew, some actually reduced their activities, and then expanded this narrower activity. Pilot projects that had several components initially subsequently might have focused on one key aspect that had proved especially beneficial and that could be delivered at relatively low cost. Instead of trying to support an entire program, one successful component was identified and built into the core organizational funding stream. The authors of the Model of Sustainability say that it is dynamic, but do not provide a way to consider this in their construct. In testing the theoretical model, several distinct measures of expansion and evolution should be delineated.

Replication Many of the award winning organizations reported that they had been contacted by other organizations and asked for information on how to replicate the service. The projects had sent materials, hosted visitors, and made site visits. One site, the Senior Services of Seattle/King County, has developed a sophisticated replication program. All sites receive training from the parent site prior to providing the service and using the software. Then, through the web-based software, the parent site gathers demographic information and scores on a variety of validated tests at baseline, six months, and 12 months, for all participants at all sites. However, except for this one project, none of the other nineteen had gathered precise data on actual replications or the number of people served at new sites. There appears to be no incentive to do so, nor a data system readily available to facilitate such tracking without special effort. Therefore, other than anecdotal information, there is no systematic knowledge about whether or not replications have actually happened, or about the ways in which replications have deviated from original program innovations. If diffusion is to be a researched phenomenon, the field needs to define data that should be collected and agree on methods and metrics for doing so.

Reconceptualization of economic viability   Financing was the greatest challenge to the majority of sites, but most were able to find creative ways to manage. The meaning of financially 'self-sufficient' was not necessarily the standard interpretation. While there was an emphasis on cost-effectiveness of the service, most projects were not income producing. Many were run on a shoestring and creative ways were found to keep them afloat (e.g. use of volunteers with very lean administrative staffs). Respondents acknowledged that perceived community benefit also played a powerful role in sustainability. Many of the projects were initiated through a grant or other external funds as a relatively small pilot. Over time, services were institutionalized within existing funding streams in larger organizations because the service was perceived as part of the organization's core values and mission. Embedding the service in the larger corporate structure provided financial stability for the most viable services and programs.

Interestingly, the projects that seemed to be having the greatest trouble finding future funding were those that were started by universities. Grants were available to start the projects and conduct specific research, but the university was not in a position to pick up the projects once started. University generated programs may be difficult to sustain because they depend on research dollars that are project and time limited. In contrast, once demonstrated to be effective, projects started by community agencies found a way to inculcate pilot projects into their mainstream operations. Although being part of a large organization was hypothesized to have a greater chance of achieving sustainability, we found that organizational size was less relevant than core mission when considering sustainability in academically driven programs. For a university, the core activity is teaching, not service, so the option of continuing a service, even if demonstrated to be valuable, does not fit within the primary mission or mainstream operations of the institution. In brief, as the model of sustainability is applied, the way in which financing is measured must be refined to capture these nuances.

Marketing and communication   These concepts are missing from the sustainability model, but are very important in both continuation and expansion. Publicizing the project took two thrusts: actions to let seniors know about the service, and activities to share the experience with the professional provider and academic communities. Community-based publicity was used to recruit seniors. In addition, many of the projects were shared with professionals through presentations at national or local meetings and through papers written for professional peer-review or invitational journals. Most of the projects produced some form of report, ranging from a progress report to a foundation that had given them a grant to a performance report for an agency with whom they contracted to a piece for the annual report of the parent organization. Such reports were used to document the value of the project and to showcase it in the community or client base. Yet, very few organizations (only two noted in our study) had a special department or person designated specifically for marketing. Typically, the visionary person who had created and implemented the program led the marketing effort by interacting with the community. This leader was also the person who made presentations or wrote papers for dissemination to professionals.

In addition to direct marketing activities, a frequent unsolicited comment during the interviews was the value that the organization had received by winning the Archstone Award recognition. This external recognition was used by many of the projects in their quest for securing funding. In short, a measure of visibility, marketing, and communication should be added to the model.

Sustainability and diffusion   Our initial comment about the diffusion literature was that sustainability was a prerequisite for expansion. It may be that it is indeed more useful to consider the two concepts together rather than try to distinguish them, i.e. sustainability may be the first or second stage of diffusion, and diffusion or expansion requires sustainability. The survey of the Archstone Award winners indicated that both concepts needed to be considered simultaneously.

Dissemination of evidence–based guidelines: CDC Chronic Disease Management Project

Chronic health conditions such as obesity, diabetes, congestive heart failure, and chronic obstructive pulmonary disease have reached near epidemic proportions across the US, especially among minority and rural populations.[55] As reflective of changing demographics, the projected burden and economic cost of diabetes alone is staggering – costing approximately $100 billion per year.[56–58] Despite the development of practice guidelines and the implementation of disease management and disease prevention programs, the rates of diabetes continue to rise.[56,59] State and community health leaders have been encouraged to partner with health-care providers, health organizations and community health centres in evaluating the effectiveness of diabetes prevention and management guidelines.[55]

The literature is replete with reports on the efficacy of evidenced-based clinical practice guidelines for the prevention and management of chronic diseases in both clinical and community settings.[60] However, these guidelines have had limited effect in changing physician behaviour and are not widely used outside of research settings.[61-63] There are a few notable exceptions that counter this pessimistic view of the failure of guidelines to be widely disseminated to intended audiences. The best example is the NCI Planet Web site http://cancercontrol.cancer.gov.rtips/index.asp which provides a user-friendly way of accessing evidence-based intervention programs and products. The Agency for Health Quality and Research, the repository for clinical guides, recognizes the problem of the plethora of guidelines, and has established a Putting Prevention into Practice Program[64] to improve the delivery of appropriate clinical preventive services.

To improve the quality of chronic care, the MacColl Institute for Healthcare Innovation developed a chronic care model to identify practical and supportive evidence-based interactions by suggesting system changes in multiple dimensions of care: patient, health-care system, and community.[65,66] These include patient self-management, delivery system redesign, decision support, clinical information systems, leadership and health system organization, and community outreach. Research to date documents primarily its use across a variety of health-care organizations, with limited understanding of utilization in small practices and communities, especially in rural areas.[67]

A multitude of expert-generated advisory guidelines exist on diabetes prevention and disease management which address what health-care providers should be doing for patients with known or potential diabetes, and how communities can also prevent or reduce risks.[4,60,68-70] These guidelines summarize best practices for disease prevention, screening, diagnosis, treatment intervention, self-management support, disease complication prevention, and referral. Within the area of disease prevention and management over 248 'guidelines' are listed for diabetes alone.[60] With expert consultation, the Texas Diabetes Council has reviewed existing guidelines and programs, developing a Diabetes Tool Kit with professional and patient education materials.[71]

Little is known about the dissemination of guidelines in rural and underserved settings. Although presumed challenges have been identified (e.g. problems with access to services), which may be attenuated by teleheath technology, there is also the potential for closer network connections which may facilitate the diffusion of innovative best practices which are seen as advantageous.[72] Since guidelines are not routinely carried out in community or clinical settings or, at best, are poorly coordinated,[73] it is important to understand individual, community and system factors that affect: (1) adoptability in real world settings; and (2) application and dissemination to more diverse populations and settings than included in original research studies.

Implementation, dissemination and sustainability of clinical and community disease prevention and disease management practice guidelines

As part of a newly funded CDC Prevention Research Center at the Texas A&M University School of Rural Public Health System, we propose to examine the factors that facilitate the implementation, adherence to core principles, diffusion and sustainability of evidence-based disease prevention and chronic disease management practices in rural and underserved communities. The two guiding research questions are: (1) Why are community and clinical practice guidelines, which are designed to improve health, not better utilized? (2) What strategies for better guideline implementation, adherence, and dissemination in especially vulnerable populations (including poor rural populations) are most effective?

The proposed research draws several research traditions together to advance prevention research. Principles and methods of community health development, diffusion of innovation studies, and behavioural change research are combined with newer emphases on translational and sustainability research to address a growing but potentially modifiable health problem. Overlaid with a concern for rural and underserved populations, this project can contribute to prevention science by identifying multiple influences and intervention points for traditionally ignored populations.

In formulating our goals and activities, we needed to continually remind ourselves that in a dissemination study, the appropriate goal is to document current practices and test strategies for enhancing dissemination, rather than focusing on the effectiveness of the existing guidelines. Drawing on some of the same behavioural change principles delineated in the beginning of this paper, we noted the importance of involving community partners in prioritizing activities, determining barriers to current implementation, and designing easy and practical solutions.

Toward this end we have identified three basic goals and ten specific activities as depicted in Figure 14.2.

Consistent with Rogers,[46] we see diffusion as a process unfolding over time. Our model bridges community and clinical settings and highlights the fact that interventions can (and should) occur in each setting and at each point along the diffusion process. For clarity, in our conceptualization, implementation includes both adoption and adherence to recommended guidelines. Dissemination refers to implementation in different settings within one county or across our counties of interest. Sustainability is the long-term adoption by clinical or community organizations.

Translational research is essential for increasing the likelihood that evidence-based practices are actually adopted and spread widely to populations at risk and ultimately improving population health.[38,74] The project is designed to refine appropriate and culturally competent methods to implement and sustain diabetes prevention and control guidelines in rural and underserved areas. Prevention research is further advanced by taking a more comprehensive view than usual of best practices at the self-management, health-care and community level and designing strategies for facilitating stronger linkages among the various stakeholders. The emphasis on community partnership has the potential for achieving results that are more robust, sustainable, and generalizable.

We will attempt to facilitate the diffusion process by engaging in small field experiments testing the trialability of the selected guideline (see Table

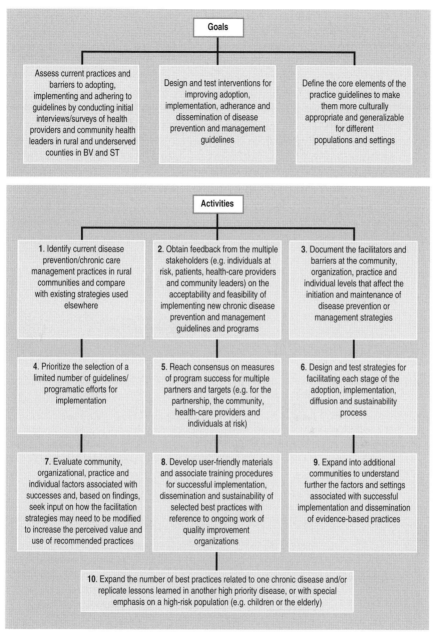

Fig. 14.2   Goals and activities.

14.1 for representative activities by domain and stage of diffusion). Our major approach is to design and test, using a PDSA (Plan-Do-Study-Act) format, interventions to facilitate the diffusion process based on several overarching themes drawn from general principles of community health development, diffusion of innovation, and behavioural change research.[66,75]

This includes helping organizations select guidelines with more favourable attributes (e.g. those with already-identified, easy, step-by-step processes) or providing technical assistance (TA) in simplifying the guidelines by breaking them down into component parts or employing simple-to-use flowcharts and reminder systems. It might also include providing TA to help communities develop better linkages across care settings (e.g. incorporating diabetes content into more socially oriented case management activities). Another intervention might involve helping a clinical practice set up a tracking and monitoring system based on existing protocols, starting with the establishment of registries and working toward more formal systems for tracking preventive services. Yet another might involve designing a template so that communities can develop their own community resource brochures. If follow-up is a problem, we envision providing TA on strategies for developing a sustainability plan. Potential intervention strategies are outlined in Figure 14.3.

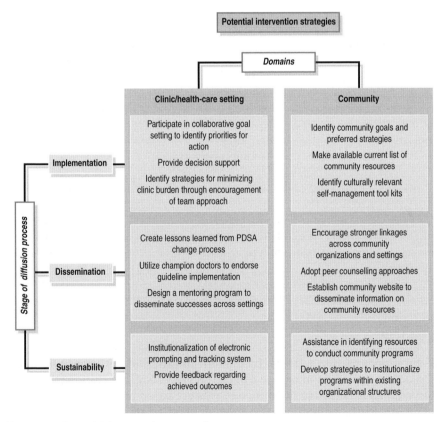

Fig. 14.3 Potential intervention strategies.

NATIONAL BLUEPRINT: SUCCESSFUL PARTNERSHIPS AND TRANSLATIONAL RESEARCH ACTIVITIES

Our previous commentary describes several research projects designed to increase the knowledge base about research applications that can make a difference in the lives of people and their communities. Focusing attention on conceptual, methodological and intervention issues surrounding research translation, sustainability and dissemination, we often point to challenges due to lack of conceptual clarity or methodological rigor, or painful slowness in research translation.

We can also point to several 'natural' successes in the physical activity field. In 2000, the Robert Wood Johnson Foundation (RWJF) sponsored a conference of nearly fifty organizations with expertise in health, social and behavioural sciences, epidemiology, gerontology/geriatrics, clinical science, public policy, marketing, medical systems, community organizations, and environmental issues. The outcome was reported in a document called The National Blueprint: Increasing Physical Activity Among Adults Age 50 and Older.[76] The Blueprint outlined both the challenges and broad strategies related to increasing physical activity among mid-life and older adults. Through leadership of its Director, Wojtek Chodzko-Zajko, the National Blueprint Office[77] has served as a stimulus for several concrete partnerships and activities that build a true bridge between research and practice. To help translate public health recommendations to practice, key public health and physical activity stakeholder organizations (e.g. Centre for Disease Control and Prevention, American College of Sports Medicine) have come together to endorse a set of best practices for physical activity programs and behavioural counselling in older adult populations.[8] There are built-in plans to disseminate these guidelines to key professional and community organizations and to develop tools for enhancing implementation. Another key accomplishment is a partnership between medical organizations, University researchers, and private industry to develop an evidence-based turnkey tool kit that can be disseminated in doctors' offices, putting a concrete tool in the hands of busy health-care providers.[78] A third accomplishment involves a landmark relationship between a fitness association (International Council of Active Ageing) and primary care physicians to assist a participating physician's referral of their older patients to age-friendly fitness and wellness organizations. Research on what makes a facility age-friendly has been condensed into a list of essential elements that guide both facilities and older consumers and their families.[79]

SUMMARY

The promotion of translational research requires careful attention to the types of conceptual and methodological papers raised in this article. There is also a need for a basic paradigm shift from academic research endeavors to campus-community partnerships, and infrastructure support to assist in these efforts. We lament the lack of (or perceived lack of) mechanisms currently available to help shift empirical research into the hands of practitioners. Researchers generally are not trained, encouraged, or 'incentivized' by their institutions or grant funding agencies to take time away from their RCTs and publishing to turn their research into products for dissemination. Without special mechanisms or initiatives (e.g. the Active for Life initiative), it is a rare investigative team that is able to turn their research findings into translatable and sustainable programs within the time and fiscal constraints of the original grant award. We strongly urge funding agencies and review bodies (including National Institute of Health) to build effectiveness research and dissemination efforts into their research expectations and funding criteria. Research translation, dissemination, and sustainability should be the ultimate objective of intervention research, above and beyond academic publications of the major intervention outcomes.

By the same token, we need to continue to work to bring innovative and apparently effective community programs to the attention of the research community, as a means of building bridges between research and practice in the reverse direction. By doing so, collaborations can be built to get community programs already in place more fully evaluated, and disseminated through scientific as well as practice channels. This type of 'two-pronged' approach is essential if we are to realize significant gains in physical activity at the population level.

References

1. Mokdad AH, Marks JS, Stroup DF, Gerberding JL. Actual causes of death in the United States, 2000. JAMA 2004; 291(10):1238–1245.
2. US Department of Health and Human Services. Healthy People 2010: Understanding and improving health, 2nd edn. [Online]. 2000 [cited 2004 Jul 20]; Available from: URL: http://www.health.gov/healthypeople/Document/tableofcontents.htm. Washington, DC: US Government Printing Office.
3. US Department of Health and Human Services. Steps to a healthier US. A program and policy perspective: The power of prevention [Online]. 2003 [cited 2004 Jul 20]; Available from: URL: http://www.healthierus.gov/steps/summit/prevportfolio/power/index.html.
4. Centers for Disease Control and Prevention. Physical Activity [Online]. 2004 [cited 2004 Jul 20]; Available from: URL: http://www.cdc.gov/nccdphp/dnpa/physical/index.htm. Atlanta, GA: US Department of Health and Human Services.
5. Morey MC, Sullivan RJJ. Medical assessment for health advocacy and practical strategies for exercise initiation. American Journal of Preventive Medicine 2003; 25(3 Suppl 2):204–208.
6. National Institute on Aging. Exercise: A guide from the National Institutes on aging [Online]. 2003 [cited 2004 Jul 20]; Available from: URL: http://www.nia.nih.gov/exercisebook/index.htm.
7. Singh MA. Exercise comes of age: Rationale and recommendations for a geriatric exercise prescription. Journals of Gerontology. A: Biological Sciences and Medical Sciences 2002; 57(5):M262–82.
8. Cress E, Buchner D, Prohaska T, Rimmer J, Brown M, Macera C et al. Best practices for physical activity programs and behaviour counseling in older adult populations. Journal of Aging and Physical Activity 2005; 13(1)61–74.

9. Active Living Network: Building a national coalition for active communities [Online]. 2004 [cited 2004 Jul 20]; Available from: URL: http://www.activeliving.org/index.php.

10. Partnership for Prevention. Creating communities for active aging [Online]. 2001 [cited 2004 Jul 20]; Available from: URL: http://www.prevent.org/publications/Active_Aging.pdf.

11. US Department of Health and Human Services. Promoting physical activity: A guide for community action [Online]. 1999 [cited 2004 Jul 20]; Available from: URL: http://www.cdc.gov/nccdphp/dnpa/pahand.htm.

12. King AC, Rejeski WJ, Buchner DM. Physical activity interventions targeting older adults: a critical review. American Journal of Preventative Medicine 1998; 15(4):316–333.

13. King AC, Castro C, Wilcox S, Eyler AA, Sallis JF, Brownson RC. Personal and environmental factors associated with physical inactivity among different racial/ethnic groups of US middle and older-aged women. Health Psychology 2000; 19(4):354–364.

14. King AC, Bauman A, Calfas K, eds. G. Innovative approaches to understanding and influencing physical activity. American Journal of Preventive Medicine 2002; 23(2 Suppl.)51-106.

15. Sallis JF, Owen N. Ecological models. In: Glanz F, Lewis M, Rimer BK, eds. Health behaviour and health education: Theory, research, and practice, 3rd edn. San Francisco, CA: Jossey-Bass; 2002:462–484.

16. Smedley BD, Syme SL, eds. Promoting health: Intervention strategies from social and behavioural research. Institute of Medicine. Washington, DC: National Academy Press; 2001.

17. Li F, Fisher KJ, Bauman A, Ory MG, Chodzko-Zaiko W, Harmer P, et al. Neighborhood influences on physical activity in middle-aged and older adults: A multilevel perspective. Journal of Physical Activity and Aging 2005; 13(1):87–114.

18. World Health Organization. WHO launches annual Move for Health day as global initiative to promote benefits of physical activity [media release]. [Online] 2003 Feb 17 [cited 2004 Aug 02]; Available from: URL: http://www.who.int/mediacentre/releases/2003/pr15/en. Geneva: World Health Organization.

19. AARP. Be Active for Life [Online]. 2003 [cited 2004 Jul 20]; Available from: URL: http://www.aarp.org/activeforlife/.

20. President's Council on Physical Fitness and Sports. The President's Challenge [Online]. 2004 [cited 2004 Jul 20]; Available from: http://www.presidentschallenge.org/home_adults.aspx.

21. Behavioural Risk Factor Surveillance System [Online]. 2002 [cited 2004 Jul 20]; Available from: URL:http://www.cdc.gov/brfss/.

22. Centers for Disease Control and Prevention. Improving nutrition and improving physical activity. [Online]. 2004 [cited 2004 Jul 20]; Available from: URL:http://www.cdc.gov/nccdphp/bb_nutrition/index.htm. Atlanta, GA: US Department of Health and Human Services; 2004.

23. Center on an Aging Society. Obesity among older Americans. Washington, DC: Georgetown University, Institute for Health Care Research and Policy; 2003.

24. Agency for Healthcare Research and Quality and the Centers for Disease Control. Physical activity and older Americans: Benefits and strategies [Online]. 2002 [cited 2004 Jul 20]; Available from: URL: http://www.ahrq.gov/ppip/activity.htm.

25. Crankshaw E, Rabiner D, O'Keeffe J. An overview of programs and initiatives sponsored by DHHS to promote healthy aging. A background paper for the blueprint on aging for the 21st century technical advisory (TAG) meeting [Online].

2003 [cited 2004 Jul 20]; Available from: URL: http://aspe.hhs.gov/daltcp/CaregiverEvent/programs.htm. Washington, DC: U.S. Department of Health and Human Services.

26. Chodzko-Zajko WJ, ed. National blueprint: Increasing physical activity among adults age 50 and older. Journal of Aging and Physical Activity 2001; 9(2 Suppl 1):S2–18.

27. Agency for Healthcare Research and Quality and the Centers for Disease Control. Physical activity and older Americans: Benefits and strategies [Online]. 2002 [cited 2004 Jul 20]; Available from: URL:http://www.ahrq.gov/ppip/activity.htm.

28. Crankshaw E, Rabiner D, O'Keeffe J. An overview of programs and initiatives sponsored by DHHS to promote healthy aging. A background paper for the blueprint on aging for the 21st century technical advisory (TAG) meeting. Assistant Secretary for Planning and Evaluation [Online]. 2003 [cited 2004 Jul 20]; Available from: URL:http://aspe.hhs.gov/daltcp/CaregiverEvent/programs.htm. Washington, DC: U.S. Department of Health and Human Services; 2003.

29. Inter City/County Management Association. Active living for older adults: Management strategies for healthy and livable communities [Online]. 2003 [cited 2004 Jul 20]; Available from: URL: http://www.leadershipforactiveliving.org/pdf_file/Active_Living_for_Older_Adults.pdf.

30. Ory MG, Hoffman M, Hawkins M, Sanner B, Mockenhaupt R. Challenging Aging stereotypes: Designing and evaluating physical activity programs. American Journal of Preventive Medicine 2003; 25(3 Suppl 2):164–217.

31. US Department of Health and Human Services. Physical activity and health: A report of the Surgeon General [Online] 1996 [cited 2004 Jul 20]; Available from: URL: http://www.fitness.gov/execsum.htm. Atlanta, GA: US Department of Health and Human Services, Centers for Disease Control and Prevention, National Center for Chronic Disease Prevention and Health Promotion.

32. Ory MG, Jordan P, Bazzarre T. Behavioural change consortium: Setting the stage for a new century of health behaviour change research. Health Education Research 2002; 17(5):500–511.

33. Glasgow RE, Vogt TM, Boles SM. Evaluating the public health impact of health promotion interventions: The RE-AIM framework. American Journal of Public Health 1999; 89(9):1322–1327.

34. Klesges LM, Estabrooks PA, Dzewaltowski DA, Bull SS, Glasgow RE. Beginning with the application in mind: Designing and planning health behaviour change interventions to enhance dissemination. Annals of Behavioural Medicine 2005 (29 Suppl.):66–75.

35. Dzewaltowski DA, Estabrooks PA, Glasgow RE. The future of physical activity behaviour change research: What is needed to improve translation of research into health promotion practice? Exercise Sports Science Review 2004; 32(2):57–63.

36. Glasgow RE, Klesges LM, Dzewaltowski DA, Bull SS, Estabrooks PA. The future of health behaviour change research: What is needed to improve translation of research into health promotion practice? Annals of Behavioural Medicine 2004; 27(1):3–12.

37. Re-aim.org. [Online]. 2004 [cited 2004 Jul 20]; Available from: URL: http://www.re-aim.org.

38. Glasgow RE, Lichtenstein E, Marcus A. Why don't we see more translation of health promotion research to practice? [Online]. 2003 [cited 2004 Jul 20]; Available from: URL: http://www.re-aim.org/2003/abstracts/a03-gr-ajph.html.

39. Glasgow RE. Practical, practice and policy relevant trials. Current Diabetes Reports 2004; 4(2):111–112.

40. Bacher TE. Finding the balance: Program fidelity and adaptation in substance abuse prevention. Conference edition [Online]. 2002 [cited 2004 Jul 20]; Available from: URL: http://modelprograms.samhsa.gov/pdfs/FindingBalance1.pdf. Washington, DC: Center for Substance Abuse Prevention, US Department of Health and Human Services.

41. Bellg AJ, Borrelli B, Resnick B, Hecht J, Minicucci DS, Ory MG, et al. Enhancing treatment fidelity in health behaviour change studies: Best practices and recommendations from the NIH Behaviour Change Consortium. Health Psychology 2004; 23(5):443–451.

42. Castro FG, Barrera M, Martinez C. The cultural adaptation of prevention interventions: Resolving tensions between fit and fidelity. Prevention Science 2004; 5(1):41–45.

43. Altman DG. Sustaining interventions in community systems: On the relationship between researchers and communities. Health Psychology 1995; 14(6):526–536.

44. Katz DL. Representing your community in community-based participatory research: Differences made and measured. Preventing chronic disease: Public health research, practice, and policy [serial online] 2004; 1(1):1–4. Available from: URL: http://www.cdc.gov/pcd/issues/2004/jan/03_0024.htm.

45. Glasgow RE, Ory MG, Klesges LM, et al. Practical and relevant measures of health behaviours for primary care settings. Ann Fam Med. 2005; 3:73–81.

45. Ory MG, Klesges LM, Glasgow M. Measures of behaviour change for primary care settings: Rationale, selection criteria and recommendations for brief measures to be utilized in prescription for health research studies. Report prepared for Prescription for Health National Program Office with support of the Robert Wood Johnson Foundation; 2004.

46. Rogers E. Diffusion of innovations, 5th edn. New York, NY: Free Press; 2003.

47. Johnson K, Hays C, Center H, Daly C. Building capacity in sustainable prevention innovations: A sustainability planning model. Evaluation and Program Planning 2004; 27(2):135–139.

48. Weiss H, Coffman J, Bohan-Baker M. Evaluation's role in supporting initiative sustainability. Harvard Family Research Project [Online]. 2002 [cited 2004 Jul 20]; Available from: URL: http://www.ksg.harvard.edu/urbanpoverty/Sitepages/UrbanSeminar/Strategies/Weiss.pdf.

49. Shediac-Rizkallah M, Bone L. Planning for the sustainability of community-based health programs: Conceptual frameworks and future directions for research, practice and policy. Health Education Research 1998; 13(1):87–108.

50. Cutler I. End Games: The challenge of sustainability. Copies are available from the author at icutler@cornerstone.org; 2000.

51. David T. Reflections on sustainability [Online]. 2002 [cited 2004, Jul 20]; Available from: URL: http://www.tcwf.org/reflections/feb_2002: California Wellness Foundation.

52. Pluye P, Potvin L, Denis JL. Making public health programs last: Conceptualizing sustainability. Evaluation and Program Planning 2004.

53. Goodman RM, McLeroy KR, Steckler AB, Hoyle RH. Development of level of institutionalization scales for health promotion programs. Health Education Quarterly 1993; 20(2):161–178.

54. Evashwick C, Ory MG. Organizational characteristics of successful innovative programs sustained over time. Journal of Family and Community Health 2003; 26(3):177–193.

55. Murphy D. Diabetes prevention and control: A public health imperative. In: Promising practices in chronic disease prevention and control: A public health framework for action. Atlanta, GA: US Department of Health and Human Services; 2003:1–19.

56. American Diabetes Association. Study shows sharp rise in cost of diabetes nationwide [Online]. 2004 [cited 2004 Jul 20]; Available from: URL: http://www.diabetes.org/for-media/2003-press-releases/02-27-03.

57. Boyle JP, Honeycutt AA, Narayan KM, Hoerger TJ, Geiss LS, Chen H, et al. Projection of diabetes burden through 2050. Diabetes Care 2001; 24(11):1936–1940.

58. Centers for Disease Control and Prevention. National Diabetes Fact Sheet. General information and national estimates on diabetes in the United States. Atlanta, GA: US Department of Health and Human Services; 2003.

59. National Center for Health Statistics. Health, United States, 2003 [Online]. 2003 [cited 2004 Jul 20]; Available from: URL: http://www.cdc.gov/nchs/hus.htm.

60. Agency for Health Research and Quality. National Guideline Clearinghouse™ [Online]. 2004 [cited 2004 Jul 20]; Available from: URL: http://www.guideline.gov/.

61. Cabana MD, Rand CS, Powe NR, Wu AW, Wilson MH, Abboud P-AC, et al. Why don't physicians follow clinical practice guidelines? JAMA 1999; 282(15):1458–1465.

62. Institute of Medicine. Committee on Quality Health Care in America. Crossing the quality chasm: A new health system for the 21st century. Washington, DC: National Academy Press; 2001.

63. McGlynn EA, Asch SM, Adams J, Keesey J, Hicks J, DeCristofaro A, et al. The quality of health care delivered to adults in the United States. The New England Journal of Medicine 2003; 348(26):2635–2645.

64. Agency for Healthcare Research and Quality. About PPIP. Put prevention into practice, May 2000 [Online]. 2000 [cited 2004 Jul 20]; Available from: URL: http://www.ahrq.gov/ppip/ppipabou.htm.

65. Wagner EH, Austin BT, Von Korff M. Organizing care for patients with chronic illness. Milbank Quarterly 1996; 74(4):511–544.

66. Wagner EH, Austin BT, Davis C, Hindmarsh M, Schaefer J, Bonomi A. Improving chronic illness care: Translating evidence into action. Health Affairs 2001; 20(6):64–78.

67. Wagner EH, Glasgow RE, Davis C, Bonomi AE, Provost L, McCulloch D, et al. Quality improvement in chronic illness care: A collaborative approach. Joint Commission Journal on Quality Improvement 2001; 27(2):63–80.

68. American Diabetes Association. Clinical Practice Recommendations 2003. Diabetes Care 2003; 26(Suppl 1):S1–S156.

69. National Committee for Quality Assurance. NCQAs Quality Plus Program [Online]. 2004 [cited 2004 Aug 03]; Available from: http://www.ncqa.org/Programs/Accreditation/Qpoverview.pdf.

70. US Prevention Task Force. Recommendations for healthcare system and management education interventions to reduce morbidity and mortality from diabetes. American Journal of Preventive Medicine 2002; 22(4 Suppl 1):10–14.

71. Texas Diabetes Council. Texas Department of Health. Diabetes tool kit [Online]. 2004 [cited 2004 Jul 20]; Available from: URL: http://www.tdh.state.tx.us/diabetes/healthcare/toolkit.htm.

72. Gamm L, Hutchison L, Dabney B, Dorsey A, eds. Rural healthy people 2010: A companion document to healthy people 2010, Volumes 1 and 2. College Station, TX: The Texas A&M University System Health Science Center, School of Rural Public Health, Southwest Rural Health Research Center; 2003.

73. Glasgow RE, Davis C, Funnell M, Beck A. Implementing practical interventions to support chronic illness self-management in health care settings [Online]. 2003 [cited 2004 Jul 20] Available from: URL: http://www.re-aim.org/2003/bios/biosk_Glasgow.html: Joint Commission Journal on Quality and Safety.

74. Narayan KM, Gregg EW, Engelgau MM, Moore B, Thompson TJ, Williamson DF, et al. Translation research for chronic disease: The case of diabetes. Diabetes Care 2000; 23:1794–1798.
75. Chin MH, Cook S, Drum ML, Jin L, Guillen M, Humikowski CA, et al. Improving diabetes care in Midwest community health centers with the Health Disparities Collaborative. Diabetes Care 2004; 27(1):2–8.
76. Robert Wood Johnson Foundation. National blueprint for increasing physical activity among adults 50 and older: creating a strategic framework and enhancing organizational capacity for change. Journal on Aging and Physical Activity 2000; 9(Suppl):S5–S28.
77. National Blueprint: Increasing physical activity among adults fifty and older [Online]. 2004 [cited 2004 Jul 20]; Available from: URL:http://www.agingblueprint.org.
78. First Step to Active Health [Online]. 2004 [cited 2004 Jul 20]; Available from: URL:http://www.firststeptoactivehealth.com.
79. International Council on Active Aging [Online]. 2004 [cited 2004 Jul 20]; Available from: URL: http://www.icaa.cc.

CHAPTER **15**

The way forward in the design and development of effective behaviour change programs

Shane A. Thomas
Colette Browning

We now turn to a discussion of what we now know following the sterling efforts of our collaborators in this work. We propose to first discuss the findings of each of the contributions in specific detail. We then propose to draw out common themes from these contributions and then finally assess the overall state of knowledge of behaviour change and to discuss important current and future developments in the application of this knowledge in viable and sustainable programs.

MODIFYING DIETARY AND EATING BEHAVIOUR

Dixon and Paxton note that promoting healthy eating involves modifying existing behaviours rather than discouraging the behaviour altogether as is the case with smoking. The multiple determinants of dietary behaviour mean that there are multiple opportunities and channels for intervention. The broad *public health nutrition interventions* covered in this chapter focus on dietary factors related to specific diseases such as diabetes, cancer and cardiovascular diseases. They include social marketing approaches, point of sale and food industry interventions, and worksite, school-based and primary care interventions. While these approaches focus on promoting less consumption of fats, more consumption of fruit and vegetables and achieving a healthy weight, the growing 'obesity epidemic' has focused attention on obesity prevention through healthy food choices as well as increased physical activity. The chapter also includes an examination of selective prevention interventions for disordered eating in adolescent girls.

Dietary behaviour interventions that have used *social marketing/mass media approaches* over an extended time have yielded the strongest evidence for behaviour change. These interventions have often been restricted to a single community and the generalizability of their effects has not been established. *Food industry interventions* involve supplying healthy alternatives on menus or promotions in supermarkets at point of sale. The authors cite recommended factors that contribute to the effectiveness of point of sale and food industry interventions including embedding the program in broader social marketing/mass media approaches, tailoring the message and type of promotion to the needs of target groups, incorporating behaviourally oriented models in the programs, involving staff in the development and implementation of the intervention, promoting the sale of healthy foods through cheaper pricing and ensuring that the program runs for at least 12 months.

Effective *healthy eating interventions in schools* include curriculum support, skills training for teachers, changes in canteen practices (including healthy choices and cheaper low fat snacks), active participation in cooking and supermarket tours and stakeholder involvement including parents and health industry representation. Strategies need to be targeted to the developmental needs of the child and grounded in theory and research. Evidence for the effectiveness of *worksite diet and weight loss interventions* show modest but positive effects on dietary behaviour. Many workplace studies use no control group, and non-randomized designs. There are a few examples of published randomized controlled trials of worksite nutrition interventions that have demonstrated significant improvements in diet and in cardiovascular disease risk factors. The most successful interventions incorporate a model such as the socioecological model, use multi-level strategies including mass media, target individual behaviours and the environment (for example, food service changes such as including cheap low-fat snacks), and involve staff, their families and managers in the development and implementation of the intervention. *Primary care settings* provide an opportunity for ongoing personalized interventions and are effective when high-risk patients are targeted but are high cost compared to community-based interventions. Dixon and Paxton suggest that in order to strengthen the evidence base in the field there is a need for well-designed studies '. . . that include adequate sample size, control groups, documentation of intervention intensity and duration, use of appropriate measures of impact, and follow-up over time'. Cost-effectiveness data also needs to be collected.

A number of common elements comprise the more effective public health nutrition interventions. These include targeting both individual behaviour change as well as modifying environments (e.g. include healthy food choices); incorporating a behaviour change or health promotion model in the intervention; involving stakeholders in the design and implementation of the intervention; using broad social marketing approaches; tailoring the message to account for individual and group differences in acceptability and targeting individuals at high risk for diseases.

Selective prevention programs for *disordered eating* typically focus on providing information and coping strategies to counteract weight loss behaviours to young adolescents, usually are conducted in school settings and focus on individual behaviour change. Their success has been modest. Dixon and Paxton argue that given the social pressures to be thin are so pervasive, interventions need to incorporate broader approaches that go beyond the role of the individual in disordered eating.

PROMOTING SEXUAL HEALTH AND REDUCING RISK BEHAVIOURS

Pitts examined interventions aimed at improving sexual health and reducing risk behaviours. The common elements of effective interventions to prevent sexually transmissible infections include incorporating behaviour change models and behavioural skills training, promoting condom use, using personal sexual health plans, tailoring and targeting of the intervention to specific groups and using peer educators and community opinion leaders in the implementation of the intervention. Interventions directed at the individual include the A (Abstinence), B (Behaviour change including be faithful or partner reduction) and C (Condom use) approach and more recently the C (Condoms), N (needles) and N (negotiating skills) approach. A review of 20 risk reduction programs found that most used behaviour change theories (mainly social learning and social cognition models) and 12 reported positive effects including increased condom use.

Group interventions through peer education have been used widely with young people and have been found to have some positive effects including changing attitudes towards postponing sexual activity. Modifying sexual risk for HIV among groups such as gay men through promotion of condom use has been highly effective. The efficacy of strategies such as negotiated safety approaches where HIV-negative gay men in a committed relationship do not use condoms is open to debate. Interventions directed at young homeless people and at women at high risk for cervical cancer have been successful in terms of increased condom use.

Large-scale community interventions to prevent HIV such as those conducted through prime time television series in South Africa have high brand-awareness and message-impact. National multi-sectoral HIV prevention programs such as those in Uganda have demonstrated reductions in HIV prevalence. Pitts concludes that 'The extent to which individual behaviour change is supported by structural and social change will determine success and good health for all'. She argues for better data on sex and sexual health, legislative change in countries where various sexual practices are illegal, and more emphasis on the positive aspects of sexual expression in sexual health interventions.

PREVENTING HARM RELATED TO ALCOHOL AND DRUG USE

In this chapter Toumbourou used developmental and motivational theories to examine the effectiveness of the various interventions. He argues that substance abuse has been associated with early developmental distress. Further it is motivated by efforts to: Manage the body and emotions, conform to social norms and to establish individual and peer identity.

Evidence from experimental and well-controlled small trials shows that interventions aimed at reducing early developmental stress at the individual, group and community level are effective. Successful examples include early years prevention, preventative case management (individual), parent education and improving school environments (group) and harm reduction strategies (community). Similarly interventions aimed at addressing normative conformity motives have been shown to reduce substance use and related harms. The more effective approaches include normative feedback (individual), 12-Step groups and at the community level, minimum age restrictions and community mobilization. Mentorship, (individual), parent education, family therapy and therapeutic communities (group) have been successful in encouraging healthy individuation. Interventions designed to encourage healthy self-management of pain, arousal and physical health have been less successful. At the individual level pharmacotherapies have resulted in efficacy being maintained in real-world service delivery contexts. However health promotion approaches, restrictions on advertising, genetic counselling and emotional competence training still require formative evaluation.

Toumbourou points out that harmful substance abuse is not restricted to disadvantaged communities. In disadvantaged communities developmental distress may be more common while in more affluent communities efforts need to be directed at the development of healthy individuation. We need to recognize the different drivers of substance abuse in different communities. He argues for interventions that '. . . address the motivational profile of substance misuse within specific communities'.

PROMOTING PHYSICAL ACTIVITY

Morris and Choi focused on physical activity intervention in community and primary care settings. They concluded that community-based and primary care interventions were equally effective in initiating behaviour change but the effects were short-lived.

In primary care settings most interventions are based on theoretical frameworks and models such as the health belief model, social cognition theory, the theory of planned behaviour and the stages of change model. Primary care interventions focus more on self-management approaches rather than changing environments as in the case in community-based interventions. Behavioural or motivational counselling is often incorporated in primary care interventions, however the evidence supporting the effectiveness of counselling is limited. Interpretation of the evidence is limited by variations in the reported length of counselling sessions and the protocol reported may not be explicit. While various combinations of approaches are equally effective in initiating behaviour change in most primary care based interventions the behaviour was not generally maintained over the long-term.

Community interventions targeted at specific groups and large-scale interventions are highlighted by Morris and Choi. As is the case with primary care interventions most are based on theoretical frameworks and models. However they also incorporate environmental considerations and the establishment of partnerships with local government and community stakeholders. Most community interventions attract people who are already active and want to be more active. They have not been as successful in attracting sedentary people. Morris and Choi suggest that individual approaches such as counselling could be incorporated in community-based interventions to shift motivations.

They concluded that future research in the area should focus on maintenance strategies and outcome measures that provide specific information on what aspects of physical activity have changed including whether changes have been maintained beyond the end of the intervention. They also argue for a re-examination of the role of motivation in the maintenance of physical activity. Motivation can be increased by the incorporation of specific opportunities to increase motivation through personal reassessment of goals and providing more opportunity for social interaction through physical activity.

SMOKING PREVENTION AND CESSATION

The effectiveness of smoking prevention and cessation interventions has been widely documented. Interventions at the individual, small group and community levels were examined in this chapter by Bittoun and Browning.

Under intervention approaches targeted at the individual, telephone counselling has been the most effective approach. There seems to be no evidence that hypnotherapy and acupuncture are effective in smoking cessation. Similarly the evidence for the effectiveness of individual behaviour change approaches is limited by lack of detail about the intervention protocols. A Cochrane review of nicotine replacement therapy (NRT) found that this approach was up to twice as effective as a placebo in achieving smoking cessation over a six-month period. However only 30 to 40% of people still do not smoke after one year after a combination of counselling and NRT. Combination NRT treatments allocated according to levels of dependency seem to show some promise but more research is needed to assess effectiveness of these treatments. There is limited evidence for the efficacy of other drug treatments such as bupropion.

Small group approaches including group behaviour therapy and family therapy have been found to be no more effective than individual counselling. Incorporating cognitive or behavioural skills appears to have little impact on the effectiveness of small group interventions for smoking cessation. The role of the immediate social environment, including peers and family, in smoking initiation and cessation requires further research.

The success of community-based interventions that incorporate individual, social and environmental factors in the design are becoming more popular but evidence for their effectiveness is modest according to a recent Cochrane review. For example evaluation of the large-scale US Community Intervention Trial for Smoking cessation (COMMIT) found that while smoking prevalence overall had reduced, there was no difference between the prevalence of smoking between the intervention and comparison communities at follow-up.

In countries such as Australia where a systematic approach to tobacco control has been implemented, smoking rates have decreased. In Australia governments and the Cancer Council have collaborated to deliver mass media campaigns, telephone counselling, the introduction of smoke-free environments and increased taxes on cigarettes to address the problem. However smoking rates have plateaued recently and attention is now focused on particular groups such as young people, those with mental health problems and indigenous groups.

DEPRESSION

Lindner notes in her chapter that the most common interventions for depression include pharmacological and psychological therapies and education and awareness-based approaches. Many reported interventions include groups with a co-morbid condition such as a chronic illness or pain. Lindner concludes that the evidence for the overall effectiveness of most of the approaches is sparse.

Antidepressant medication is the most common treatment for depression but there are problems with non-adherence. There is a need for more research in the causes of non-adherence. Lindner argues that psychological treatment for depression should address non-adherence issues as well as the depression itself. In terms of the effectiveness and safety of antidepressants the level of evidence is not high. Cognitive behaviour therapy (CBT) is the most common form of psychological treatment for depression. However its efficacy has been questioned and the individual components of the therapy are not well-researched. Some new approaches at the individual level include telephone counselling and computer delivery of treatment. There is some evidence that computer delivery is effective in reducing depressive symptoms and also cost-effective and CBT via telephone has been shown to reduce symptoms over a six-month period. There are few evaluated group interventions for depression and this may be because the condition precludes attendance at group sessions. Group approaches include CBT and psychotherapy and both approaches have limited evidence for their effectiveness. Community interventions have focused on education about depression, acceptance of depression and promoting opportunities to seek help. Again the evidence for the effectiveness of these approaches is limited.

INSOMNIA

Greenwood notes that while much needs to be done in determining the effectiveness of treatments for insomnia, the real problem is in convincing individuals, health professionals and policy makers that sleep disorders are a serious health problem in need of intervention. Further if help is sought the sources of help are rarely equipped to treat sleep problems.

Interventions for insomnia include drug therapies, psychological approaches including stimulus control, sleep restriction, sleep hygiene education, relaxation training and cognitive restructuring, self-help approaches, and mass media and Internet approaches. He concludes that while interventions at the individual and small-group level are well-developed, there is little activity at the public health intervention level. Community based and mass media approaches are rare in the literature but Greenwood argues for further development of these approaches.

Drug therapies for sleep disorders, while common, are '... ineffective and dangerous'. Greenwood argues for psychological approaches that have a good evidence-base. For example CBT for insomnia has been shown to be effective for individuals and in small group settings. However psychological treatments are not readily sought by the community perhaps due to their high cost and limited availability. Greenwood argues for a cost-effective self-help approach. However, in reviewing the literature on self-help approaches he concludes that 'The literature reviewed ... does not provide quality evidence about the efficacy of self-help approaches for insomnia'. There is a need for trials that compare self-help approaches with standard therapist led interventions. The self-help approach needs to include similar components to those used in therapist-led interventions. Greenwood also suggests that the impact of some therapist contact in self-help approaches needs to be evaluated as well as determining what type of people would best benefit form self-help approaches.

PROBLEMATIC GAMBLING

Jackson's chapter notes that interventions for problematic gambling vary according to the characteristics of the subpopulation of interest (e.g. 'normal' problem gambler, emotionally disturbed gamblers or those with impulse control problems associated with neurological dysfunction) and the goal of the intervention. Jackson concludes that there is a 'paucity' of data about the effectiveness of prevention programs and treatment interventions. He concludes that '... much more is known about interventions and associated behavioural changes which are aimed at individuals, less about small groups and very little about communities'. He highlights a number of methodological problems in evaluating the outcomes of interventions. These include sample selection (often heterogeneous and with psychiatric co-morbidity), variation in treatment outcome (abstinence vs. reduced frequency or improved functioning), failure to report refusal to enter program or drop-out rates, confounding of different treatment effects, unknown reliability and validity of change measures. Definitions of relapse are not clear, and follow-up periods are variable.

Problem gambling intervention models at the individual or small group level include the medical model, the behavioural model and the cognitive model. Community-based models that provide services through community health centres have used counselling and support for the gambler and their family. Hospital inpatient and outpatient models and self-help approaches are also part of the intervention suite for problem gambling. The interventions are mainly focused on the individual with few examples of small group or community based interventions.

Self-help approaches such as Gamblers Anonymous have shown low success rates based on a two-year abstinence criterion, but commentators concede that such a criterion may underestimate the impact of GA. There is some evidence that behavioural treatments such as desensitization, and controlled gambling and cognitive therapy are effective. There is criticism of these approaches and there is growing evidence for the effectiveness of multi-modal approaches that recognize the co-occurrence of problems such as depression and family and social problems. Pharmacological interventions have been effective in the case of pathological gambling.

Jackson presents a model developed by him and Thomas of influences on gambling behaviour and outcomes with a range of intervention foci. Using this model, interventions can be targeted at the propensity to gamble, the supply of gambling products and the negative outcomes to the individual, family and community.

CRASH AND INJURY PREVENTION

Fildes and Pronk note that an evidence-based approach to injury prevention had its beginnings in the 1960s when Haddon categorized injury prevention into a number of components including preventing the crash, preventing the injuries and minimizing trauma. This evidence-based approach has led to the use of seat-belts, improving roads and the safety of cars, reducing drink-driving and improvements in enforcement methods and community knowledge. The biggest improvements in road safety have come through engineering and enforcement interventions rather than through education.

Individual approaches include fines and licence demerit points for law-breakers that can lead to licence suspension, vehicle interlocks and impounding and driver rehabilitation courses. There is evidence that motor vehicle sanctions such as impounding of vehicles of unlicensed drivers can lead to reductions in unlicensed driver fatalities and removal of unroadworthy vehicles from the road. Rehabilitation programs for drink driving combined with licensing sanctions have been shown to be effective in reducing alcohol-related crashes and multi-modal treatments are more effective than single modal approaches.

Some examples of group interventions include road safety education, young driver education, programs that promote safe walking routes to school, safe walking for seniors and fleet safety programs. Evaluations of these programs are limited. Community interventions include mass-media programs around drink driving, speeding and fatigue. Speed cameras have been effective in reducing average speed and numbers exceeding the speed limit as well as casualty crashes. A meta-analysis of mass media campaigns found a 15% reduction in crashes after the campaigns. However many studies do not allow a cost–benefit analysis to be conducted. Effective campaigns need to incorporate a theoretical framework, incorporate emotional persuasion, combine the advertising with enforcement and be implemented at the local level.

In looking for a way forward in road safety Fildes and Pronk contrast the traditional safety models with a model where safety is seen as a health problem. Traditional models assume that a degree of road trauma is acceptable in maintaining high levels of mobility. In contrast the Swedish *Vision Zero* and the Netherlands *Sustainable Safety* places preventing death and serious injury above other considerations. While this approach may lead to reduced mobility and increased travel time, individuals and the community will benefit from reduced health costs. Fildes argues that under this new approach interventions need to be integrated system-wide and involve engineering approaches as well as driver behaviour. Investment in infrastructure would need to be increased and changes in community attitudes to road safety and mobility promoted. Fildes also recommends that the quality and detail of crash data collected by police and insurance companies needs to be improved to support this new approach to road safety.

SELF-MANAGEMENT AND CHRONIC ILLNESS

Weeks and Swerissen note that the management of chronic illness has emerged as a significant health-care issue in most countries especially as populations age. Self-management of chronic illness is a participatory approach to chronic illness that involves partnerships between the individual, their family and health professionals to manage the condition. A number of programs now exist that teach the skills of self-management to people with chronic illnesses. Most programs incorporate behaviour change models. Evidence suggests that these programs are effective in terms of improving health status, increasing positive health behaviours, decreasing use of health services, increasing adherence to treatment regimens and are cost-effective.

Randomized controlled trials have shown that the benefits of self-management programs are related to improvement in self-efficacy and improvements in self-efficacy are a common outcome across a range of programs and chronic illnesses. Similarly increases in physical activity are a common outcome of programs. The inclusion of action plans in asthma self-management has been shown to be a key determinant of perceived control of symptoms.

Weeks and Swerissen highlight a number of shortcomings in the literature. Methodological weaknesses of studies include self-recruitment, lack of randomization and lack of specification of outcome measures. There is a need to examine the effectiveness of the different elements of the programs and to further examine the effectiveness of programs in different settings and across social and cultural groups. They call for further examination of the effectiveness of self-management programs in '. . . mainstream health care settings as part of the overall delivery of treatment, care and support'.

WHAT WERE THE COMMON THEMES IN THE REVIEWS?

While the chapters are obviously specific to the domains reviewed by their authors, we consider that a number of common themes and considerations emerged in them concerning the design and development of effective interventions. These were:

- Know the target audience and the drivers of behaviour that pertain to specific groups within the target populations(s).
- Tailoring of programs to individuals and like groups is necessary: one size does not fit all.
- Use a recognized behaviour change/health promotion model to inform the intervention program logic.
- Peer education is a useful and effective method of delivery of intervention programs.
- Involve stakeholders in program design.
- Clear specification of intervention components is necessary.
- Outcome measures need to be defined and incorporated into program delivery to monitor program outcomes and improve targeting.
- Cost-effectiveness needs to be measured and reported.
- There is currently more evidence on effectiveness of individual interventions than population level interventions in some areas.
- Translation of research evidence to diverse settings and populations is a key issue.
- Integrating behaviour change approaches into mainstream health care is a desirable end.

We now take up some of these themes in our concluding and overview discussion.

THE WAY FORWARD

It is obvious that favourable research outcomes do not automatically translate themselves into viable and sustainable interventions or into funded programs to deliver them. As Marcia Ory and her colleagues note elsewhere in this volume (and in other writings[1]) the translation of successful behavioural research into practice is, in itself, a burgeoning area of enquiry. The research work in this area has identified that there are many barriers to the uptake and implementation of new and successful interventions. The systematic review movement, i.e. the Cochrane Collaboration, the Campbell collaboration and the many evidence-based practice centres and interest groups, addresses the issue of availability of good quality information concerning the efficiency and effectiveness of interventions, provided of course, the relevant research has actually been performed, has been able to be located and was actually reported in the review. However, systematic review does not address the other barriers to successful translation and uptake. It merely organizes the information in a systematic fashion, but even then, not necessarily in a form that is accessible to practitioners. The existence of pertinent systematic and critical reviews is the equivalent of an enabler to the 'contemplation' stage in Prochaska and DiClemente's Model of Stages of change in terms of enabling contemplation of the need to change the behaviour of the organization and staff delivering the evidence-based service. The transition into later stages of implementation of program change is impacted by a range of factors other than the mere availability of the necessary evidence base. One might consider the availability of the evidence base to be a necessary but not sufficient condition for program change. What then is needed to be done to create viable programs from research evidence?

Haines and Donald's volume on 'Getting research findings into practice' is a compendium of papers on barriers to uptake of research findings into practice and how to address them. In Haines and Donald's volume, Grimshaw et al.'s analysis of 41 systematic reviews of changing provider behaviour provides a very useful analysis of key findings in this literature. Their main findings were that:

- Passive dissemination of research findings was most unlikely to result in provider behaviour change, i.e. you need a purpose-built program to achieve change.
- Educational outreach and systems that involve structured reminders for clinicians about targeted changes in current practice seem to work well. We know from both the decision support and behaviour change literatures that both training and tools to support adherence to desired clinical pathways are very effective ways of achieving behaviour change and maintaining program integrity and adherence.[2-5]
- Multi-faceted programs based on a local needs analysis of local barriers to implementation are most likely to be effective.

In our experience, a further major barrier to the implementation of successful programs based upon research evidence is the paucity of information contained and reported in many of the research studies and their associated reviews. This problem has recently been recognized and taken up by researchers and editors of learned journals. Two major relevant developments merit discussion. These are the CONSORT and the Behavior Change Consortium (BCC).

A large group of bioscientist researchers and journal editors have collaborated in the CONSORT (Consolidated Standards of Reporting Trials) project.[6-8] CONSORT is a very useful attempt to improve standards of the reporting of randomized control trials. It consists of a set of standards and an associated checklist that acts as a guide to researchers and editors concerning exactly what should be reported in papers describing the design and outcomes of RCTs. The CONSORT project came into being because of concerns about the standards of reporting of RCTs. Anyone who has attempted to conduct a meta-analysis of such studies will readily attest to the low level of compatible information reported across different trials.[9,10] Even at the crudest levels of analysis it is frequently very difficult to construct a viable analysis because of the wide variation in reporting practices across different studies and journals. CONSORT has been embraced by a wide and growing range of journals and this is to be applauded.

In a more specialized domain, the BCC has attempted to address the issue of different reporting standards of studies of behaviour change programs. The BCC was established as a consequence of US NIH funding of a program of research on 'Innovative Approaches to Disease Prevention through Behaviour Change' from 1997 onwards. Volume 17 Issue 5 of the *Journal Health Education Research* contains a compendium of the work of members of the consortium. The BCC consists of NIH staff and the research investigators from the projects funded under the NIH program as well as several co-sponsoring private foundations. However, while the concept of the BCC has been widely endorsed, there are nevertheless some critics of the content of the focus of the BCC. Connelly, for example, has argued that the BCC ought to incorporate a wider consideration of social context variables and socioeconomic factors in their studies. Connelly's call, while pertinent to the BCC, is indicative of much wider issues in the design and reporting of intervention studies that are in no way unique to the BCC. The BCC is a useful and worthy venture that shares many of the same goals as the CONSORT program.

While we endorse the thinking behind the CONSORT and BCC initiatives, there is also further room for development of the concepts and implementation of these interesting developments. In terms of practical use of the data and findings from intervention studies in the social and behavioural domains, there remain many gaps. Program designers would be hard pressed to find even basic costing information in most published studies, even basic information that would allow the construction of basic costing estimates. For example, information such as the following is rarely reported:

- What was the distribution of hours that was spent by the program staff and the participants engaged in the actual interventions?
- What was spent in time and materials to develop the program interventions and associated materials?
- Following development costs what did it actually cost per head to deliver the program?

Glasgow et al.'s paper[10] discusses these and other issues in the reporting of intervention research. Thus while the typologies and standards engendered in projects such as CONSORT are very useful, there remains further avenues for substantial improvement and elaboration of them. We need standards, but we need reporting standards with content that assists program designers and developers to translate the research findings into viable and sustainable programs. At present, we do not consider that this is the case, but activities such as CONSORT and BCC are important steps in the right direction. We consider that on top of the many challenges faced by program designers the inadequacy of the scope and nature of the information reported in many intervention studies is, in itself, a major barrier to successful program uptake. In the translational research agenda, we need to pay much closer attention to the link between what information program designers and funders need to effect their programs and the information that is collected and reported by scientists studying behaviour change phenomena. We need to study formally and better the information needs of program designers and funders in order that we can advise scientists as to what they need to collect and report in their studies to maximize their usefulness. As we stated at the outset of this discussion 'It is obvious that favourable research outcomes do not automatically translate themselves into viable and sustainable interventions nor into funded programs to deliver them'.

This book commenced with a challenge by some of our colleagues involved in the funding of health and human services programs as to what usefully could we tell them about behaviour change research and how this could be practically applied in program design and implementation. So what can we tell our colleagues?

We think we can tell them that there is a vast array of behaviour change research published in the various domains targeted by this text. We consider that the contributors to this volume have made a very good fist of the remarkably arduous task set them. Although they are leading academics and practitioners, many have told us that this is the most difficult and arduous assignment that they have undertaken. The current state of the art in each of the domains is very well reviewed in each of the chapters. We consider that other researchers and program designers in these domains will find them to be very useful.

In terms of the state of the nation of behaviour change research in general, we can tell them that although the level of effort has been vast, it has not been coordinated and this has resulted in a wide range of studies with quite varied approaches to reporting and conduct of the studies. We consider that programs such as the Cochrane and Campbell collaborations service important functions in selecting the very best evidence available and summarizing its key features. However, we consider that they do not deliver the kind of information that a hard-nosed program designer or program funder needs to investigate the feasibility of developing new services or changing old ones. The CONSORT and BCC initiatives are also useful and important initiatives. Nevertheless, it is obvious that there are large gaps in the research evidence base in terms of the typology we proposed at the commencement of this project to our collaborators. While research funding is a whole different kettle of fish, we consider that there is scope for research funding agencies to employ more encompassing and targeted strategies to ensure that the results of the work they fund is reported in a manner that is consistent with standards that promote the transfer and uptake of this work. After all, in intervention research, the ultimate goal is to extract the essence of 'what works' in order that it may be then applied in an effective and efficient manner within the community that has funded the work.

We are very grateful to our collaborators in this vast project and to those who posed those hard questions to us at the commencement of this journey. We have not fully answered them, but we consider we now have much better insight into how they could be answered. We consider that well-targeted translational research is one of the answers. Another answer is the more intelligent collection, analysis and reporting of intervention study data. So the overall result for the behaviour change behemoth is 'has tried hard but could do better'. We look forward to continued participation in the behaviour change area in the future and to the contributions of our many colleagues.

References

1. Evashwick C, Ory M. Organizational characteristics of successful innovative health care program sustained over time. Family and Community Health 2003; 26(3):177–193.
2. Bucknall TK, Thomas SA. Clinical decision making behaviours of critical care nurses. Australian Journal of Advanced Nursing 1995; 23:10–17.
3. Bucknall TK, Thomas SA. Nurses' reflections on problems associated with decision making in critical care settings. Journal of Advanced Nursing 1997; 25(2):229–237.
4. Considine J, Ung L, Thomas SA. Clinical decision using the National Triage Scale: How important is postgraduate education? Accident and Emergency Nursing 2001; 9:101–108.
5. Thomas SA, Wearing AJ, Bennett M. Clinical decision making for nurses and health care professionals. Sydney: Harcourt Brace Jovanovich; 1991.
6. Ioannidis JP, Evans SJ, Gotzsche PC, O'Neill RT, Altman DG, Schulz K, et al. Better reporting of harms in randomized trials: An extension of the CONSORT statement. Ann Intern Med 2004; 141(10):781–788.
7. Moher D, Schulz KF, Altman DG. The CONSORT statement: Revised recommendations for improving the quality of reports of parallel-group randomised trials. Lancet 2001; 357(9263):1191–1194.
8. Altman DG, Schulz KF, Moher D, Egger M, Davidoff F, Elbourne D, et al. The revised CONSORT statement for reporting randomized trials: Explanation and elaboration. Ann Intern Med 2001; 134(8):663–694.
9. Belle SH, Czaja SJ, Schulz R, Burgio LD, Gitlin LN, Jones R, et al. Using a new taxonomy to combine the uncombinable: Integrating results across diverse interventions. Psychology and Aging 2003; 18(3):396–405.
10. Glasgow RE, Klesges LM, Dzewaltowksi DA, Bull SS, Estabrooks P. The future of behaviour change research: What is needed to improve translation of research into health promotion practice? Annals of Behavioral Medicine 2004; 27(1):3–12.

Index